Anatomic Kinesiology

Anatomic Kinesiology

Third Edition

Gene A. Logan

Wayne C. McKinney

cb

Wm. C. Brown Company Publishers
Dubuque, Iowa

PHYSICAL EDUCATION

Consulting Editor

Aileene Lockhart
Texas Woman's University

Contents

Preface

The objective of this book is to present subject matter from anatomic kinesiology in a functional manner so it can be both understood and knowledgeably applied in teaching-coaching situations. There are reciprocal relationships between the theory of kinesiology, the use of that theory in practice, and the quality of teaching-coaching in physical education. Kinesiology should be a daily "working tool" for the physical educator.

Confusion often exists concerning the relationship of theory to practice. Arthur Schopenhauer, noted nineteenth-century philosopher, indicated that theoretical subject matter in any discipline must have a logical basis. If the theory cannot be applied in practice, it is not good theory. The subject matter of kinesiology in the areas of anatomic kinesiology and biomechanics has withstood the tests of time and critical analysis. When kinesiology theory is utilized in the teaching-coaching of neuromuscular skills, the physical educator is better equipped to help students attain their potentials as performers.

Now in its third edition, the book known in the first edition as *Kinesiology* was changed in the second edition to *Anatomic Kinesiology*. This was done to better reflect its emphasis on applied anatomy related to the study of human motion. The professional physical educator must have an understanding of anatomic kinesiology in order to: (1) prescribe exercises, and (2) critically analyze motions of performers during sport, dance, and exercise.

The book is divided into three parts. These parts are presented in progressive sequence. Part One, "Fundamentals of Motion," presents basic anatomic kinesiology concepts regarding human motion. These concepts must be understood prior to the study of Part Two, "Applied Myology." "Application of Kinesiology Theory," presented in Part Three, is based on comprehension of the subject matter in the first two parts of the book.

Planes of motion, selected anatomic landmarks, and joint motions are presented in Part One. Since most kinesiology students have had a prerequisite course in human anatomy, no attempt has been made to duplicate and discuss all anatomic and bony landmarks in this book. These have been delimited to include only those most important to developing an understanding of anatomic kinesiology.

A detailed discussion of *applied myology* is included in Part Two. There the emphasis is on aggregate or group muscle action. The myology for each joint motion is discussed. Figures to illustrate the spatial relationships of the muscles at each joint are included, along with figures which show surface anatomy. In addition, following discussion of the motions possible at each joint, a figure is included which details muscle involvement as well as proximal and distal attachments (lines of pull) for each muscle. There is considerable emphasis in this part, including many examples, on the differences between concentric and eccentric contractions.

Part Three is designed to show the student how kinesiology theory may be applied in practice. Techniques for analyses of performance skills are presented. These analytic techniques are confined to those applicable directly to the teaching-coaching process. These are noncinematographic and basic cinematographic analyses. Advanced analytic techniques as used in intermediate cinematographic analysis and research are not presented in this book. Example analyses are presented on two levels: (1) the basic cinematographic analysis project as it should be conducted by the student involved in professional preparation in physical education, and (2) noncinematographic and basic cinematographic analytic techniques as they should be used by the professional physical educator. Part Three also includes a discussion of improvement of individual performances through the development of strength, muscular endurance, flexibility, and cardiovascular endurance.

The extensive bibliography includes references in anatomic kinesiology and biomechanics as well as related areas. In addition, the selected references and recommended readings at the end of each chapter will help the student pursue the topics presented and serve as a starting point for a review of the literature useful in the development of a kinesiology project.

Acknowledgment is made to Don Anderson, U.S.C. Athletic News Service; Dr. Dick Perry, U.S.C. Athletic Director; Dick Bank and Phil Bath of Visual Track and Field Techniques; Robert E. Pritchard of Lafayette Instrument Company; and Sue Seyferth, Director of University Publications at California State University at Long Beach, for their assistance in obtaining various photographs used throughout the text. In addition, the authors wish to acknowledge all of the *exceptional athletes* who appear in the photos in this book.

Bill Armstrong provided the plane of motion drawings in Part One. Philip J. Van-Voorst provided the anatomic landmark drawings in Part One and the surface anatomy drawings in Part Two. The remaining anatomic drawings in Part Two were done by Gene A. Logan.

Acknowledgment is made to the following individuals for their assistance as models in numerous figures throughout the book: Gareth Burk, Bonus Frost, Tom Hodge, Henry Jackson, the late Bill Lamberson, Ardie McCoy, Jon McKinney, Mike McKinney, Ruth Miller, Andrea Morris, Sue Schuble, and Jan Stevenson.

The authors are also grateful to Dr. L. Dennis Humphrey, Professor of Physical Education at Southwest Missouri State University, and to Dr. Jerry Stockard, Assistant Professor of Physical Education at Pittsburg State University in Kansas, for their professional critiques over the years. Finally, the invaluable assistance of Shirley A. Minger in preparing the manuscript is appreciated.

The content of the book, together with possible errors, is the sole responsibility of the authors.

Gene A. Logan, Ph.D.
Wayne C. McKinney, Ph.D.

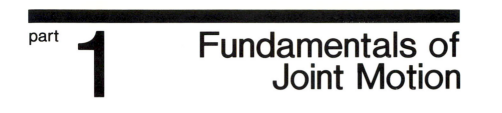

part **1**

Fundamentals of Joint Motion

1 Study of Human Motion

The word "kinesiology," like many scientific terms in the English language, was developed by utilizing two Greek verbs. The prefix, *kinein,* means "to move," and the suffix, *logos,* means "to discourse." Therefore, kinesiology is generally defined as the study of motion (Atwater 1980).

For the physical educator with teaching and/or coaching responsibilities at the elementary school, secondary school, or university level, kinesiology specifically means the study of the diversified human motions one observes in the fields of sport, dance, and exercise. One of the major objectives of physical education is to improve the performance and physiologic efficiency levels of students in these areas. Knowledge and understanding of kinesiology help provide the physical educator with the "working tools" to meet that important professional objective.

Kinesiology as a formal area of study in physical education is most commonly directed toward helping the student gain a functional understanding of *normal* human motion. There are other fields, such as physical medicine and physical therapy, along with the specialized area known as adapted physical education, which place the emphasis on studying, analyzing, and helping with human motion problems of an abnormal, pathologic, or traumatic origin. Study emphasis in this book is on the area of *normal* human motion. The reader is referred to the Bibliography for references on medical kinesiology.

An understanding of the many ramifications of human motion is derived primarily when one gains knowledge about the interrelationships between human anatomy and physics. The merger of these two academic areas helps provide the structural basis for kinesiology. *Anatomic kinesiology* is the study of the human organism's musculoskeletal system primarily. This part of kinesiology has also been termed "applied anatomy," "functional anatomy," and "structural kinesiology." The application of pertinent subject matter from physics to human motion is known as *biomechanics.* Specifically, studying and analyzing humans in motion, sport object motion, and the forces acting upon these animate and inanimate bodies is biomechanics. (The older term for biomechanics is "mechanical kinesiology.") The combination of knowledge from these two areas (applied anatomy/biomechanics) allows physical educators to analyze and study the development of internal forces within humans, the effects of internal and external forces on the human body, and the motion of the sport objects and implements handled by performers. *Anatomic kinesiology is the basic concern of this book.* The reader is directed to the Bibliography for many excellent references on biomechanics.

Professional preparation in physical education has two major bases: (1) technical, and (2) scientific. The technical aspects (techniques) relate primarily to skill development and understanding the *how* and *what* regarding sport, i.e., students are taught *how* to perform skills from numerous sports and activities and *what* they should do in a variety of situations within physical education. If preparation in physical education were to stop at that point, the student would simply be a *technician.* Such a person, trained in the techniques dimension only, would have to rely almost exclusively upon a pragmatic approach to the teaching-coaching process. Trial and error at the expense of students' development would be utilized until something was found which worked. The students are the losers in such a situation under that type of "coach."

Technicians coach sports. They are overwhelmed with such things as offenses and defenses, winning and losing, and their own egos. *Professional physical educators coach people who participate in athletics.* Therein lie tremendous differences, especially within the realm of athletics for athletes in educational environments.

The term "professional" implies that the physical educator not only knows how and what to do in regard to teaching-coaching but also is cognizant of *why* specific instructions are given to students in order to produce positive adaptations and improve performance in sport, exercise, or dance. It is the scientific basis of the professional preparation process which helps the physical educator answer the many questions related to the "why" of human motion.

No student should ever be put into an exercise, drill, or performance situation unless the physical educator is fully aware of the total effect of such participation upon the individual student. An academic background in the scientific basis of human motion including such courses as anatomic kinesiology, exercise physiology, motor learning, sports medicine, biomechanics, and sport psychology, can help the physical educator make that type of professional judgment. *Teaching-coaching is an art based upon a scientific understanding of humans in motion.*

The student of kinesiology planning to enter the physical education profession as a teacher-coach should gain functional knowledge and skill of noncinematographic (fig. 1.1) and cinematographic (fig. 1.2) techniques utilized to analyze human motion. *Disciplined analytic technique,* without and with film, is one of the "tools" the physical educator must work with on a daily basis (Dillman and Sears 1978) (Northrip, Logan, & McKinney 1979).

Anatomic kinesiology is a scientific subject which has the potential for assisting the physical educator to undertake analyses of sport skills and make accurate decisions concerning the physical conditioning process for students and student-athletes. A systematic and accurate analysis of a performer executing a skill must always precede any instruction. The starting point for such an analysis is functional knowledge of joint motion including such things as accurate motion terminology for descriptive purposes, potential ranges of motion

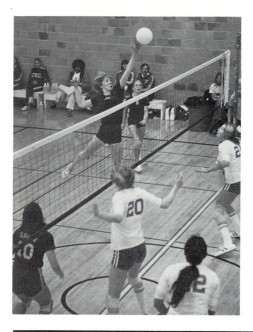

Figure 1.1. A coach must rely upon a disciplined noncinematographic analysis technique if critical adjustments of individual and team performances are to be made. Courtesy *USC Athletic News Service.*

at each joint, and details of musculoskeletal involvement. The study of anatomic kinesiology helps one gain this knowledge which can lead to accurate definition of motion problems of students. These problems cause students to be inefficient performers, as evidenced by force dissipation, loss of angular and linear velocities, and a number of other biomechanic factors. A total analysis must include considerations from anatomic kinesiology and biomechanics.

Accurate analysis of a student's motion problem by the physical educator is analogous to a physician's diagnosis of an illness. Analysis is the starting point for teaching-coaching, just as an accurate diagnosis is a start for the cure of a patient. The *quality* of teaching-coaching is in direct proportion to the *scientific accuracy* of the analysis; therefore, anatomic kinesiology has a direct bearing on the improvement of performances and helping students reach their potentials in sport and dance.

It is a generally accepted fact that development of physical fitness of students and student-athletes is an important professional obligation of the physical educator in the school situation. As someone entrusted with the development of physiologic fitness, the physical educator is expected to be an *expert* on all facets of strength, muscular endurance, flexibility, and cardiovascular endurance development. The professional background for this expertise comes from formal course work in such areas as anatomic kinesiology and exercise physiology.

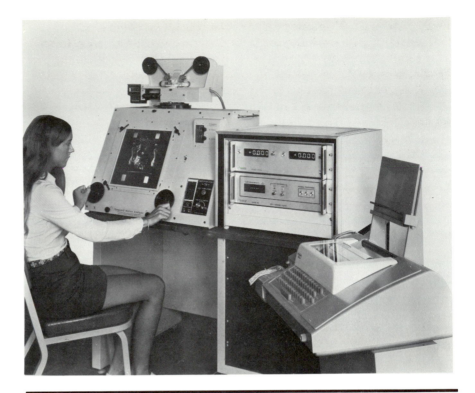

Figure 1.2. Utilization of the Vanguard Motion Analyzer, data transfer system, and computer for cinematographic analyses. Courtesy Vanguard Instrument Corporation, Melville, L.I., N.Y.

Anatomic kinesiology provides much of the myologic, osteologic, and neurologic background that enables the physical educator to prescribe appropriate fitness activities for classes, athletic teams, and individuals at diversified levels of physiologic fitness. Prescribing appropriate conditioning exercises and activities to meet the requirements of students is a moral, ethical, and legal obligation of the physical educator. Assigning exercises potentially harmful to certain students is inexcusable. Thus, the physical educator is professionally obligated to analyze the potential effects of an exercise or activity on students *before* having them participate in such exercises, drills, or performance activities. A person without a background in anatomic kinesiology theory would find it very difficult to undertake such an analysis. Communicating and applying that theory to students in practice is part of the art of teaching noted previously. Functional knowledge of kinesiologic theory, therefore, can contribute positively to qualitative and quantitative aspects of the teaching and learning processes in physical education.

Atwater, Anne E. "Kinesiology/Biomechanics: Perspectives and
    Trends," *Research Quarterly for Exercise and Sport,* 51 (March,
    1980), 193–218.
Dillman, Charles J., and Sears, Ronald G. (Eds.). *Proceedings
    Kinesiology: A National Conference on Teaching.* Urbana-
    Champaign: University of Illinois, 1978.
Northrip, John W.; Logan, Gene A.; and McKinney, Wayne C.
    Introduction to Biomechanic Analysis of Sport (Second Edition).
    Dubuque, Iowa: William C. Brown Company Publishers, 1979.

**Recommended
Reading**

2 Basic Musculoskeletal Concepts

A course in human anatomy is a prerequisite to the study of anatomic kinesiology at most colleges and universities. That course is necessary to provide a general study of systemic anatomy without overemphasizing any particular area such as osteology or myology. The relationships among the various anatomic systems should be understood prior to the study of human motion involving both anatomic kinesiology and exercise physiology.

The purposes of this chapter are to present and review some basic musculoskeletal concepts, a knowledge of which is essential to learning about anatomic kinesiology. Analysis positions, reference terminology, and anatomic landmarks are presented in this chapter.

Analysis positions

The *anatomic position* as shown in figures 2.1, 2.2 and 2.3 serves as one of the major reference positions for analytic kinesiology. This position can be utilized as reference for all joint motions. However, it is most commonly used for the motions at the shoulder, elbow, radio-ulnar, wrist, and hand articulations. If the human body (cadaver or skeleton) is hung from a point in the center of the superior aspect of the skull, it will hang with the shoulder joints laterally rotated with the remaining joints in the upper limbs extended. The ankles would be plantar flexed. The latter is not the case in the weight bearing situation shown in figures 2.1, 2.2, and 2.3.

The *attention position* is another reference for starting joint motion analyses (fig. 3.1). It is usually utilized as the reference position for all joint motions except those of the upper limb. The main difference between the anatomic and attention positions lies in the upper limbs. In the attention position, the shoulder joints are medially rotated to the point that the palmar surfaces of the hands are in contact with the lateral aspects of the thighs. All other joints are in the same positions as shown for the anatomic position in the weight bearing situation. The attention position has been used for centuries by the military, and it is utilized frequently as the starting stance by gymnasts as they begin their routines.

Performers in sport and dance move their bodies in a complex sequence of motion on land, through the air, and in water. They rotate their bodies through various planes and often dive inverted through the air to the earth. The motion capabilities, combinations, and sequences for the human body are infinite. However complex the series of motions may be during a performance, the physical

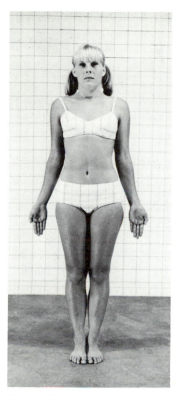 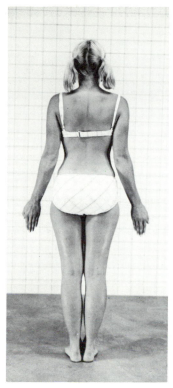 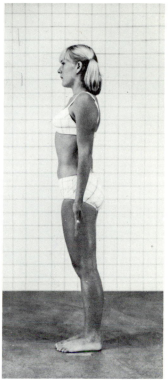

Figure 2.1.   **Figure 2.2.**   **Figure 2.3.**

Figure 2.1. Anatomic position (anterior) (Andrea Morris).

Figure 2.2. Anatomic position (posterior).

Figure 2.3. Anatomic position (lateral).

educator analyzing it must define the planes and joint motions by utilizing the anatomic and/or attention position as the reference point. All definitions of joint motions for kinesiologic analyses are based on these two analysis positions.

There are six basic terms which need to be understood. For the most part these are used to *describe relative position* of one anatomic structure to another segment, bone landmark, joint, or to the total body. These terms are also used in many different ways in the study of anatomic kinesiology and analyses of human motion. The general reference points used here as examples are the traditional planes of motion described in Chapter Three:

Reference terminology

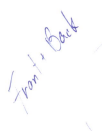

Middle

Front + Back

Top

Bottom

Medial. The cardinal anteroposterior plane shown in figure 3.1 is the midline or medial aspect of the body. Any structure positioned relatively close to the midline of the body is medial, e.g., the sternum (figure 2.19) is medial to the arm or upper limb. Relative positions of all body parts are described in this manner.

Lateral. This term is used in the same context as "medial," but it is used to describe the opposite position. To continue the above example, the upper limb is lateral to the sternum. Anatomic landmarks should be learned in regard to their relative positions to each other. For example, the trochanters of the femur as shown in figure 2.11 are located laterally and medially to each other. The greater trochanter is lateral in relation to the lesser trochanter and the center of the hip joint. It is important to know these kinds of relative spatial relationships.

Anterior. The lateral plane of motion shown in figure 3.6 is the general reference line for differentiating between what is anteriorially or posteriorially positioned on the body. ("Ventral" is a synonym for anterior.) Anterior can be used in a wide variety of ways. As one example, palpation of the belly of the biceps brachii muscle and its tendon in the anatomic position would validate the fact that the tendon has an anterior relationship to the center of the elbow joint. The location of muscle-tendons to joints has important implications in terms of the function of muscles during contraction to joint motion.

Posterior. This term is used in the same context as "anterior" relative to the lateral plane, but in the opposite manner. ("Dorsal" is a synonym for posterior.) Posterior can be used extensively to describe relative positions of large and small body parts. As one example, the coranoid and olecranon processes are located on the ulna as shown in figure 2.26. Their relative position would be described as follows: the olecranon process is posterior to the coranoid process. Also, the olecranon process is posterior to the center of the elbow joint (fig. 2.25). A muscle-tendon attached to the olecranon process would have a posterior spatial relationship to the elbow joint.

Superior. This term, like the others above, is used to describe relative position. It is not used in a qualitative context. In the anatomic position, the skull is superior to the feet. That denotes position only. It is not a statement regarding the relative value of skull-brain over feet. Superior can be used to describe relative position of any body structure. As an example, the ulna olecranon process is located superior to the ulna styloid process (fig. 2.26).

Inferior. This term is utilized to describe anatomic parts as the opposite of superior, e.g., the styloid process of the ulna is inferior to the olecranon process. *The tendons of the extrinsic muscles of the feet are described as being either inferior or superior to the interphalangeal and metatarsophalangeal joints* (fig. 2.5).

The reference terms are often used in conjunction with each other to describe exact locations of body structures. Examples are shown in figure 2.12 regarding the iliac spines on the iliac crests of the pelvic girdle.

The learning of anatomic kinesiology can be much easier if locations of bone landmarks and joint muscle-tendon relationships are known. Understanding joint motion will be facilitated by knowing exactly where the internal force of muscle contraction is being applied to the bone levers.

Anatomic landmarks

The illustrated landmarks in this chapter have been delimited to include only those used most frequently as attachment points for muscles, leverage mechanisms for tendons, and those which serve important functions related to joint and body segment motions. A minimum review list of bones and skeletal landmarks appears in figure 2.4. Each of the landmarks cited in figure 2.4, as well as those labeled in the remaining figures in this chapter, should be studied

FOOT	Talus, calcaneus, navicular, cuboid, medial, lateral and intermediate cuneiforms, tuberosity of fifth metatarsal, sustentaculum tali
LEG	Fibula—lateral malleolus, styloid process, head Tibia—medial malleolus, anterior border-medial surface, tibial tuberosity, medial and lateral condyles
THIGH	Femur—medial and lateral condyles, linea aspera, lesser trochanter, greater trochanter, head, neck
PELVIS	Pelvis—ilium, ischium, pubis—pubic crest, crest of ilium, anterior and posterior, superior and inferior spines, ischial tuberosity, acetabulum, iliopectineal eminence
SPINE	Vertebrae—cervical, thoracic, lumbar—body, transverse and spinous processes—atlas and axis
CHEST	Ribs, Sternum—body, manubrium, and xiphoid process
SHOULDER GIRDLE	Scapula—spine, acromion process, infra and supraglenoid tubercles, superior border, vertebral border, inferior angle, glenoid fossa, coracoid process, superior angle, subscapular fossa, supraspinatous fossa, infraspinatous fossa and lateral angle clavicle—deltoid tubercle, trapezoid line-ridge
ARM	Humerus—greater tubercle, lesser tubercle, head, anatomical neck, surgical neck, medial and lateral epicondyles, olecranon fossa, trochlea, capitulum, deltoid tuberosity, intertubercular groove
FOREARM	Ulna—olecranon process, coranoid process, styloid process, trochlear notch Radius—head, neck, radial tuberosity, styloid process
HEAD	Skull—mastoid process, zygomatic arch, mandible, maxilla, superior nuchal line, occipital protuberance
HAND	Navicular, lunate, capitate, triangular, pisiform, greater multangular, lesser multangular, hamate

Figure 2.4. Selected bones and skeletal landmarks.

with care. The student should know the exact locations on the bones relative to the anatomic parts involved. Furthermore, it is important to know the positions of the landmarks relative to joint centers in the immediate vicinity. The reference terms cited above should be used to help conceptualize and describe these anatomic landmarks, as well as their relationships to other anatomic structures, to each other, and to joint centers.

It is further recommended that the bones and landmarks also be studied on a fully articulated skeleton. Pictures in a textbook do not provide a three dimensional format for viewing the interrelationships of the skeletal structures. Three dimensional conceptualization leads to a better understanding of locations of anatomic landmarks. This is necessary for two important reasons: (1) to understand the lines-of-pull of muscles from attachment to attachment and, (2) to have a basis for understanding the spatial relationships of muscles and muscle groups to the joints they cross. The *spatial relationship concept* is discussed in detail in Chapter Five.

Muscles have a line-of-pull from one bone attachment point to another attachment point. The tendons of the muscles attach to these specific points, and that is where the internal force generated by the muscle during contraction is applied. Many of these attachment points are included in the figures of this chapter. Attachment points simply indicate muscle location for the application of force.

There are several terms related to these muscle attachments which need to be understood. The muscle attachments themselves are important only when used in relation to descriptions of the line-of-pull and force application of the muscle. These muscle attachments have specific names, depending upon body location.

The most common terms used for muscle attachments are *proximal and distal attachments*. These terms have replaced *origin* and *insertion,* because these older terms conveyed a misconception regarding motion.

The often stated idea to the effect that all origins are relatively stable and all insertions instable during motion is misleading. Muscles have the potential of reversing their pull at either end. For example, during the pull-up exercise one sees a reversal of the traditional idea of attachment movement within the biceps brachii, brachialis, and brachioradialis muscles at the elbow. The forearm is relatively stable as the upper arm flexes toward the forearm during the upward phase of the pull-up. Here it can be seen that the origin, or proximal attachment, of the biceps brachii in particular is actually the moving end. The same phenomenon is occurring in regard to the other muscles most involved for elbow flexion against resistance. The distal attachments remain stable so the humerus can move toward the forearm during the pull-up exercise. The opposite movement and stabilization involving attachments is seen during a "biceps curl" exercise. Motion can be in any direction, depending upon (1) which attachment is relatively more stable at the time of contraction, and, (2) the performance objective.

The terms *proximal attachment* and *distal attachment* are used in some cases to describe muscle-bone attachments in the upper and lower limbs only. They are used for all muscle attachments in this book; however, the reader is provided below with alternate terms for muscles located entirely on the trunk. In describing lines of pull for those muscles, the alternate terms may make it easier to conceptualize the lines of pull and force application of muscles on the trunk.

Proximal attachments are located near the trunk of the body. This replaces the term *origin*. As an example of proximal attachments, figure 2.23 shows the coracoid process and supraglenoid tubercle of the scapula. These are designated as the proximal attachments of the biceps brachii muscle, due to their proximity to the trunk.

Distal attachments are located farther from the trunk of the body than proximal attachments. *Distal attachment* replaces the term *insertion*. With the body in the anatomic position, it can readily be noted by palpation that the distal attachment of the biceps brachii is farther from the trunk than the proximal attachments. It is the radial tuberosity (fig. 2.25) inferior to the elbow joint.

Terms which can be used for the muscle attachments involving muscles located on the trunk and cervical spine-head segments are: (1) *superior attachment,* (2) *inferior attachment,* (3) *medial attachment,* and (4) *lateral attachment.* These are presented and defined in this book so the reader may use these terms if he or she desires.

Using the analysis positions, it can be observed that proximal and distal attachment usage can be confusing when describing the lines of pull of muscles located entirely on the trunk. *Therefore, for muscles lying vertically on the trunk, the terms superior attachment and inferior attachment can be used.* An example of this usage would be in reference to the large rectus abdominis muscle which has a vertical line of pull. Its superior attachment would be on the cartilage of ribs 5–7 and the xyphoid process (fig. 2.19). The inferior attachment is on the superior aspect of the pubic crest (fig. 2.12).

For muscles with a line of pull relatively horizontal or diagonal to the earth located on the trunk, the terms medial and lateral attachments can be used. As an example, the external oblique muscle of the abdomen has a medial bone attachment on the anterior half of the iliac crest and the pubic crest (fig. 2.14). The lateral attachment is on the inferior border of the lower eight ribs (fig. 2.19). This muscle, like the rectus abdominis, can be palpated directly.

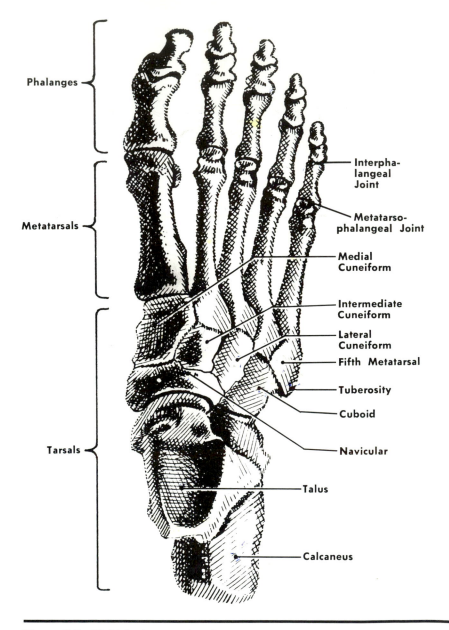

Phalanges

Metatarsals

Tarsals

Interpha-
langeal
Joint

Metatarso-
phalangeal Joint

Medial
Cuneiform

Intermediate
Cuneiform

Lateral
Cuneiform

Fifth Metatarsal

Tuberosity

Cuboid

Navicular

Talus

Calcaneus

Figure 2.5. Right foot—superior view.

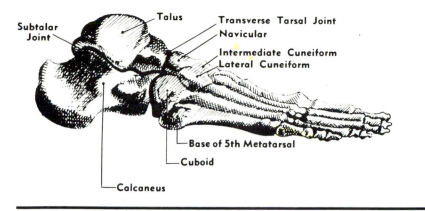

Figure 2.6. Right foot—lateral view.

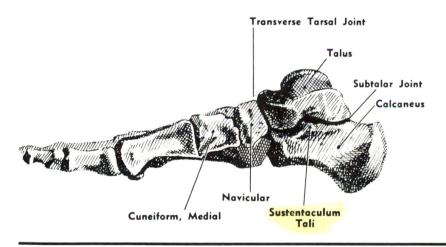

Figure 2.7. Right foot—medial view.

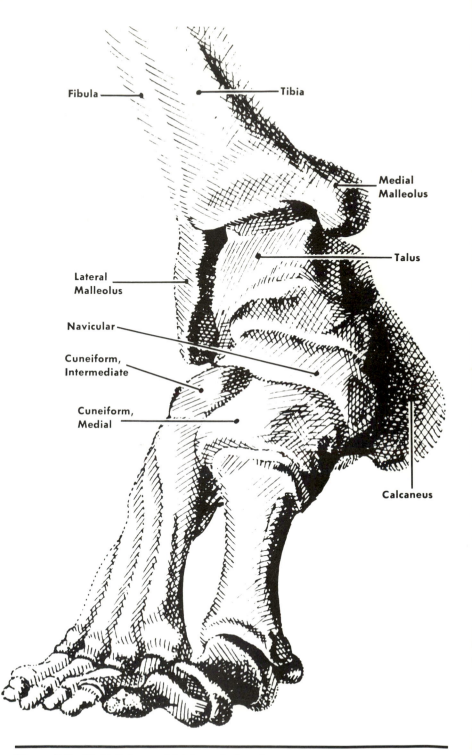

Figure 2.8. Right Talocrural joint—anterior view.

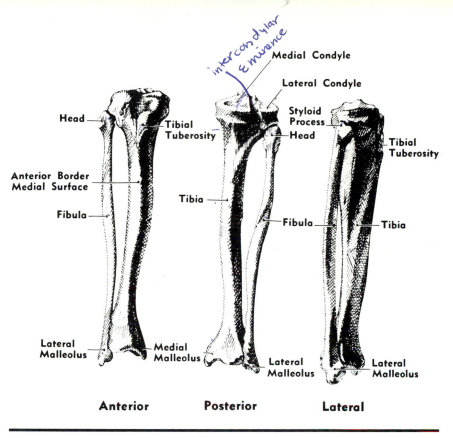

Figure 2.9. Skeletal landmarks of the tibia and fibula.

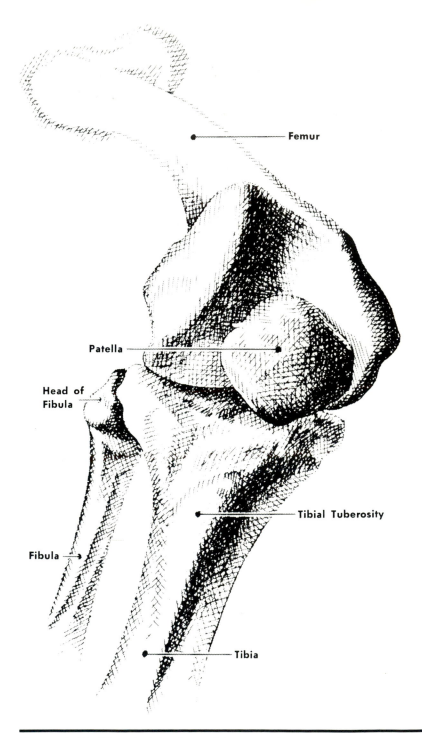

Figure 2.10. Flexed right knee joint—anterior view.

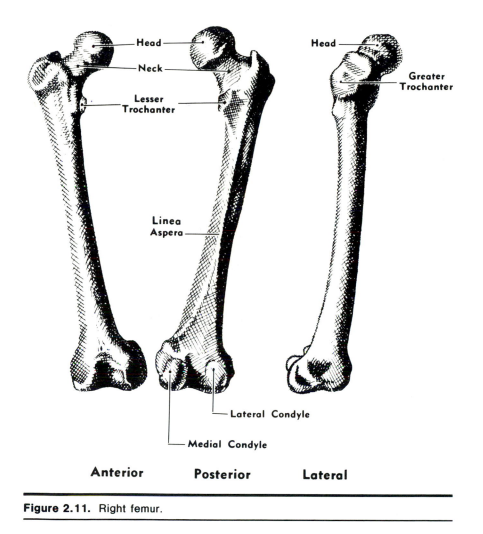

Head

Neck

Lesser
Trochanter

Head

Greater
Trochanter

Linea
Aspera

Lateral Condyle

Medial Condyle

Anterior   **Posterior**   **Lateral**

Figure 2.11. Right femur.

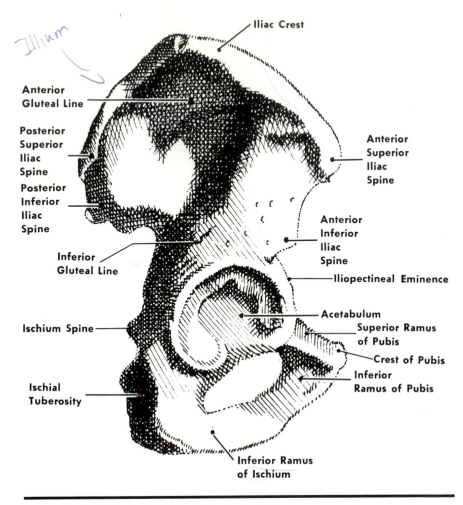

Illium

Iliac Crest

Anterior Gluteal Line

Posterior Superior Iliac Spine

Posterior Inferior Iliac Spine

Inferior Gluteal Line

Ischium Spine

Ischial Tuberosity

Anterior Superior Iliac Spine

Anterior Inferior Iliac Spine

Iliopectineal Eminence

Acetabulum

Superior Ramus of Pubis

Crest of Pubis

Inferior Ramus of Pubis

Inferior Ramus of Ischium

Figure 2.12. Right half pelvic girdle—lateral view.

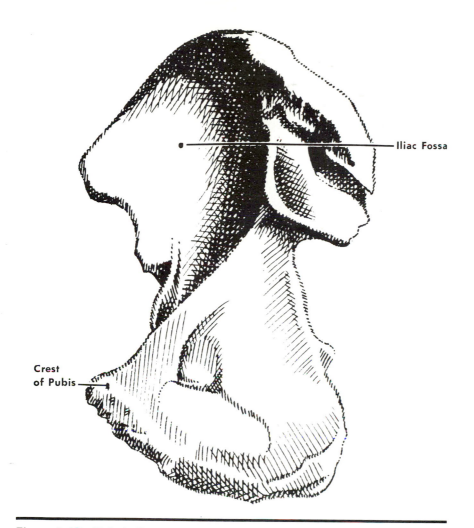

Iliac Fossa

Crest
of Pubis

Figure 2.13. Right half pelvic girdle—medial.

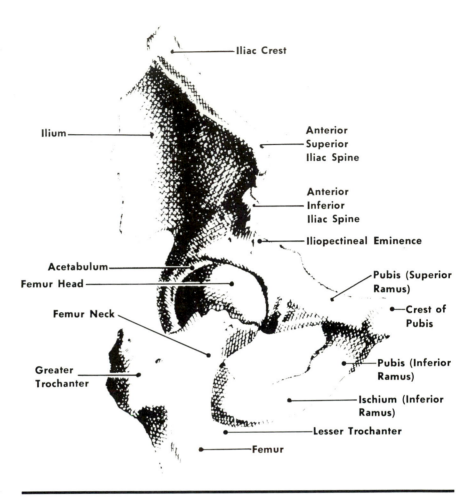

Figure 2.14. Right hip joint—lateral view.

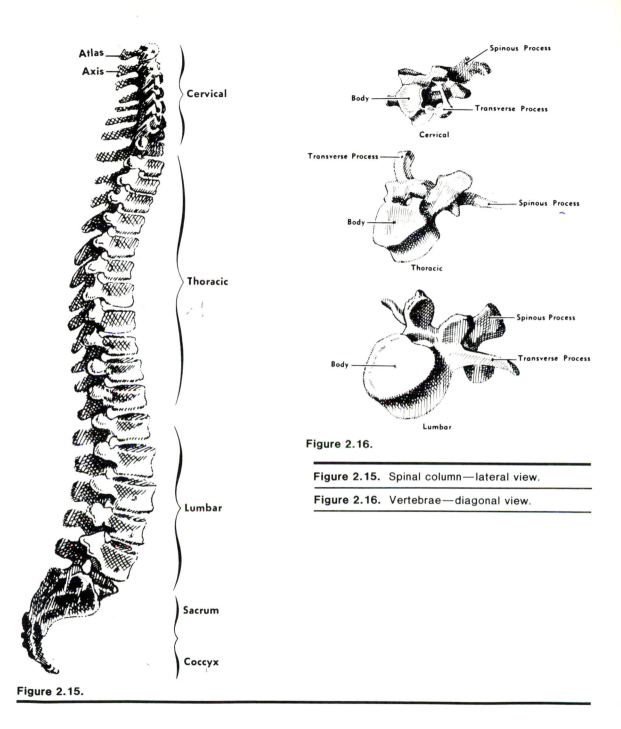

Atlas
Axis
Cervical

Spinous Process
Body
Transverse Process
Cervical

Transverse Process
Body
Spinous Process
Thoracic

Thoracic

Spinous Process
Body
Transverse Process
Lumbar

Lumbar

Sacrum

Coccyx

Figure 2.16.

Figure 2.15. Spinal column—lateral view.

Figure 2.16. Vertebrae—diagonal view.

Figure 2.15.

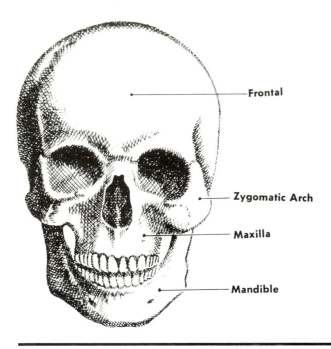

Figure 2.17. Skull—anterior view.

Frontal

Zygomatic Arch

Maxilla

Mandible

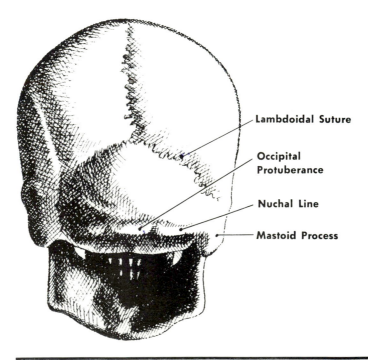

Figure 2.18. Skull—posterior view.

Lambdoidal Suture

Occipital Protuberance

Nuchal Line

Mastoid Process

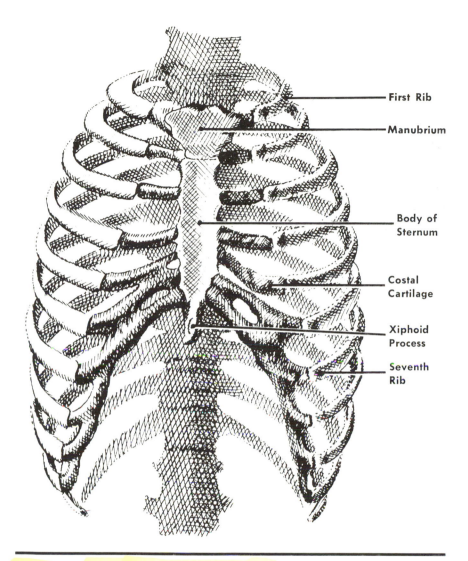

First Rib

Manubrium

Body of
Sternum

Costal
Cartilage

Xiphoid
Process

Seventh
Rib

Figure 2.19. Skeletal landmarks of the rib cage—
anterior view.

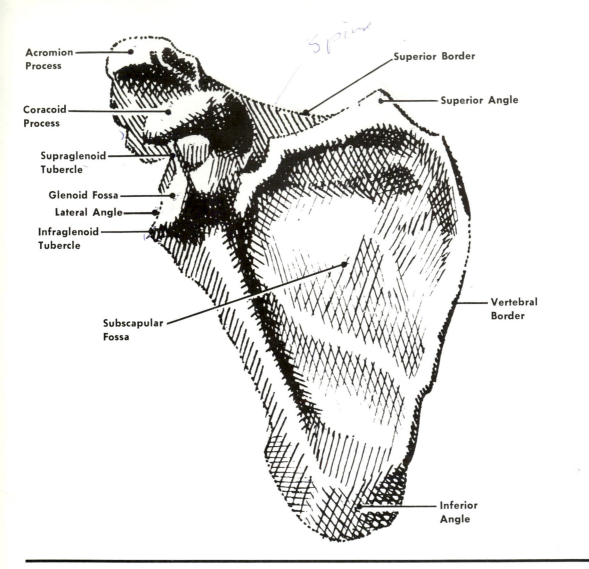

Acromion Process

Coracoid Process

Supraglenoid Tubercle

Glenoid Fossa

Lateral Angle

Infraglenoid Tubercle

Subscapular Fossa

Spine

Superior Border

Superior Angle

Vertebral Border

Inferior Angle

Figure 2.20. Skeletal landmarks of the right scapula—anterior view.

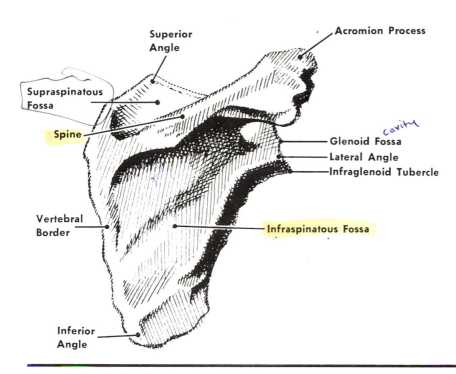

Figure 2.21. Skeletal landmarks of the right scapula—posterior view.

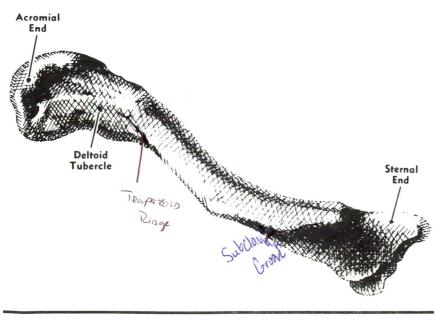

Figure 2.22. Right clavicle—anterior view.

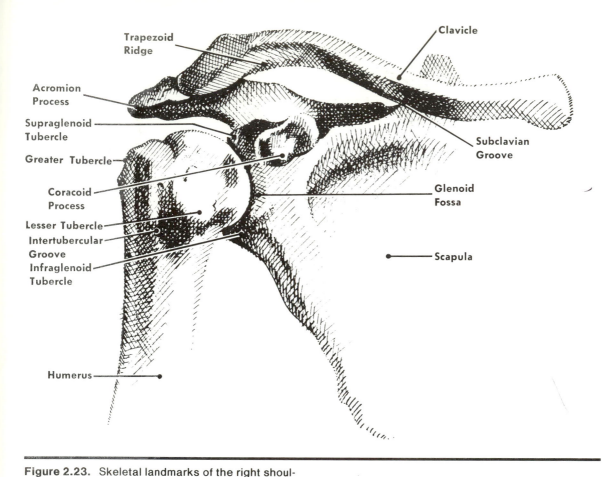

Figure 2.23. Skeletal landmarks of the right shoulder joint—anterior view.

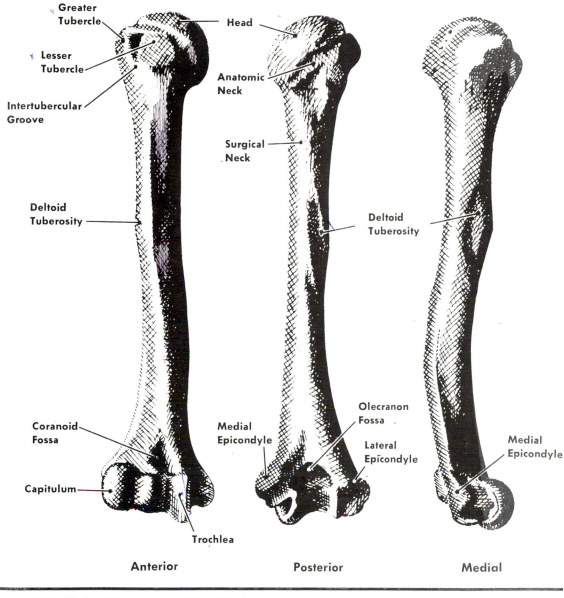

Greater Tubercle

Lesser Tubercle

Intertubercular Groove

Deltoid Tuberosity

Coranoid Fossa

Capitulum

Trochlea

Head

Anatomic Neck

Surgical Neck

Deltoid Tuberosity

Olecranon Fossa

Medial Epicondyle

Lateral Epicondyle

Medial Epicondyle

Anterior

Posterior

Medial

Figure 2.24. Skeletal landmarks of the right humerus.

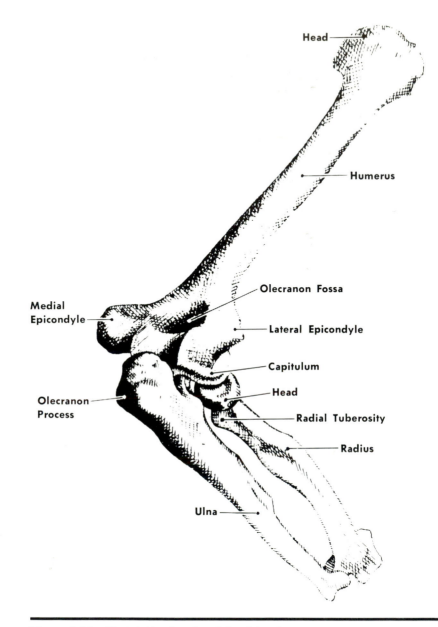

Head

Humerus

Olecranon Fossa

Medial
Epicondyle

Lateral Epicondyle

Capitulum

Head

Olecranon
Process

Radial Tuberosity

Radius

Ulna

Figure 2.25. Skeletal landmarks of the right elbow
joint in a flexed position—diagonal view.

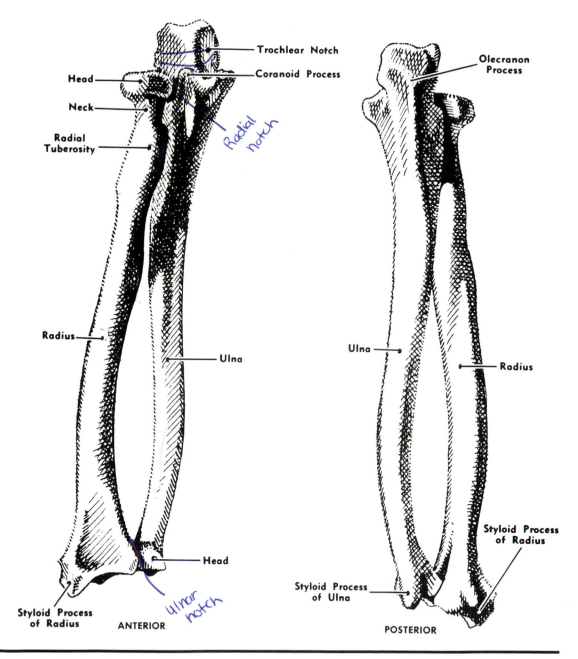

Trochlear Notch

Coranoid Process

Head

Neck

Radial Tuberosity

Radial notch

Radius

Ulna

Styloid Process of Radius

Head

Ulnar notch

ANTERIOR

Olecranon Process

Ulna

Radius

Styloid Process of Radius

Styloid Process of Ulna

POSTERIOR

Figure 2.26. Right radius and ulna.

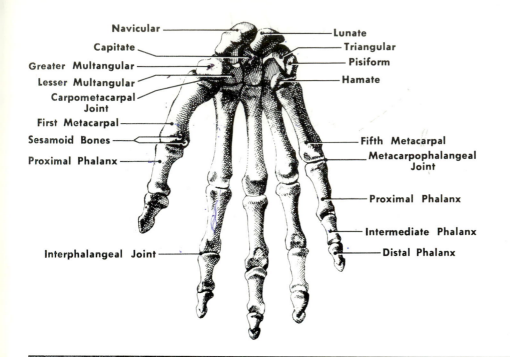

Navicular
Lunate
Capitate
Triangular
Greater Multangular
Pisiform
Lesser Multangular
Hamate
Carpometacarpal
Joint
First Metacarpal
Fifth Metacarpal
Sesamoid Bones
Metacarpophalangeal
Joint
Proximal Phalanx
Proximal Phalanx
Intermediate Phalanx
Interphalangeal Joint
Distal Phalanx

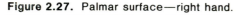

Figure 2.27. Palmar surface—right hand.

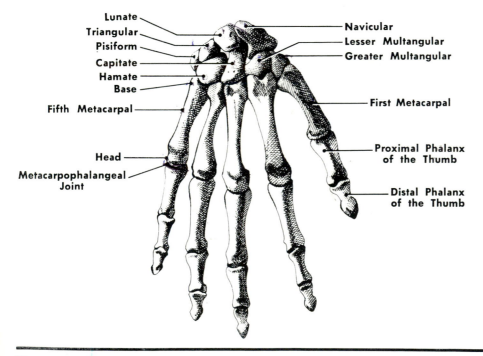

Lunate
Navicular
Triangular
Lesser Multangular
Pisiform
Greater Multangular
Capitate
Hamate
Base
Fifth Metacarpal
First Metacarpal
Proximal Phalanx
of the Thumb
Head
Metacarpophalangeal
Joint
Distal Phalanx
of the Thumb

Figure 2.28. Dorsal surface—right hand.

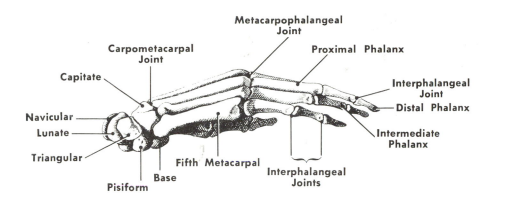

Figure 2.29. Right hand—ulnar view.

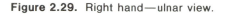

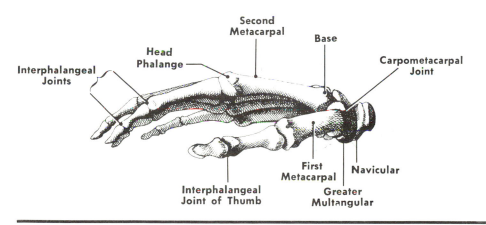

Figure 2.30. Right hand—radial view.

Gray, Henry. *Anatomy of the Human Body.* Philadelphia: Lea & Febiger, 1973.

Logan, Gene A. *Adaptations of Muscular Activity.* Belmont, Calif.: Wadsworth Publishing Company, 1964.

————. *Adapted Physical Education.* Dubuque: Wm. C. Brown Company, Publishers, 1972.

Peck, Stephen Rogers. *Atlas of Human Anatomy for the Artist.* New York: Oxford University Press, 1951.

Selected references

3

Planes
of
Motion

Basic locomotor activities performed by humans, such as walking, jogging, and running, most commonly result in linear motion of the total body. The cause of this motion is a perfectly timed series of rotational or angular motions within the joints at the ankle, knee, and hip primarily. All motions within the articulations or joints of the body are rotary in nature, i.e., joints and their attached limbs or body segments turn through a number of degrees dependent upon the anatomic configuration of the articulation. The motion potential in each joint differs considerably; therefore, each has a measurable *range of motion* in degrees, with specific limitations. Each limb or body segment is moved by means of internal forces developed by muscle contractions through all or a portion of its range of motion, through a *plane of motion.*

A plane of motion is defined as an imaginary two-dimensional surface through which a limb or body segment is moved. To best conceptualize a plane, it may be imagined as a circular windowpane which dissects an area of the body or the center of a joint (fig. 3.1). The rotation of the joint through a plane of motion occurs around an imaginary line or axis of motion through and perpendicular to the plane of motion, i.e., a body segment moving through a plane revolves around an axis. There is a ninety-degree relationship between a plane of motion and its axis.

To conceptualize a theoretical plane and axis at a joint, one must first make an *estimate* concerning the location of the center of the joint. The plane and axis both pass through the center of the joint with the axis of rotation lying perpendicular to the plane of motion as noted. The exact center of a joint cannot be determined scientifically unless radiologic filming techniques are utilized, and this is not feasible for numerous reasons, except in rare research situations.

Joint centers can be estimated with relative accuracy on film and videotape by utilizing one's knowledge of joint anatomy, including bone and muscle relationships as well as the motion capabilities of the joint. As an example, the ankle joint is formed by the articulation between the talus and tibia (figure 2.8). This joint has two motion capabilities: (1) dorsiflexion and (2) plantar flexion. (Joint motions are defined in Chapter Four.) These motions move the foot segment through an anteroposterior plane of motion around an axis of rotation perpendicular to that plane. The axis of rotation can be visualized by drawing an imaginary line through the medial malleolus to the lateral malleolus. The foot turns through an anteroposterior plane of motion as it dorsiflexes and plantar flexes. The theoretical plane would be anterior and posterior through the center of the ankle joint formed by the talus and tibia.

A simpler method of visualizing a plane with its axis of rotation is to tie a low weight object such as a ring on a piece of string six to eight inches in length. The other end of the string is then tied to the center of a pencil. The weighted string should be moved to allow it to turn or rotate through 360 degrees around the center of the shaft of the pencil. The pencil simulates the axis of rotation, and the weighted string enables one to picture mentally the plane of motion. Flexion and extension of the elbow, as a joint motion example, constitutes the same axis-plane relationship, except the elbow motion is limited to approximately 150 degrees through its plane due to joint structure and surrounding tissue mass. (fig. 3.3).

Traditional planes of motion

For centuries anatomists and kinesiologists have recognized, in the literature on this subject, the existence of three anatomic reference planes. These traditional planes of motion are: (1) anteroposterior or saggital plane, (2) lateral or frontal plane, and (3) transverse or horizontal plane. The term *cardinal* is used at times in connection with these planes. When this expression is used it means that the discussion is centered on only the two vertical planes (anteroposterior and lateral) as they are shown in figures 3.1 and 3.6.

When the anatomic position is assumed these two planes meet at a theoretical point within the body known as the *center of gravity* (refer to figure 2.1). The center of gravity of the total body shifts continuously as one performs in sport and dance. In some activities such as high jumping, diving, and pole vaulting, the theoretical point for the center of gravity can lie outside the body.

The center of gravity of the total body is where the weight of the body is concentrated. *It is a mathematic construct not a reality.* Centers of gravity may be calculated for each body segment, as well as for the total body, in order to study such phenomona as segment displacement patterns and equilibrium. However, these calculations are not made during kinesiologic analyses at the non-cinematographic and basic cinematographic levels. For these analytic techniques, which are used on a daily basis, it is not necessary or feasible to calculate mathematically the location of the center of gravity. However, scientific study of centers of gravity of the human body and its segments during motion is of prime concern to many research investigators in the fields of anatomic kinesiology and biomechanics.

The general position of the center of gravity for the total body in the anatomic position was described above. This point for adult males is approximately 56 to 57 percent of their total height. Usually this is near the level of the umbilicus at a central point within the body. Due to greater distribution of subcutaneous adipose tissue in adult females around the anterior, lateral and posterior pelvic-hip area, the center of gravity lies at approximately 55 percent of their total height.

The terms *horizontal* and *vertical* tend to be somewhat confusing when used in connection with planes of motion. Since these terms are usually used to indicate a position relative to the surface of the earth, they can be misleading in regard to sport movements. As an example, the transverse plane is a horizontal plane (to the earth) when the individual is in an upright position. The axis of motion is vertical. Performers do not always assume upright positions, and this is where confusion can exist. When the performer is supine and suspended in air, as during a dive, the transverse plane becomes a vertical plane, and the axis of motion becomes horizontal. To avoid this type of communication problem, the terms *horizontal* and *vertical* are not used herein to depict planes of motion of performers in relation to the earth. *The reference for planes is the body itself.*

Anteroposterior or sagittal plane of motion

The cardinal anteroposterior plane divides the body into equal, bilateral segments (fig. 3.1). This theoretical plane bisects the body through the center of the skull, spinal column, rib cage, pelvis, and lower limbs. Motions through the cardinal

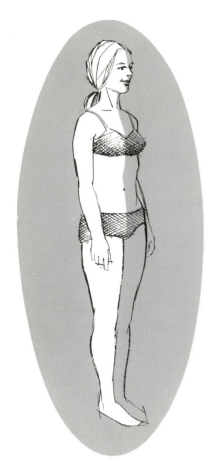

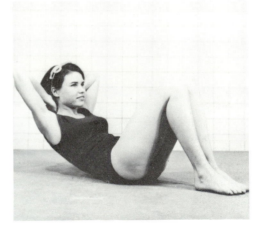

Figure 3.2.

Figure 3.1. Cardinal anteroposterior plane of motion.

Figure 3.2. Hook-lying sit-up—an exercise through the cardinal anteroposterior plane of motion (Ruth Miller).

Figure 3.1.

anteroposterior plane involve the cervical, thoracic, and lumbar regions of the spinal column. Motions through this plane occur, for example, during a sit-up exercise (fig. 3.2).

Anteroposterior plane motions are not restricted to movements involving the spinal column. When the term *cardinal* is not used with this or any other traditional plane, it means that the motion being described causes the joint or limb to move in a plane *parallel* to the cardinal plane of motion. An example of this would be the biceps curl weight-training exercise shown in figure 3.3. The weight and lower half of the arm move through an anteroposterior plane as the elbow is flexed and extended. In this illustration, the anteroposterior plane being traversed is parallel to the cardinal, anteroposterior plane of motion.

The long jumper shown in figure 3.4 is flexing her left hip and knee joints through anteroposterior planes parallel to the cardinal anteroposterior plane. These joint motions, with others, are important for the long jumper at take-off, because they help determine the critical angle of take-off and subsequent trajectory for the flight of the body. Maximum distance in flight is determined, in part, by the efficiency of these anteroposterior plane motions. For example, extreme hip flexion would tend to lift the body too much vertically and increase

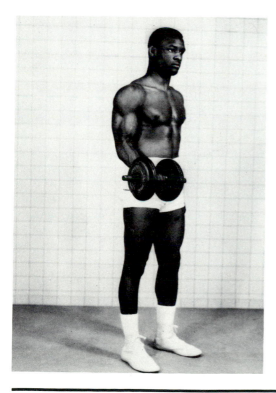

Figure 3.3 Biceps curl—movement through an anteroposterior plane of motion (Ardie McCoy).

the take-off angle. That would also decrease horizontal speed and adversely effect the distance of the jump. In all sport skills, there are optimum joint motions through appropriate planes at correct velocities to produce the desired results.

The balance beam in women's gymnastics is a very demanding piece of apparatus, because it is only 10.16 centimeters wide. This dictates that several anteroposterior plane motions must be executed precisely by an elite performer during a routine or she will lose her equilibrium. The gymnast in figure 3.5 is shown moving several major joints and segments through anteroposterior planes: (1) left hip joint—extension, (2) right hip joint—flexion, (3) lumbar-thoracic spine—hyperextension, (4) cervical spine—hyperextension, and (5) both shoulder joints—flexion. The spinal motions are through the cardinal anteroposterior plane, and the other motions noted are through anteroposterior planes parallel to the cardinal plane.

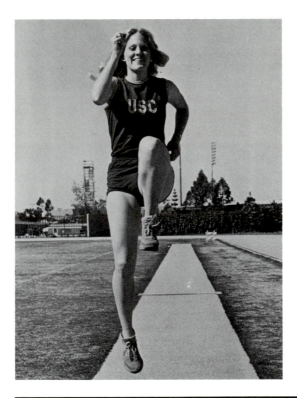

Figure 3.4. Anteroposterior plane motions at the left hip and knee are important to long jump performance as demonstrated by Sandy Crabtree. Courtesy *U.S.C. Athletic News Service*—Michael R. Harriel.

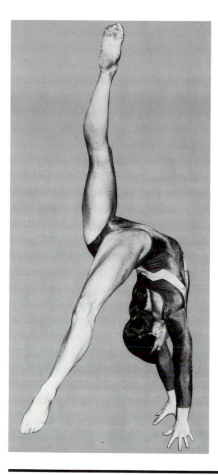

Figure 3.5. Gale Wyckoff, USC gymnast, executing a balance beam skill which requires several joint motions through anteroposterior planes. Courtesy *USC Athletic News Service.*

Lateral or frontal plane of motion

This cardinal plane divides the body into anterior and posterior halves. It bisects the body laterally through the ear, shoulder, spinal column, pelvis, hips, knees, and ankles (fig. 3.6).

Motion capabilities through the lateral plane are somewhat limited in relation to the other planes of motion. Body areas involved are the upper and lower limbs, cervical, and lumbar-thoracic spinal regions. The jumping-jack calisthenic exercise as shown in figure 3.7 is a good example of upper and lower limb segments moving through the lateral plane of motion.

Numerous calisthenic exercises utilize the lateral plane motions at the shoulder and hip joints as well as the spinal column. The "thrust phase" of the elementary back stroke in swimming utilizes powerful shoulder and hip joint lateral plane motions (adductions) to propel the body forward in the water. Motions of the upper and lower limbs through the lateral plane are often used to enhance body stability or equilibrium both in moving and nonmoving situations. The gymnast in figure 3.8 has moved her upper limbs through the lateral plane during a floor exercise routine. This helps her maintain equilibrium over a relatively small, unilateral weightbearing base of support (the toes of her left foot).

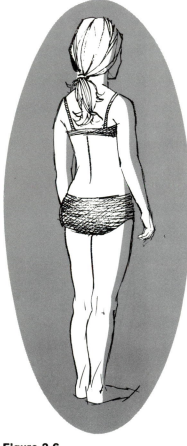

Figure 3.6.

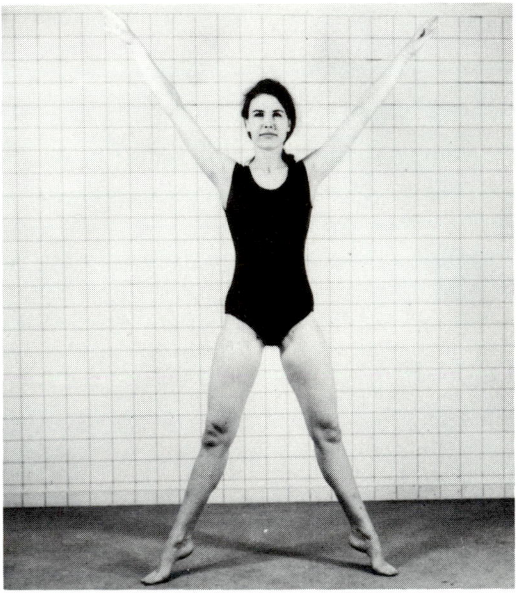

Figure 3.7.

Figure 3.6. Cardinal lateral plane of motion. From Northrip, Logan, and McKinney. *Introduction to Biomechanic Analysis of Sport.*

Figure 3.7. Jumping jack—a movement through the cardinal lateral plane of motion (Ruth Miller).

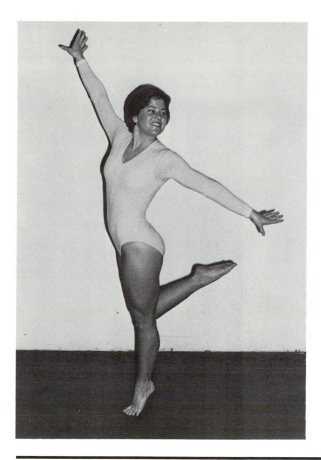

Figure 3.8. Holley Donaldson, USC gymnast, abducts both shoulder joints moving her upper limbs through the lateral plane of motion to maintain equilibrium during a floor exercise routine. Courtesy *USC Athletic News Service.*

Transverse or horizontal plane of motion

The cardinal transverse plane of motion theoretically divides the body into superior and inferior halves when the individual is in the anatomic position. This plane is shown in figure 3.9. The position of the cardinal transverse plane differs slightly in the average adult male and female. As noted, the transverse plane for the adult female lies at a point slightly below the umbilicus. The reason for this lies in the fact that adipose tissue distribution following sexual maturation of women is usually below the iliac crests posteriorly and laterally. Adipose tissue is also distributed anteriorly and inferior to the umbilicus. This means that the center of gravity is slightly lower in the average adult female than in the average adult male. Men have a higher center of gravity and cardinal transverse plane

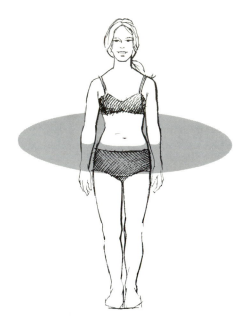

Figure 3.9. Cardinal transverse plane of motion.
From Northrip, Logan, and McKinney. *Introduction
to Biomechanic Analysis of Sport.*

due to the fact that adipose tissue, if any excess is found on the trunk, is usually immediately superior to the iliac crests. This causes the cardinal transverse plane to separate the superior and inferior halves of the "ideal" male body at the umbilical level.

The "twisting motions" of the spinal column (rotations) are performed through the cardinal transverse plane of motion (fig. 3.10). There are numerous calisthenic type exercises for flexibility development which depend upon spinal column rotations. In addition, there are many ballistic sport skills, gymnastic routines, and diving maneuvers wherein spinal column rotations through the cardinal transverse plane are absolutely basic to acceptable performance levels (fig. 3.8).

Rotations through a transverse plane are also possible within joints other than the spinal column. The medial and lateral rotations, as examples, at the hip and shoulder joints, while in the anatomic position are through transverse planes. The bench press is another example of an exercise performed through a transverse plane with the axis longitudinal to the body (fig. 3.11).

Diagonal planes of motion

Description of motions during analyses of sport skills is very limited when restricted to the movements strictly defined by the three traditional planes of motion. Therefore, to add to motion terminology and enhance the accuracy of motion description in the area of analytic kinesiology, Logan and McKinney introduced the diagonal planes of motion in 1970. These planes and the motions

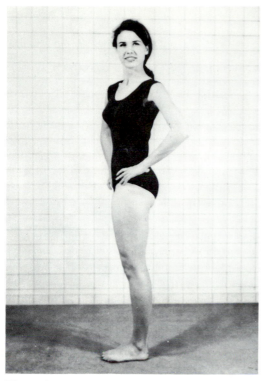

Figure 3.10.

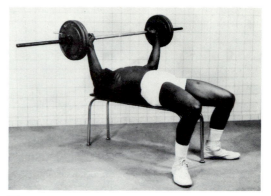

Figure 3.11.

Figure 3.10. Spinal rotation—a movement through the cardinal transverse plane of motion (Ruth Miller).

Figure 3.11. Bench press—an exercise through a transverse plane (Ardie McCoy).

through the diagonal planes were established to be utilized with, not to replace, the three traditional planes of motion.

The diagonal planes are: (1) *high diagonal* for upper limbs at the shoulder joints, (2) *low diagonal* for upper limbs at the shoulder joints, and (3) *low diagonal* for lower limbs at the hip joints. In regard to diagonal plane motion at the hip joint, the muscular and ligamentous structures do not allow motion through a high diagonal plane which would be analogous to shoulder joint motion. A high diagonal plane of motion for an upper limb is shown in figure 3.12. The corresponding low diagonal plane of motion of the *opposite* upper limb is shown in the same illustration. A low diagonal plane of motion for the left *lower limb* is shown in figure 3.13. Figure 3.14 is a composite of the three diagonal planes at the hip and shoulder joints.

It is interesting to note that sports which tend to utilize the traditional planes of motion the most are the so-called "judged sports." Many times these sports, such as gymnastics, diving, and portions of weight-lifting, have their bases for scoring in aesthetic factors. Perhaps there is a relationship between this type of activity and formal programs of physical education. Through 1927 the formal programs seen extensively in the past throughout Germany, Sweden, and in America had as their bases movement patterns associated with traditional planes of motion which were described by and borrowed from anatomists.

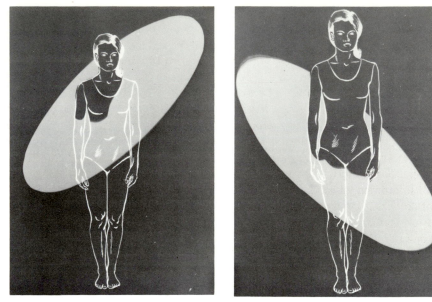

Figure 3.12.   **Figure 3.13.**

Figure 3.12. High diagonal plane of motion for the
left shoulder joint.

Figure 3.13. Diagonal plane of motion for the left
hip joint.

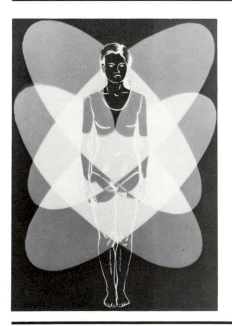

Figure 3.14. Composite of diagonal planes at both
hip and shoulder joints.

Many sport motions do not conform precisely to movement through the anteroposterior, lateral, and transverse planes of motion. On the other hand, activities such as marching, wands, and calisthenics include numerous motions through the traditional planes. Physical education programs utilizing these formal activities in the latter part of this century in America would not be too popular. Instruction in a wide variety of sports is the trend.

The longitudinal axis of the body is the reference point for diagonal limb motions, i.e., a limb moving through a diagonal plane moves in an arc oblique or diagonal to the cardinal anteroposterior plane. It is a commonly observed fact that there are numerous times in sport when the upper and lower limbs move diagonally through planes toward or away from the longitudinal axis of the body. Most throwing, striking, and kicking techniques employ these motions. The act of "crossing the legs" while seated or standing requires a diagonal motion of one lower limb involving the hip joint. Since these planes and motions are so common, it was deemed necessary to identify them formally. This was done to enhance skill analysis, motion description, and the communication process related to the teaching and learning of neuromuscular skills.

Structural observations of the shoulder and hip joints provide some of the rationale for diagonal planes of motion. These joints are classified as enarthrodial (ball-and-socket) joints. This means that these joints have motion capabilities of a multiaxial nature. Motion is not restricted to the three traditional planes only. The hip joint arrangement of the head of the femur (ball) being received into the acetabulum of the pelvis (socket) allows the lower limbs to be moved diagonally. This is analogous to an automobile-trailer hitch arrangement, and the reader is familiar with the versatility of motion of a trailer when one tries to back it into a parking space. For a closer analogy to the versatility of motion within the hip and shoulder joints, imagine that the trailer is hitched to an airplane flying through the air. Depending upon the external forces, the airborne trailer can move in any direction! It is not restricted to up-and-down (anteroposterior), back-and-forth (lateral), or limited rotation around its longitudinal axis (transverse) motions. The same can be said of the hip and shoulder joints. They can be moved in any direction. The shoulder joint structure involving the head of the humerus (ball) articulating with the glenoid fossa of the scapula (socket) allows the same motion versatility as the hip joint. Therefore, the bone structure of these joints allows the limbs to be moved diagonally as well as through the three traditional planes of motion.

Muscular observations of the shoulder and hip joints provide additional rationale for diagonal planes of motion. Muscle contraction provides the internal force to move the body segments. The muscles are attached proximally and distally to bones, and the tendons of muscles cross joints at a point either anterior, posterior, medial, or lateral to the joint center. The *lines-of-pull* and *spatial relationships* of muscles and muscle groups to joints are important considerations affecting the motion capabilities of any joint.

The arrangement of the muscles at the hip joint indicates that several powerful muscles have *diagonal lines-of-pull.* The gluteus maximus (lower fibers), three large adductor muscles, and other muscles of the hip have the capability, by virtue of lines-of-pull and spatial relationship to the center of the hip joint, of moving the lower limb diagonally. The pectoralis major, latissimus dorsi, teres major, deltoid, and other muscles have diagonal lines-of-pull at the shoulder joint; therefore, they are optimally placed to exert their contractile forces on the upper limbs and move them through diagonal planes, if desired.

The multiaxial nature of the shoulder and hip joints allows the limb levers to be pulled diagonally during muscle contraction when the proximal attachments of the muscle group are momentarily stabilized, allowing the force to be exerted distally. This diagonal bone-muscle arrangement allows the performer to apply more force to a sport object if desired. In addition, this arrangement allows for more functional dissipation of force during the follow-through phases of ballistic motions such as those involving throwing, striking, and kicking skills (figure 3.16).

Another reason that diagonal motions are the rule for most ballistic actions is that pendular levers (the limbs) revolving on multiaxial articulations do involve angular momentum. As an attempt is made to move a limb through a range of motion in one plane, there is also a tendency for a lever or limb to describe a circular action. Therefore, the limb moves in an arc diagonal to the longitudinal axis of the body because the joint involved is also literally moving through space. This action is possible due to the multiaxial bony configuration and spatial relationship of the muscles to the shoulder and hip joints.

What problems would be encountered by a performer if the shoulder and hip joints were only structured to execute motions through the three traditional planes? Right-handed baseball or softball hitting will serve as an example of some of the problems one would encounter. First, the bat could not be gripped initially with both hands. The stance is assumed, and the bat is held in the left hand. The left shoulder joint and limb is moved through the anteroposterior plane (flexed) to the level of the shoulder where motions are possible through a transverse plane involving the shoulder joint. The bat is then moved through the transverse plane (horizontal adduction) to a position of readiness to await the pitch. The bat can now be gripped with the right hand. The spinal column is also rotated through the cardinal transverse plane during the stance. The pitch is delivered. There is a weight shift involving lateral plane motion of the left hip joint, and the bat and upper limbs are moved through a transverse plane at the shoulder to the point of impact with the ball. It is rather obvious that such motion limitations would greatly inhibit effective performance as it is known. The necessary force, angular velocities, and other components would not be generated, and the "traditional plane hitter" would always have to make contact with a ball out of the strike zone! Obviously, humans do utilize motions through traditional as well as the diagonal planes to perform skills; therefore, it is recommended that physical educators analyze and describe all skills using traditional and diagonal plane motion nomenclature.

High diagonal plane of motion (shoulder)

Figure 3.15 shows a baseball pitcher utilizing high diagonal plane motions involving the left shoulder joint. The left arm would follow the plane during release, and the follow-through would be diagonally across the pitcher's longitudinal axis.

The highly skilled pitcher in figure 3.16 shows the typical diagonal plane motion of the throwing limb during the follow-through phase of the skill. Variations on this motion pattern through a diagonal plane for almost all of the ballistic throwing and striking skills involving shoulder joints are dependent upon the direction of spin applied to the sport object. If "back spin" has been applied to the baseball (sport object), the throwing limb motion through the diagonal plane as seen in figure 3.16 is observed. Spin application to sport objects is critical in most sports, and it can ultimately determine the skill level the performer can attain in his or her sport specialty.

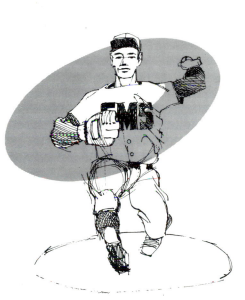

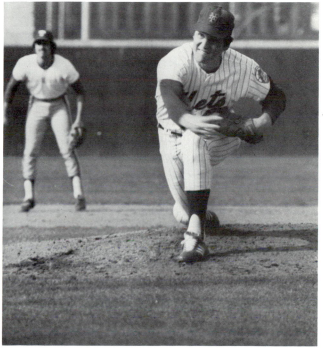

Figure 3.15.   **Figure 3.16.**

Figure 3.15. High diagonal plane of motion—left shoulder joint.

Figure 3.16. Diagonal adduction of the right shoulder joint of Tom Seaver, former USC pitcher. Roy Smalley, former USC shortstop, has started moving by plantar-flexing both ankle joints. Courtesy *USC Athletic News Service*.

High diagonal plane motions occur at any degree *above* the transverse plane at the shoulder joint, i.e., the plane is determined by the angle traversed by the upper limb during the motion. A person throwing a sport object such as a ball or javelin "over the top" would be using a very high diagonal plane. The term many coaches give for the diagonal plane being used by the pitcher in figure 3.15 is *three-quarters overhand.* "Overhand," regardless of the angle or degree of motion traversed by the shoulder joint and limb, is considered to be a high diagonal plane. A true "sidearm" motion is through a transverse plane at the shoulder joint, and this is not an anatomically or biomechanically sound way to perform throwing or striking motions. Throwing by using shoulder joint motions which bring the upper limb through the transverse plane can cause considerable stress due to centrifugal force, and this can lead to injuries to the "rotary cuff" of the shoulder and to other structures and articulations in the throwing limb.

Low diagonal plane of motion (shoulder)

The upper limb moves through this plane of motion when performers execute some "underhand" skills. Usually, but not in all cases, the low diagonal plane is traversed when considerable force or velocity is desired by the performer. The low diagonal planes are *below* the transverse plane at the shoulder joint. Figure 3.17 shows a discus thrower utilizing a low diagonal plane of motion using the right shoulder and upper limb.

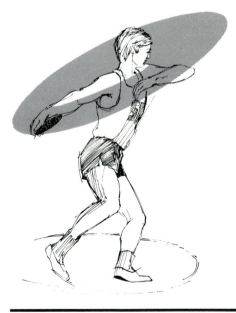

Figure 3.17. Low diagonal plane of motion—right shoulder joint. From Northrip, Logan, and McKinney. *Introduction to Biomechanic Analysis of Sport.*

Simple anteroposterior, pendular motions of the shoulder joint and upper limb are observed commonly when force and velocity are not prime objectives. A discus thrower, for example, throws through a low diagonal plane to attain maximum velocity and to give the discus the proper type of aerodynamic release and trajectory. It would be very inefficient for the athlete to release a discus underhand while flexing the shoulder and moving the limb through an antero-posterior plane of motion. A *slow* pitch softball pitcher, on the other hand, might throw underhand using anteroposterior plane motions. However, good *fast* pitch softball pitchers utilize low diagonal plane motions.

Golf is a game which demands extensive use of low diagonal plane motions involving the shoulder joints. As seen in figure 3.18, the golfer is utilizing diagonal abduction of the left upper limb and diagonal adduction of the right upper limb. These motions through low diagonal planes are necessary to transfer effectively the summated forces from the contraction of muscles to the sport implement (golf club) and subsequently apply those forces to the sport object (golf ball).

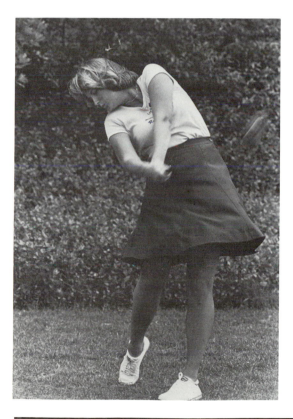

Figure 3.18. Denise Strebig, USC golfer, demonstrates the utilization of low diagonal plane motions involving both upper limbs during a golf shot. Courtesy *USC Athletic News Service.*

Low diagonal plane of motion (hip)

Figure 3.19 shows a soccer player using the diagonal plane of motion for a kick involving the right hip joint and lower limb. This type of movement pattern is observed rather commonly among soccer kickers and punters, and it is being applied more often among American football kickers and punters who are interested in more force application to the ball resulting in greater heights and distances. It should be noted, however, that low diagonal plane motions involving the hip joint do not have to be ballistic in nature. The crossing of one's legs while seated, or the scissors kick of the side stroke in swimming, involve motions through the low diagonal plane at hip joints performed at a low velocity.

As indicated, the hip joint is multiaxial in nature. Therefore, it has a tremendous potential range of motion. This potential is most commonly reduced due to the lack of flexibility within the noncontractile tissue surrounding the hip joints. Dance directors, gymnastic coaches, and diving coaches have long known the value of hip flexibility to range of motion and performance. It now appears that some coaches in team sports are also increasing flexibility in their student-athletes to enhance motion at the hip joint through anteroposterior, transverse, lateral, and diagonal planes.

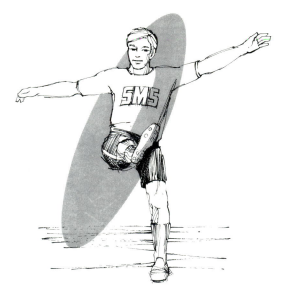

Figure 3.19. Diagonal plane of motion—right hip joint.

There are a relatively few individuals who, by virtue of special flexibility training and, perhaps, genetic or familial predisposition for flexibility, have the capability of moving the lower limb through a diagonal plane at the hip in an analogous position to the high diagonal plane at the shoulder. That plane of motion is difficult to attain at the hip joint, and it is not commonly observed. Therefore, it is not included in this text for discussion purposes. One should be aware, however, that a high diagonal plane potential at the hip joint may exist.

Recommended reading

Hellebrandt, F. A., et al. "The Location of the Cardinal Anatomical Orientation Planes Passing Through the Center of Gravity in Young Adult Women." *American Journal of Physiology* 121 (1938) :465.

Johnson, Robert E. "Comparison of Segment Ratio Weights and Centers of Gravity in the Living Human Male and Female." *Research Quarterly,* 47 (March, 1976), 105-109.

Swearingen, J. J. "Determination of Centers of Gravity of Man." *Federal Aviation Agency Report* 62-14 (August 1962) :37.

4

Joint Structure and Motion

An understanding of motion as it occurs in sport, exercise, or dance has its basis in the knowledge of motion possible in the major joints (articulations) of the body. In analyzing skill, the following factors related to motions in joints should be known: (1) the type of joints involved, (2) motions possible within these joints, and (3) the ranges of motion through which joints move during the performance. Motion occurs at joints as a result of muscles pulling on bony levers. The amount of motion possible within a joint is limited by muscle mass, connective tissue, and bony structures.

Classification of joints

Joints are classified in three major categories: (1) synarthrodial, (2) amphiarthrodial, and (3) diarthrodial. When working with human motion, the first classification is not of any great consequence because *synarthrodial joints are immovable joints,* and they are relatively rare in the body. Examples of these are found in the sutures of the skull and in articulations between the teeth and mandible or maxilla (fig. 2.17 and 2.18).

Amphiarthrodial joints are those which allow a slight amount of motion to occur. There are two major subclassifications for amphiarthrodial joints. One is *syndesmosis. A syndesmosis articulation is defined as two bones joined together by a ligament or an interosseous membrane.* The bones may or may not touch each other at the actual joint. An example of this type of joint is the coraco-clavicular joint. The other amphiarthrodial classification is known as *symphysis* or *synchondrosis. This type of joint is typified by two bones joined together by a fibrocartilage.* The symphysis pubis is an example of this articular arrangement.

There are seven types of *diarthrodial,* or freely movable, joints. Each of these joints has a different type of bony arrangement. This is one factor which determines the motions possible by the joint: (1) *arthrodial* (gliding) joints consist of two plane, or flat, bony surfaces which butt against each other. There is very little motion possible in any one articulation of this type. More often, there is a series of arthrodial articulations which have the capacity to summate motion. Prime examples of these joints are found between the vertebral facets. This arrangement allows for flexion, extension, lateral flexion, and rotation in the spine. (2) A *ginglymus* (hinge) joint is a uniaxial articulation, i.e., the articular surfaces of a hinge joint are shaped to allow motion in one plane only. An example of this type of joint is the elbow. The elbow allows flexion and extension only through an anteroposterior plane of motion while in the anatomic position. (3) A *trochoid* (pivot) joint is also a uniaxial articulation. One example, the atlantoaxial joint, has a bony pivot-like process which turns in a bony ring. Another example of a pivot joint is found at the proximal end of the radio-ulnar joint. (4) An *ellipsoid* joint is a biaxial ball-and-socket joint. It is ovoid in shape. An example of this type of joint is found at the articulations between the carpals and radius. The motions allowed within an ellipsoid joint are flexion, extension, abduction, and adduction. Any joint having the combination of these four movements also has a fifth movement, circumduction. (5) A *condyloid* (knuckle) joint is a biaxial articulation. It is also a ball-and-socket structure. One bone with an oval concave surface is received into another bone with an oval convex surface. Examples of a condyloid joint are found at the second, third, fourth, and fifth metacarpophalangeal joints. Flexion, extension, abduction, and adduction are the four basic motions allowed at the knuckle joints. The interphalangeal joints have the same bony configuration; however, the ligamentous structures surrounding the interphalangeal joints do not allow the joints to be abducted or adducted. Flexion and extension are the only motions possible within the interphalangeal joints. (6) An *enarthrodial* joint is a multiaxial ball-and-socket joint. It is characterized by having a bony, rounded head received into a rounded, concave articular surface. A ball-and-socket joint of this type allows flexion, extension, abduction, adduction, diagonal abduction, diagonal adduction, and rotation. Rotation seen within an enarthrodial joint is medial and lateral around the longitudinal axis of the bone. Examples of enarthrodial joints are found at the hip and shoulder joints. (7) The *saddle joint* is a unique, triaxial joint. The carpometacarpal joint of the thumb is the sole example in the body. The two articulating surfaces at this joint are reciprocally concave and convex. This bony arrangement allows flexion, extension, abduction, adduction, and a slight amount of rotation within this joint (Moore, 1949).

Diarthrodial joint structure

Since most motion is permitted at freely movable joints, an understanding of the structural components of a diarthrodial joint is necessary. The outer surfaces of the articulating bone are covered with a firm, smooth, and highly elastic material known as *hyaline cartilage*. This tissue is also called articular cartilage. Hyaline cartilage does not have a blood vascular network or nerves. As a result, there is very little, if any, ability for it to regenerate in case of injury. The hyaline cartilage serves two functions: (1) to absorb shock within the joint, and (2) to allow a greater freedom of motion within the joint by reducing the friction factor.

A freely movable joint has what is known as a *joint cavity*. It must be remembered that a joint cavity is a *potential* opening within the joint as opposed to a real opening. In a functional movable joint in a live human being, there is no appreciable space within the joint. A real joint cavity will appear within a joint when ligamentous and other connective structures surrounding the joint are elongated to their extreme, provided the surrounding musculature is relaxed. This condition may or may not be traumatic.

A freely movable joint has a sleevelike structure which serves as a "housing" for the joint. This is the *synovial membrane*. This vascular connective tissue completely surrounds the joint cavity. The synovial cells within the membrane secrete a viscous fluid known as synovial fluid. Thus, the major function of the synovial membrane is to provide joint lubrication. The synovial fluid also has a tendency to lubricate and nourish the hyaline cartilage.

Movable joints have an *articular capsule.* This is a fibrous structure or tissue surrounding the synovial membrane. The articular capsule functions, in part, to hold the articulating bones together. This capsule may be thought of as the outer "housing" of the joint, because it has a direct relationship with stronger articulating structures known as the capsular ligaments.

Ligaments are integral parts of freely movable joints. They consist of fibrous tissue which reinforces the articular capsule. *Ligaments hold bones together.* Due to this function, ligaments serve as a major limiting factor to the degree of motion possible within freely movable joints. Ligaments must be stretched to improve flexibility.

Although ligaments regulate the extremes of joint motion, the muscles actually maintain the integrity of the joint. Strength of muscle groups surrounding a joint is directly proportional to the stability of a joint. Tendons are extensions of muscles as they cross most joints. As a result, one should not think of muscles and tendons as separate entities. A tendon serves to narrow the attachment of the muscle; consequently, the muscle will have a place at which to exert force on the bony lever. *A muscle belly and its tendon is one functional unit and will be discussed as such through this book.*

Joint motion definitions

Each motion of the human body has been carefully defined. This has been done to enable physical educators and other interested professionals to communicate precise and scientific descriptions of motion in concise and consistent terms. The joint motion nomenclature presented in this chapter must become a part of the student's vocabulary. These terms are utilized when describing motion to professional peers either verbally or in writing; they should also be used to accurately verbalize motions for students in the teaching-coaching situation.

Vernacular motion terminology tends to be very confusing, especially when used without benefit of some form of concurrent visual demonstration. Does "cocking the wrist" mean the same as "twisting the wrist" when, for example, these terms are used by a badminton instructor? What precise wrist motion is desired? There are six possible motions of the wrist joint, and ambiguous slang terms used by instructors often add to the difficulty of learning. What does a teacher mean when he tells a student, "bend your back!" There is no precision in this type of suggestion. Does he mean forward? Backward? Laterally? Slang terms to describe motion should be used sparingly by physical educators when conveying concepts about skills to their students. Secondary school students, for example, can be taught the joint motion nomenclature presented in this chapter. Once this has been accomplished, the physical educator will find that communication of ideas regarding sport skills will be enhanced.

For the reader's convenience, four aspects of joint motion terminology are presented in this chapter, in the following order:

1. Definitions of joint motions are provided in alphabetical order;
2. The motions possible at each joint or articulation are presented, with illustrations and mean ranges of motion cited for most of the motions;
3. Joint motions are listed in tabular form with their planes of motion; and
4. Joint motion synonyms are listed to help the reader to understand joint motion terminology as it appears in most kinesiology literature.

Abduction is movement of a body part or limb away from the midline of the body. There are some exceptions to this, described later in this chapter. An example of abduction is movement of the upper limb away from the side of the body through the lateral plane of motion.

Adduction is movement of a body part toward the midline of the body. There are some exceptions to this also, and these, too, are discussed later in this chapter. An example of adduction is the return of the abducted upper limb to the anatomic position through the lateral plane of motion.

Circumduction is movement of a limb or body part in a manner which describes a cone. Circumduction involves a combination of four joint motions: (1) flexion, (2) extension, (3) abduction, and (4) adduction. Or, circumduction can be the result of diagonal abduction and diagonal adduction at the hip and shoulder joints.

Depression is downward movement of the shoulder girdle. Very little depression within the shoulder girdle can occur from the anatomic position. Depression is the return movement of the shoulder girdle from elevation to the anatomic position.

Diagonal abduction is movement by a limb through a diagonal plane across and away from the midline of the body. An example of diagonal abduction at the shoulder joint is seen in the recovery phase of the back crawl swimming stroke (fig. 4.1).

Diagonal adduction is movement by a limb through a diagonal plane toward and across the midline of the body. An example for the upper limb would be the overhand throwing action commonly used by the baseball pitcher. An example of hip joint diagonal adduction as employed by the punter in American football is seen in figure 4.2.

Dorsiflexion is movement at the ankle joint of the "top" of the foot toward the lower limb, i.e., flexion of the ankle, or talocrural, joint. Dorsiflexion action is observed in the sole of the foot trap used in soccer (fig. 4.3).

Elevation is upward movement of the shoulder girdle. The "shoulder shrug" is an example of this movement.

Eversion is movement of the sole of the foot outward. This movement takes place within the subtalar and transverse tarsal joints as opposed to the ankle joint.

Extension is any movement resulting in an *increase* of a joint angle. Most major joints are in extension while the individual is in the anatomic position.

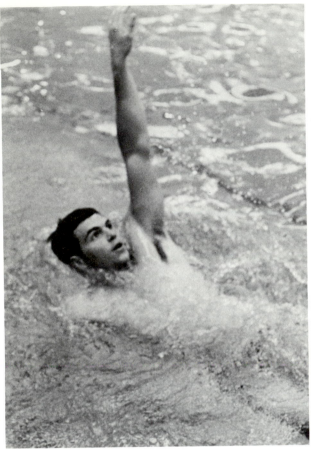

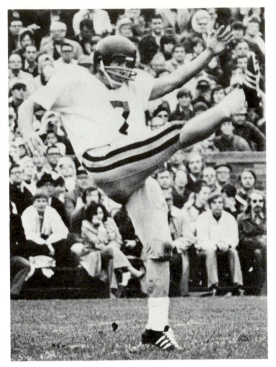

Figure 4.2.

Figure 4.1.

Figure 4.1. Diagonal abduction of the left shoulder joint by Steve Cameron, USC swimmer, during the back crawl. From Northrip, Logan, and McKinney. *Introduction to Biomechanic Analysis of Sport.*

Figure 4.2. Diagonal adduction—right hip joint by Dave Boulware, USC punter. From Northrip, Logan, and McKinney. *Introduction to Biomechanic Analysis of Sport.*

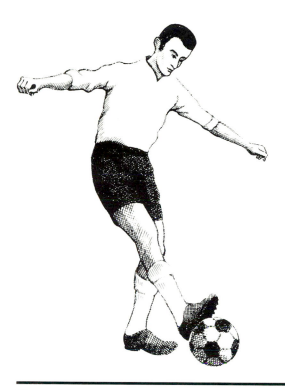

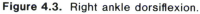

Figure 4.3. Right ankle dorsiflexion.

Complete extension of a body part approximates 180 degrees. For example, the elbow is extended 180 degrees while in the anatomic position (fig. 2.1).

Flexion is any movement resulting in a *decrease* of a joint angle. For example, when the elbow is being flexed from the 180-degree extended position the number of degrees within the joint angle is decreased as the hand moves toward the shoulder.

Horizontal abduction is movement of an upper limb through the transverse plane at shoulder level away from the midline of the body.

Horizonal adduction is movement of an upper limb through the transverse plane at shoulder level toward the midline of the body.

Hyperextension is movement of any joint beyond the joint's normal position of extension. Hyperextension of the cervical and lumbar spines, as an example, are seen during the swan dive. Hyperextension of the shoulder joints is seen in figure 4.4.

Inversion is movement of the sole of the foot medially. If both feet are inverted, the soles of the feet will be toward each other. Inversion occurs at the subtalar and transverse tarsal joints.

Lateral flexion is movement of the head and/or trunk laterally away from the midline of the body. Lateral trunk flexion is seen when a gymnast performs a cartwheel. *Reduction* is the return of the spinal column to the anatomic position from lateral flexion. These are lateral plane motions.

Opposition of the thumb is a diagonal movement of the thumb across the palmar surface of the hand to make contact with one of the four fingers. This thumb movement is commonly seen in gripping various sport implements such as golf clubs and baseball bats.

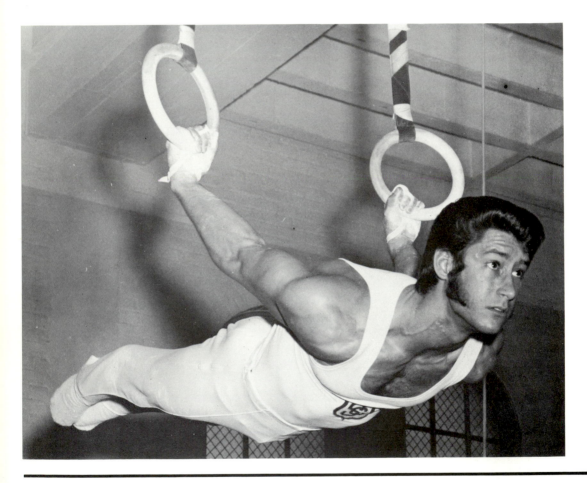

Figure 4.4. Hyperextension of both shoulder joints by Don Elshire, USC gymnast. From Northrip, Logan, and McKinney. *Introduction to Biomechanic Analysis of Sport.*

Plantar flexion is movement at the ankle joint of the sole of the foot downward. The term *plantar flexion* is an exception to the previous definition of flexion. In reality, plantar flexion is extension of the ankle. Most body movements in the vertical or erect body position begin with plantar flexion. Dancers use plantar flexion extensively for its aesthetic effect while performing (fig. 4.5).

Pronation occurs at the radio-ulnar joint. When the hand is in a position of pronation, the radius lies diagonally across the ulna. The hands, for example, are in a position of pronation while doing the push-up.

Prone position is the face-downward position by the entire body. The body does not have to be lying face downward on the ground or some other supportive surface. The prone position can be assumed, for example, in midair while rebound tumbling.

Protraction is forward movement of the shoulder girdle (abduction).

Radial flexion is movement at the wrist of the thumb side of the hand toward the forearm. As an example, the right wrist of the right-handed golfer is radially flexed during the backswing.

Retraction is backward movement of the shoulder girdle (adduction).

Rotation downward is rotary movement of the scapula with the inferior angle of the scapula moving medially and downward. The glenoid fossa is rotated downward. Downward rotation of the scapula always accompanies adduction, extension, and diagonal adduction at the shoulder joint. An example from sport

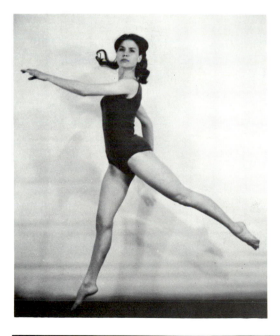

Figure 4.5. Plantar flexion of both ankle joints (Ruth Miller).

of downward rotation of the scapula takes place during the pulling phase of the back crawl stroke in swimming.

Rotation laterally is movement around the longitudinal axis of a bone away from the midline of the body. Any overhand throwing or striking motion must include lateral rotation of the humerus. For example, lateral rotation of the humerus must take place prior to executing the overhead serve in volleyball, serving a tennis ball, or throwing a baseball. This action helps to place muscles on stretch.

Rotation medially is movement around the longitudinal axis of the bone toward the midline of the body. As an example, the "snap throw" of the baseball catcher involves medial rotation of the humerus immediately prior to release of the ball.

Rotation upward is rotary movement of the scapula with the inferior angle moving laterally and upward. The glenoid fossa is being rotated upward to accommodate the head of the humerus. Upward rotation of the scapula always accompanies abduction, flexion, and diagonal abduction at the shoulder joint. An example from sport of upward rotation of the scapula occurs in basketball during the process of shooting the jump shot. The jump shot in basketball involves shoulder joint flexion; consequently, the scapula must be rotated upward.

Supination is the "palms forward" position of the hands in the anatomic position (fig. 2.1). Supination is the return movement from pronation, and it takes place at the radio-ulnar joint. When the hand is in a position of supination, the radius and ulna are parallel to each other. A flat handball serve involves supination.

Supine position is lying with the body in a face-up position. The body does not have to be lying face upward on a supportive surface. It may be suspended in air in a supine position. This is observed in diving and rebound tumbling.

Ulnar flexion is movement of the little finger side of the hand toward the forearm. Ulnar flexion in both wrists is seen at the point of impact in hitting a baseball or softball.

Joint motions

Within this section there is a discussion of all motions in selected joints. The motions are illustrated for reference purposes, and arrows are included in the figures to indicate motion direction. *Average ranges of motion* are also indicated. From the standpoint of biomechanics, all joints are constructed to rotate through a range of motion measured in degrees. The extent of any joint range of motion is dependent upon: (1) the bony structure of the joint, (2) the size of muscles surrounding the joint, and (3) the tension of the ligaments and other noncontractile tissue in the immediate joint area.

Interphalangeal joints of the toes

These joints are classified as condyloid joints. Due to the specialized nature of the ligamentous tissue surrounding these joints, flexion and extension are the only movements possible (fig. 4.6). The movement of flexion in the interphalangeal joints is through a range of 90 degrees. The toes are flexed from a

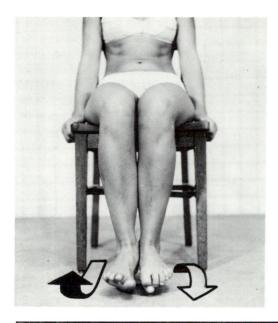

Figure 4.6. Interphalangeal joint motions: extension and flexion.

starting or extended position of 180 degrees to a completely flexed position of 90 degrees. Extension is the return from flexion, i.e., the angle is increased from 90 degrees to 180 degrees. Some hyperextension may be observed at times within these joints, especially when attempting to maintain equilibrium.

Metatarsophalangeal joints

These joints are classified as condyloid. Motions allowed are flexion, extension, abduction, and adduction. Flexion and extension are seen in figure 4.6. Ranges of motion are limited for abduction and adduction at these joints. Flexion occurs through a range of thirty-five degrees. Extension is possible through a range of eighty degrees; however, the last forty-five degrees of extension is more properly called hyperextension.

Although abduction and adduction of the toes are relatively minor motions within an analysis of a sport skill, the reference point for these motions should be noted. *The reference line for abduction and adduction within the feet and hands differs from the abduction and adduction line for other body parts.* Within the foot, the reference line for these motions runs longitudinally through the second toe.

Tarsometatarsal joints

These arthrodial joints allow a small amount of gliding movement. The joints are located between the cuneiform bones, the cuboid and proximal ends of the five metatarsals.

Transverse tarsal and subtalar joints

These joints consist of the articulations between the talus and navicular bones as well as the calcaneus and cuboid bones. The motions of inversion and eversion occur within the subtalar and transverse tarsal joints (figs. 4.7 and 4.8). The movement possible between the talus and calcaneus supplements the motions of inversion and eversion.

Talocrural joint (ankle joint)

The bones involved at this joint are the tibia, fibula, and talus. This hinge joint allows dorsiflexion and plantar flexion only (figs. 4.9 and 4.10). However, a slight amount of rotation may take place within the talocrural joint. Dorsiflexion occurs through approximately fifteen degrees, and plantar flexion occurs through approximately forty-five degrees.

Knee joint

The bones involved at this joint are the femur, tibia, and patella. This joint is a trochoginglymus, or modified hinge, joint. It is so classified because the knee joint allows flexion (fig. 4.11), extension (fig. 4.12), and slight rotation medially

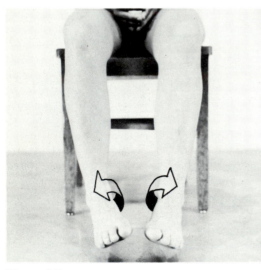
Figure 4.7.

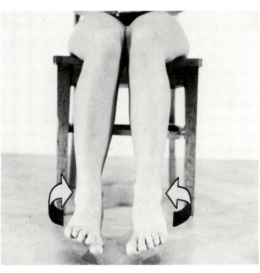
Figure 4.8.

Figure 4.7. Inversion of transverse tarsal and subtalar joints.

Figure 4.8. Eversion of transverse tarsal and subtalar joints.

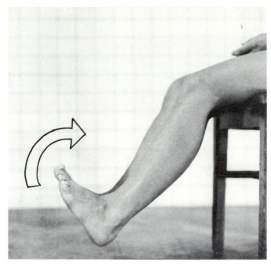

Figure 4.9.

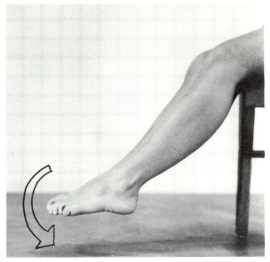

Figure 4.10.

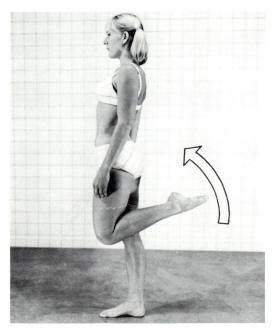

Figure 4.11.

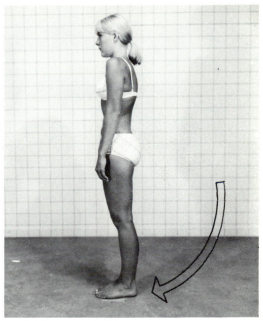

Figure 4.12.

Figure 4.9. Dorsiflexion of the ankle.

Figure 4.10. Plantar flexion of the ankle.

Figure 4.11. Knee flexion (Andrea Morris).

Figure 4.12. Knee extension.

(fig. 4.13) and laterally (fig. 4.14). The knees are extended 180 degrees in the anatomic position. The knee may be flexed through a range of 130 degrees. When the knee is flexed, slight medial and lateral rotations are possible.

The patella is a sesamoid bone lying within the quadriceps femoris tendon. It must be remembered that the posterior surface of the patella has a cartilaginous surface which articulates with the femur. The patella serves two functions within this articulation: (1) protects the knee joint and (2) increases the angle of pull of the quadriceps femoris muscle group.

Hip joint

The bones involved at this joint are the pelvis and femur. Specifically, the hip joint consists of the articulation between the head of the femur and acetabulum. The hip joint is a ball-and-socket, or enarthrodial, joint. This joint allows flexion (fig. 4.15), extension (fig. 4.16), abduction (fig. 4.17), adduction or the return from abduction as seen in figure 4.17 to the anatomic position, diagonal abduction (fig. 4.18), diagonal adduction (fig. 4.19), medial rotation (fig. 4.20), and lateral rotation (fig. 4.21).

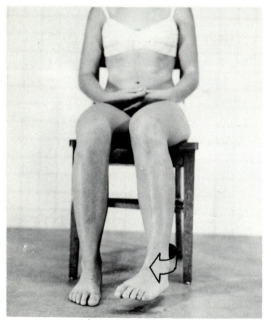 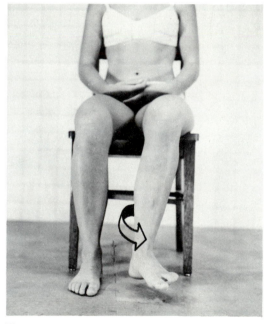

Figure 4.13.   **Figure 4.14.**

Figure 4.13. Medial rotation of the flexed left knee.

Figure 4.14. Lateral rotation of the flexed left knee.

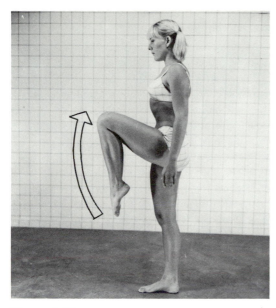

Figure 4.15.

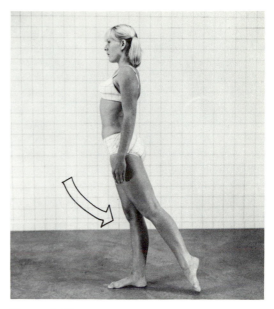

Figure 4.16.

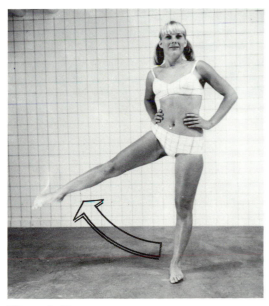

Figure 4.17.

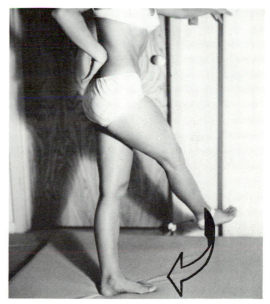

Figure 4.18.

Figure 4.15. Hip flexion—left hip joint.

Figure 4.16. Hip extension—left hip joint.

Figure 4.17. Hip abduction—right hip joint.

Figure 4.18. Diagonal abduction—right hip joint.

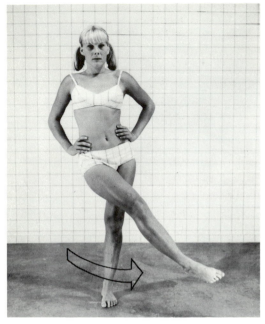

Figure 4.19.

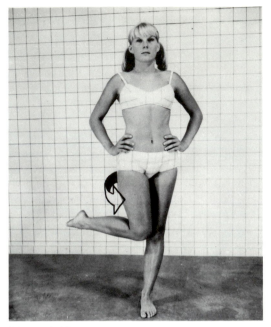

Figure 4.20.

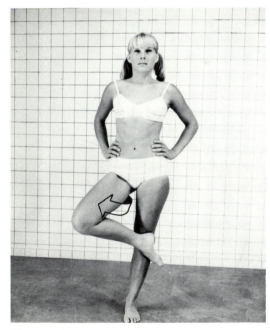

Figure 4.21.

Figure 4.19. Diagonal adduction of right hip joint.

Figure 4.20. Medial rotation of right hip joint.

Figure 4.21. Lateral rotation of right hip joint.

Experience has indicated that confusion exists when discussing the hip. In common usage, many people use the term *hip* to refer to the iliac crests. The use of the term in this manner is not completely incorrect, because the iliac crests are parts of the "hipbone," or pelvic girdle. However, the hip joint should never be confused with the entire pelvic girdle. Hip joint movements are of prime concern to the physical educator when analyzing performance. The iliac crests are also valuable anatomic landmarks while analyzing performers in sports, and they can be used extensively as such without confusion arising between iliac crest (pelvis) and hip joint motions.

The two major ball-and-socket joints of the body, the hip and shoulder joints, have similar motion. The amount of motion within these joints varies due to their differing functions. The primary purposes of the hip joint are stability and weight bearing. The depth of the acetabulum in receiving the femoral head allows for these purposes. The depth of the glenoid fossa at the shoulder is relatively shallow when compared with the acetabulum; consequently, the shoulder joint permits greater ranges of motion than the hip joint. The ranges of motion seen at the shoulder joints allow performers to execute a wide variety of neuromuscular skills. Because of the required functions of the hip joint, however, the ranges of motion are relatively less than those found in the ball-and-socket joint at the shoulder.

The average range of motion for hip joint flexion is 125 degrees. Hip flexion is shown in figure 4.15. It should be noted that the knee of the subject is also flexed in this illustration. If the knee were extended, the subject would be able to go through approximately 90 degrees of hip flexion only. Therefore, flexing the knee allows for an additional 35 degrees of hip flexion. This is the result of mechanical and spatial arrangements of the muscles on the posterior aspects of the knee and hip joints.

Hip extension is merely the return movement from flexion to the anatomic position. Hip abduction (fig. 4.17) occurs through a range of approximately forty-five degrees. Adduction of the hip is the return from abduction to the anatomic position. Diagonal abduction of the hip is shown in figure 4.18, and the extreme of diagonal adduction is shown in figure 4.19. The range of motion for diagonal abduction at the hip is approximately sixty degrees. Diagonal adduction is the return movement through the diagonal plane of motion.

Rotary movements at the hip are around the longitudinal axis of the femur. The total, combined rotary action of the hip is ninety degrees. Medial rotation takes place through forty-five degrees of motion, and lateral rotation also occurs through forty-five degrees. Medial and lateral rotation at the hip joint starts from the anatomic position.

The hip joint does not allow hyperextension to occur in the same manner as observed at the shoulder joint. The motion illustrated in figure 4.16 is erroneously called "hip hyperextension" by some people. This degree of extension of the hip joint is actually the result of concurrent anterior pelvic rotation and hyperextension of the lumbar-thoracic spine.

Pelvic girdle motions

Although terminology exists in the literature regarding pelvic girdle movement, it tends to be both ambiguous and confusing. Thus, illustrative examples and new terminology for pelvic girdle rotations are introduced. These are illustrated in figures 4.22, 4.23, and 4.24. The objective in presenting new pelvic girdle motion terminology is to provide for better communication and description in performance analyses. The iliac crests are the most important anatomic land-

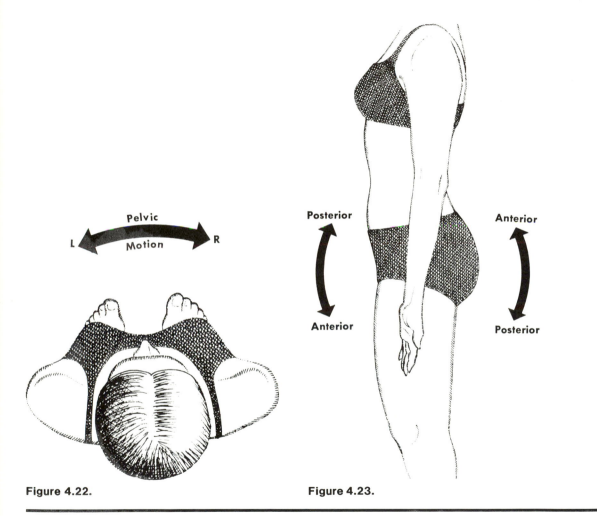

Figure 4.22.

Figure 4.23.

Figure 4.22. Transverse pelvic girdle rotation. Arrows indicate direction of pelvic movement around a longitudinal axis (top view).

Figure 4.23. Anteroposterior pelvic girdle rotation. Arrows indicate movement around a lateral axis through hip joints.

marks to observe for pelvic girdle motions. Pelvic girdle motions described are in relation to the three traditional planes of motion: (1) anteroposterior, (2) lateral, and (3) transverse. Although pelvic girdle motions can be described anatomically as a combination of movements occurring at the hip joint and/or lumbar spine, the terminology presented is in reference specifically to movement of the pelvic girdle *per se*.

Six pelvic girdle motions are introduced. Figure 4.22 shows the paired pelvic girdle motions in the transverse plane. The transverse plane is around the longitudinal axis of the body. As seen in the illustration, in the standing position *right transverse pelvic rotation* occurs clockwise, or to the performer's right, and *left transverse pelvic rotation* takes place counterclockwise, or to the performer's left. Baseball coaches often use the term "open the hips" as a coaching suggestion for hitters. For the right-handed hitter in baseball, "opening the hips" simply means a more pronounced left transverse rotation of the pelvic girdle during the preparatory phase of hitting.

Figure 4.23 shows anteroposterior pelvic movement. The axis for the anteroposterior plane is lateral, i.e., from side to side. As stated previously, the anatomic landmark for all of these pelvic movements is the crest of the ilium. In *anterior pelvic rotation* the iliac crests move forward. Conversely, *posterior*

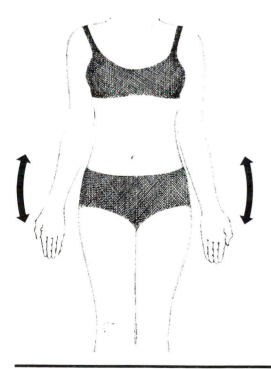

Figure 4.24. Lateral pelvic girdle rotation. Arrows indicate pelvic movement around an anteroposterior axis through center of the pelvis.

Joint structure and motion   69

pelvic rotation results in the iliac crests being moved backward. An example of posterior pelvic girdle rotation is the so-called "bump action" of the burlesque dancer.

Lateral pelvic rotation is illustrated in figure 4.24. Lateral pelvic rotation occurs either right or left through the lateral plane of motion, and the axis is anteroposterior. These motions occur when the weight is borne unilaterally or on one leg. Lateral pelvic rotations can also be seen when a performer is utilizing the hands as a base of support either hanging or in an inverted position. Lateral pelvic rotations occur during weight shifting as commonly observed in walking, running, and pivoting situations.

The spinal column

Generally, most motion within the spinal column occurs in the lumbar and cervical regions. Although the total summation of movement within the spinal column appears great, there is relatively little motion between individual vertebrae.

For kinesiologic analyses, the spinal column is thought of as having three functional units: (1) the lumbar spine and pelvic girdle, (2) thoracic spine and rib cage, and (3) cervical spine and head. Contrary to traditional study of the spinal column in the anatomic position, it is essential in kinesiology that the spinal column be considered for study in the following positions or situations: (1) in a weight-bearing position on one or both feet, (2) with the weight being borne by the hands, (3) in a non-weight-bearing position, or (4) in the water.

Lumbar motion may initiate pelvic girdle rotations or thoracic-rib cage movement. This is dependent upon which of these two body areas is stabilized at a given time. For example, when the weight of the body is borne by the feet, an attempt to touch the toes with the fingertips results in lumbar flexion (fig. 4.25). The pelvic girdle is dynamically stabilized while rotating anteriorly. The thoracic spine-rib cage moves toward the pelvis. When hanging by the hands from a horizontal bar, lumbar flexion results in the pelvic girdle being moved toward the relatively stable thoracic spine-rib cage. This is the opposite of the weight-bearing position when the weight is being borne by the feet. When un-supported, as in rebound tumbling, lumbar flexion would result in pelvic girdle movement or thoracic-rib cage movement, depending upon which of these two body parts is most stable at any given time while the body is in free flight. The moving body segment is dependent upon the part serving as the axis of the body mass.

Motions of the lumbar spine are as follows: Lumbar flexion is shown in figure 4.25; Lumbar extension is the return from lumbar flexion to the anatomic position; Hyperextension of the lumbar spine is also possible (fig. 4.26); Lateral flexion of the lumbar spine (fig. 4.27) is described as being either right or left depending upon which side of the body is being flexed through the lateral plane of motion.

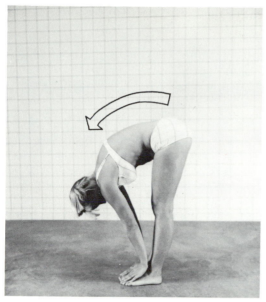

Figure 4.25.

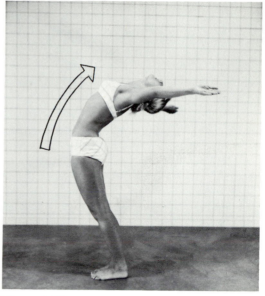

Figure 4.26.

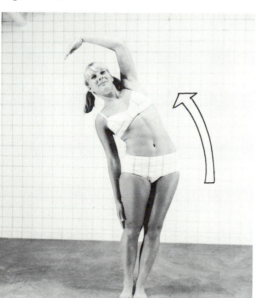

Figure 4.27.

Figure 4.25. Lumbar flexion.

Figure 4.26. Lumbar hyperextension.

Figure 4.27. Lateral flexion (right) of the lumbar spine.

Lateral flexion of the lumbar spine is always accompanied by slight spinal rotation. The normal spinal curve within the lumbar area is anteroposterior. When lateral flexion occurs in the lumbar spine, a lateral curve is induced. This superimposition of a lateral curve on an anteroposterior curve causes rotation to occur within or between the vertebrae.

Reduction is the term used to describe the motion from lateral flexion back to the anatomic position.

Spinal rotation is motion of the rib cage right or left in relation to the longitudinal axis of the body (fig. 4.28). Due to the bony arrangement of the lumbar spine, very little rotation actually occurs in this area. The two functional units, which include the pelvic girdle and lumbar spine as well as the thoracic spine and rib cage, move as a unit when the lumbar spine is flexed, extended, laterally flexed, or rotated.

The functional unit of the head and cervical spine permits a wide variety of motions. Cervical flexion (fig. 4.29) is movement of the head anteriorly. Extension is the return movement from flexion to the anatomic position. Hyperextension of the cervical spine is used frequently in sports (fig. 4.30). For example, the wrestler uses cervical spine hyperextension while "bridging." The football player who must block or tackle is taught by his coach to "keep his

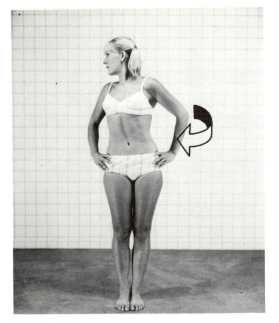

Figure 4.28.

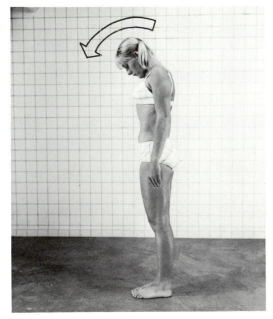

Figure 4.29.

Figure 4.28. Spinal rotation (right) of the lumbar spine.

Figure 4.29. Cervical flexion.

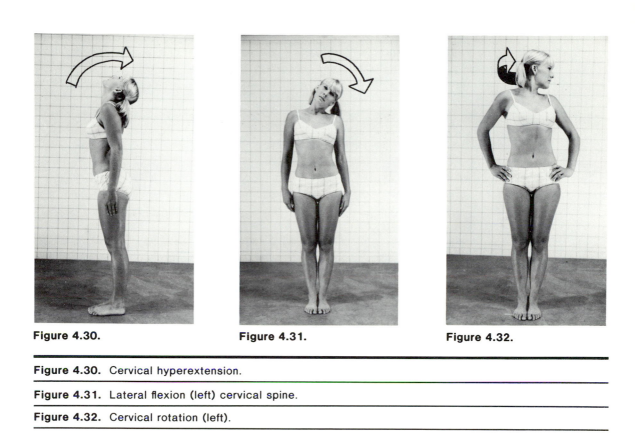

Figure 4.30.   **Figure 4.31.**   **Figure 4.32.**

Figure 4.30. Cervical hyperextension.

Figure 4.31. Lateral flexion (left) cervical spine.

Figure 4.32. Cervical rotation (left).

head up." "Keeping the head up" in this context is an example of cervical hyperextension. Lateral flexion of the cervical spine involves movement of the head to the right or left (fig. 4.31). Rotation of the cervical spine must occur with lateral flexion of the cervical spine. The same principles involving curves are involved here as in the previous discussion about the lumbar spine. Cervical spine rotation occurs around the longitudinal axis of the body (fig. 4.32). Cervical spine rotation is described as being either right or left, depending upon the direction of movement of the head in relation to the individual's body. In rebound tumbling and diving, as examples, motions occurring in the functional unit of the cervical spine and head tend to initiate movements in other parts of the body. This, of course, has its basis in neurologic reflexes active in head and neck areas.

Shoulder girdle motions

Shoulder girdle motions are as follows: (1) abduction (fig. 4.33) or protraction due to the forward movement of the shoulder girdle, (2) adduction (fig. 4.34) or retraction due to the backward movement of the shoulder girdle, (3) upward rotation (fig. 4.35), (4) downward rotation (fig. 4.36), (5) elevation (fig. 4.37), and (6) depression (fig. 4.38).

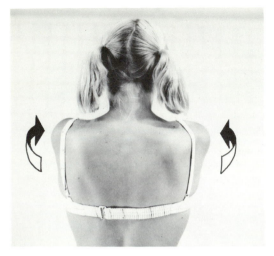

Figure 4.33.

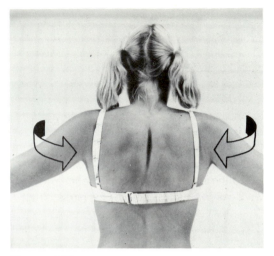

Figure 4.34.

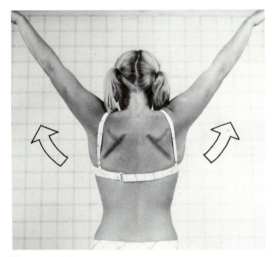

Figure 4.35.

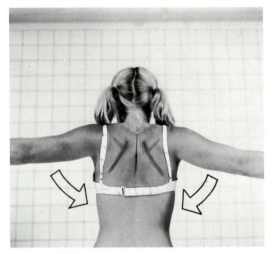

Figure 4.36.

Figure 4.33. Scapular abduction or protraction.

Figure 4.34. Scapular adduction or retraction.

Figure 4.35. Upward rotation of the scapulae concurrent with shoulder abduction.

Figure 4.36. Downward rotation of the scapulae; the vertebral border returns to the anatomic position.

When the upper limbs move upward through any plane of motion, the scapulae are upwardly rotated. Conversely, when the upper limbs are moved downward, the scapulae are downwardly rotated. While in the upward rotation position, the scapulae may be elevated, abducted, or adducted. The swimmer who uses the butterfly arm action utilizes all combinations of shoulder girdle motions. This is a very mobile area of the human body.

A girdle is designed to encompass or encircle an area. The pelvic girdle is an example of a "true girdle," because the pelvic girdle is roughly an ovoid structure. In contrast, the shoulder girdle is not a complete ovoid structure composed of bone. The shoulder girdle is interrupted anteriorly and posteriorly. The clavicles are attached to the sternum anteriorly. Posteriorly, the scapulae are attached to the spine by muscles. The interrelationship of bone and muscle in this area does form an ovoid-type or girdle structure.

The sternoclavicular joint is the most freely movable gliding joint in the body. Since the sternoclavicular joint is a part of the shoulder girdle and the scapulae are attached to the spine by muscles, there is a great amount of potential movement within the shoulder girdle. This is in direct contrast to the pelvic girdle which allows a relatively small amount of movement.

The moving bony parts of the shoulder girdle are the two scapulae and two clavicles. The articulation between each clavicle and scapula occurs at the acromioclavicular joint. During the motions of the shoulder girdle, the spine of the scapula and the clavicle maintain approximately a forty-five degree angle to each other. This constant relationship between the scapula and the clavicle

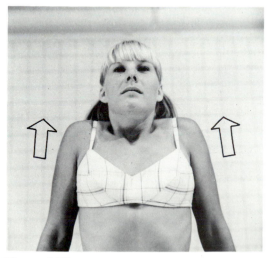

Figure 4.37.

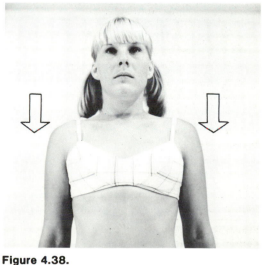

Figure 4.38.

Figure 4.37. Elevation of the shoulder girdle.

Figure 4.38. Depression of the shoulder girdle.

is possible since very little movement is observed within the acromioclavicular joint. Functionally, the acromioclavicular joint could be a solid unit without the loss of too much movement within the shoulder girdle proper. Of the three joints involved in the shoulder area, the sternoclavicular and glenohumeral joints provide the greatest potential for movement.

For purposes of discussion, the shoulder girdle is considered separately. However, the shoulder girdle area and the shoulder joint must function in conjunction with each other in a "teamwork" manner. Motions of the shoulder joint usually involve scapular action. The reciprocal action between the humerus and the glenoid fossa of the scapula allows for a wide range of motion to take place within the glenohumeral joint. The scapula is also treated as a separate entity for discussion purposes. In reality, its total movement is integrated with clavicular and humerus movements.

There are six motions possible within the shoulder girdle. Rotation of the clavicle is not included, because it is relatively slight. This rotation occurs around the longitudinal axis of the clavicle. When clavicular rotation does occur, the scapula is also moving, owing to the fact that the acromioclavicular joint is a fixed joint due to its ligamentous arrangement.

Shoulder joint motions

As indicated above, any time motion occurs at the glenohumeral joint there is concomitant action within the shoulder girdle; however, there is one skeletal deterrant which must be considered when discussing shoulder joint movements. To abduct the humerus through a 180-degree range of motion while it is medially rotated is impossible. The humerus must first be laterally rotated to allow it to move through 180 degrees of shoulder joint abduction. Lateral rotation allows the head of the humerus to clear the inferior surface of the acromion process. This action involves a concept known as "force couple action," which will be discussed in detail in Part Two.

In addition to the eight shoulder joint motions found in the literature, two additional shoulder joint motions are introduced here and described. These are diagonal adduction (fig. 4.39) and diagonal abduction. The eight traditional motions observed in the shoulder joint are (1) abduction (fig. 4.40), (2) adduction is the return from abduction to the anatomic position, (3) flexion (fig. 4.41), (4) hyperextension (fig. 4.42), (5) horizontal abduction (fig. 4.43), (6) horizontal adduction is the return action from horizontal abduction, (7) medial rotation (fig. 4.44), and (8) lateral rotation (fig. 4.45).

There are varying ranges of motion in the shoulder joint. Diagonal adduction takes place through approximately 200 degrees of motion, and diagonal abduction is simply the return from diagonal adduction. Abduction is possible through 180 degrees *if* the humerus is laterally rotated. Adduction is, of course, the return from abduction. Flexion at the shoulder joint occurs through a range of 180 degrees, and extension is the return from flexion. Horizontal adduction occurs through approximately 100 degrees, and horizontal abduction is the return action through the same range of motion. Medial rotation, which takes place along the longitudinal axis of the humerus, occurs through a range of 90 degrees.

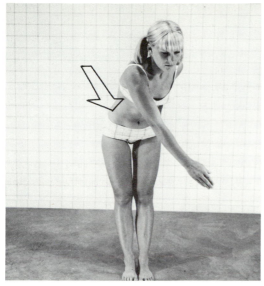

Figure 4.39.

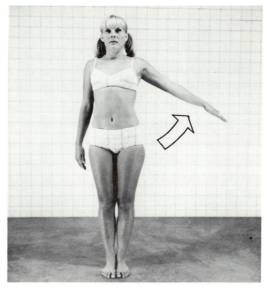

Figure 4.40.

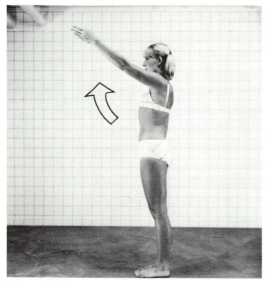

Figure 4.41.

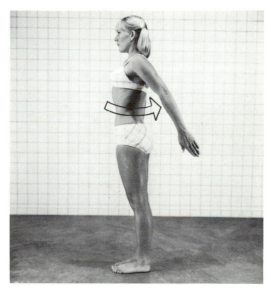
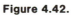

Figure 4.42.

Figure 4.39. Diagonal adduction of the right shoulder joint.

Figure 4.40. Shoulder joint abduction—left shoulder.

Figure 4.41. Shoulder joint flexion.

Figure 4.42. Shoulder joint hyperextension.

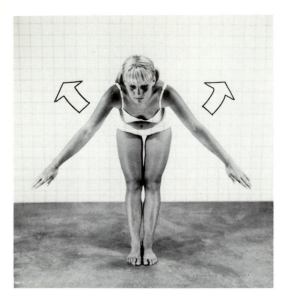

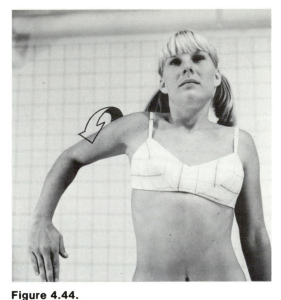

Figure 4.43.   **Figure 4.44.**

Figure 4.43. Horizontal abduction of the shoulder joints.

Figure 4.44. Medial rotation of the right shoulder.

Lateral rotation of the humerus around its longitudinal axis also moves through 90 degrees. The total range of motion of the humerus in rotary movement around its longitudinal axis is 180 degrees.

Elbow joint motions

The elbow is a hinge joint allowing flexion (fig. 4.46) and extension. In the anatomic position the elbow is in a position of 180 degrees of extension (fig. 2.1). The elbow of most individuals cannot go beyond the position of extension because of the bony projection at the proximal end of the ulna butting against the distal aspect of the humerus. Flexion of the elbow is mainly limited by the size or mass of the musculature on the anterior aspect of the upper limb. Flexion of the elbow takes place through approximately 150 degrees, and extension is the return from flexion.

Radio-ulnar joint motions

Movement of the radio-ulnar joint results in supination (fig. 4.47) and pronation (fig. 4.48) of the hand. The hands are supinated in the anatomic position. If the hands are fully pronated from the anatomic position, they move through approximately 180 degrees. The return of the hands from a pronated position is

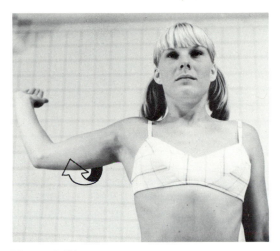

Figure 4.45.

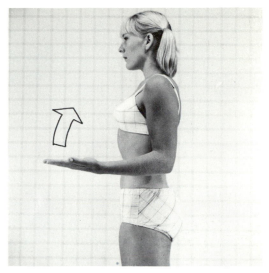

Figure 4.46.

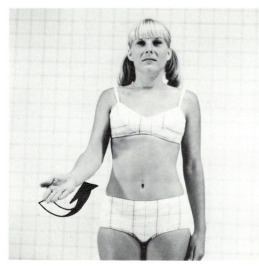

Figure 4.47.

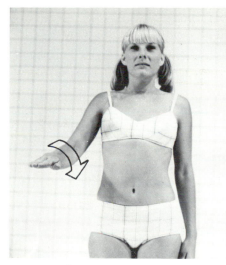

Figure 4.48.

Figure 4.45. Lateral rotation of the right shoulder.

Figure 4.46. Elbow flexion.

Figure 4.47. Supination—right radio-ulnar joint.

Figure 4.48. Pronation—right radio-ulnar joint.

supination. For purposes of kinesiologic analysis, the position of the elbow is very important in determining pronation and supination. When the elbow and radio-ulnar joints are stabilized, for example, medial and lateral rotations occurring within the shoulder joint appear to pronate and supinate the hand. Therefore, when analyzing these motions, careful observations of both the shoulder and radio-ulnar joints must be made to determine which joint is involved.

Wrist joint motions

There are six motions possible at the wrist joint: (1) flexion (fig. 4.49), (2) extension, (3) hyperextension (fig. 4.50), (4) radial flexion (fig. 4.51), and (5) ulnar flexion (fig. 4.52).

Flexion of the wrist takes place through approximately ninety degrees, and extension is a return from flexion to the anatomic position. Radial flexion takes place through twenty-five degrees. Ulnar flexion occurs through a range of approximately sixty degrees. Circumduction is the sixth motion possible at the wrist.

Thumb joint motions

There are three major joints to be considered in the thumb: (1) carpometacarpal (the saddle joint), (2) metacarpophalangeal, and (3) interphalangeal. The opposition action (fig. 4.53) is a unique function of the thumb. The motions possible

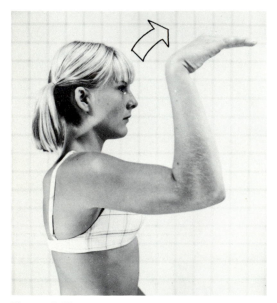

Figure 4.49.

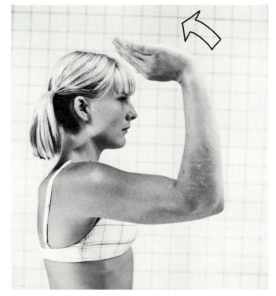

Figure 4.50.

Figure 4.49. Wrist flexion.

Figure 4.50. Wrist hyperextension.

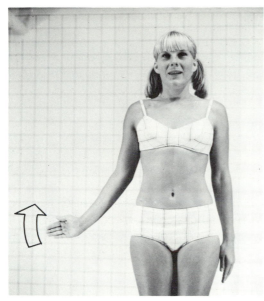

Figure 4.51.

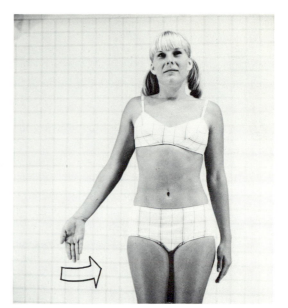

Figure 4.52.

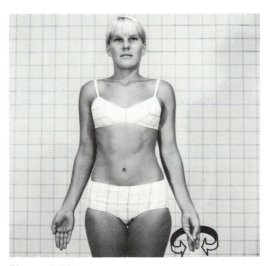

Figure 4.53.

Figure 4.51. Radial flexion of the wrist.

Figure 4.52. Ulnar flexion of the wrist.

Figure 4.53. Opposition action of the left thumb.

within the saddle joint are flexion, extension, abduction, adduction, and a slight amount of rotation around the thumb's longitudinal axis. The thumb can move diagonally across the palm of the hand and work in opposition to any of the fingers. The metacarpophalangeal joint of the thumb allows flexion and extension. The interphalangeal joint of the thumb allows flexion and extension only.

Finger joint motions

Each finger has three joints: (1) metacarpophalangeal, (2) proximal interphalangeal, and (3) distal interphalangeal. The metacarpophalangeal joints allow abduction and adduction (fig. 4.54) and flexion and extension (fig. 4.55). Each of the interphalangeal joints allows flexion and extension.

The reference structure for metacarpophalangeal abduction as shown in figure 4.54 is the middle finger. The index, third, and fourth fingers are abducted as they move away from the middle finger. Adduction involves motion toward this finger. The motions of the middle finger through the lateral plane are radial and ulnar flexions, and they are defined the same as wrist joint motions as seen in figures 4.51 and 4.52.

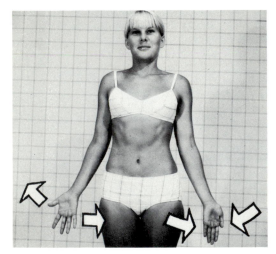

Figure 4.54.

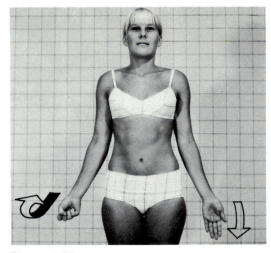

Figure 4.55.

Figure 4.54. Finger abduction (right) and finger adduction (left).

Figure 4.55. Finger flexion (right) and finger extension (left).

SEGMENT / JOINTS	MOTIONS POSSIBLE	PLANE OF MOTION
I. Foot		
A. Interphalangeal Joints	Flexion	Anteroposterior
	Extension	Anteroposterior
B. Metatarsopha-langeal Joints	Flexion	Anteroposterior
	Extension	Anteroposterior
	Abduction	Lateral
	Adduction	Lateral
C. Transverse tarsal and subtalar Joints	Inversion	Transverse
	Eversion	Transverse
II. Talocrural Joint	Dorsiflexion	Anteroposterior
	Plantar flexion	Anteroposterior
III. Knee Joint	Flexion	Anteroposterior
	Extension	Anteroposterior
	Lateral rotation	Transverse
	Medial rotation	Transverse
IV. Hip Joint	Flexion	Anteroposterior
	Extension	Anteroposterior
	Abduction	Lateral
	Adduction	Lateral
	Lateral rotation	Transverse
	Medial rotation	Transverse
	Diagonal abduction	Diagonal
	Diagonal adduction	Diagonal
V. Pelvic Girdle	Anterior rotation	Anteroposterior
	Posterior rotation	Anteroposterior
	Lateral rotation left and right	Lateral
	Transverse rotation left and right	Transverse
VI. Lumbar-Thoracic Spine	Flexion	Anteroposterior
	Extension	Anteroposterior
	Hyperextension	Anteroposterior
	Rotation left and right	Transverse
	Lateral flexion left and right	Lateral
VII. Cervical Spine	Flexion	Anteroposterior
	Extension	Anteroposterior
	Hyperextension	Anteroposterior
	Rotation left and right	Transverse
	Lateral flexion left and right	Lateral

Figure 4.56. Joint motion summary with planes of motion.

Figure 4.56. Continued.

SEGMENT/JOINTS	MOTIONS POSSIBLE	PLANE OF MOTION
VIII. Shoulder Girdle	Elevation	
	Depression	
	Upward Rotation	
	Downward Rotation	
	Abduction	
	Adduction	
IX. Shoulder Joint	Flexion	Anteroposterior
	Extension	Anteroposterior
	Hyperextension	Anteroposterior
	Abduction	Lateral
	Adduction	Lateral
	Lateral Rotation	Transverse
	Medial Rotation	Transverse
	Horizontal Abduction	Transverse
	Horizontal Adduction	Transverse
	Diagonal Abduction	Diagonal—Low and High
	Diagonal Adduction	Diagonal—Low and High
X. Elbow Joint	Flexion	Anteroposterior
	Extension	Anteroposterior
XI. Radio-Ulnar Joint	Pronation	Transverse
	Supination	Transverse
XII. Wrist Joint	Flexion	Anteroposterior
	Extension	Anteroposterior
	Hyperextension	Anteroposterior
	Radial Flexion	Lateral
	Ulnar Flexion	Lateral
XIII. Hand		
A. Interphalangeal Joints (Thumb and Fingers)	Flexion	Anteroposterior
	Extension	Anteroposterior
B. Metacarpopha-langeal Joints (Four fingers)*	Flexion	Anteroposterior
	Extension	Anteroposterior
	Hyperextension	Anteroposterior
	Abduction	Lateral
	Adduction	Lateral
C. Carpometacarpal Joint (Thumb)	Flexion	Anteroposterior
	Extension	Anteroposterior
	Abduction	Lateral
	Adduction	Lateral
	Opposition	Diagonal
	Rotation	Transverse

*The middle finger lateral plane motions are called radial and ulnar flexions instead of abduction and adduction.

Joint motions and planes

Figure 4.56 is provided as a summary listing the majority of the major joint motions. The plane of motion for each joint motion is also listed in figure 4.56.

One major motion which is not listed is *circumduction*. If a joint is capable of flexing, extending, abducting, or adducting, it can also be circumducted. Or another criterion for circumduction at a joint can be whether or not the joint is capable of being diagonally abducted and diagonally adducted. If so, it can also be circumducted.

The motion terminology presented in this chapter should become a functional part of a professional physical educator's vocabulary. As indicated, this is necessary to communicate adequately and to describe skills involving joint motions. It is also essential to know these terms to fully understand the literature in biomechanics and anatomic kinesiology. The motion terms defined in this chapter are used extensively, *but not exclusively,* by authors of kinesiology literature to describe movement. Consequently, there is a need to be cognizant of the definitions of and synonyms for terms which also appear in the literature. Some of the more common terms are included in figure 4.57.

Motion synonyms

MOTION TERMS	DEFINITIONS AND/OR SYNONYMS
I. Subtalar and Transverse Tarsal Joints	
A. Pronation of the foot	A. Eversion, talonavicular abduction plus eversion
B. Supination of the foot	B. Inversion, talonavicular adduction plus inversion
II. Talocrural Joint	
A. Dorsal flexion	A. Dorsiflexion, foot flexion
B. Extension	B. Plantar flexion, foot extension
III. Hip Joint	
A. Hyperadduction	A. Diagonal adduction
IV. Pelvic Girdle	
A. Decreased inclination	A. Posterior pelvic rotation, backward tilt, decreased tilt, backward rotation
B. Increased inclination	B. Anterior pelvic rotation, forward tilt, increased tilt, forward rotation
C. Lateral tilt	C. Lateral pelvic rotation
D. Lateral twist	D. Transverse pelvic rotation, rotation

Figure 4.57. Definitions and synonyms of motion terms.

Figure 4.57. Continued.

MOTION TERMS	DEFINITIONS AND/OR SYNONYMS
V. Spinal Column	
A. Abduction	A. Lateral flexion
B. Adduction	B. Return to the anatomic position from lateral flexion or abduction, reduction
VI. Shoulder Girdle	
A. Lateral tilt	A. Slight rotation of the scapula around its vertical axis
B. Reduction of upward tilt	B. Return to the anatomic position from upward or forward tilt, backward tilt
C. Scapular abduction	C. Protraction
D. Scapular adduction	D. Retraction
E. Upward tilt	E. Backward protruding of the inferior angle of the scapula which occurs with shoulder joint hyperextension in some individuals, forward tilt
VII. Shoulder Joint	
A. Horizontal extension	A. Horizontal abduction
B. Horizontal flexion	B. Horizontal adduction
C. Hyperflexion	C. Flexion beyond 180 degrees
D. Inward rotation	D. Medial rotation
E. Outward rotation	E. Lateral rotation
VIII. Radio-ulnar Joints	
A. Lower arm lateral rotation	A. Supination
B. Lower arm medial rotation	B. Pronation
IX. Wrist Joint	
A. Wrist abduction	A. Radial flexion, radial deviation
B. Wrist adduction	B. Ulnar flexion, ulnar deviation
X. Thumb-Carpometacarpal Joint	
A. Hyperadduction	A. Posterior motion at right angles to the hand.
B. Hyperflexion	B. Medial motion from a position of slight abduction
C. Reposition	C. Return to the anatomic position following opposition

Ahlback, Sven, and Lindahl, Olor. "Sagittal Mobility of the Hip Joint." *Acta Orthopaedica Scandinavica* 34 (Fase 4, 1964). :310-22.

Hirt, Susanne P. "Joint Measurement." *American Journal of Occupational Therapy* 1 (1974) :209-14.

Moore, Margaret Lee. "The Measurement of Joint Motion." *The Physical Therapy Review* 29 (June 1949) :1-20.

Morris, Roxie. *Anatomy Study Guide.* Mimeographed. Los Angeles: University of Southern California, 1960.

Salter, N. "Methods of Measurement of Muscle and Joint Function." *Journal of Bone and Joint Surgery* 37-B (1955). :474-91.

**Selected
references**

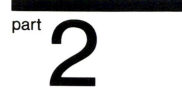

part

2

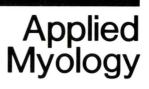

Applied
Myology

5

Aggregate Muscle Action

Aggregate muscle action means that to achieve a given joint motion, muscles work in groups rather than independently. This is a well-established scientific fact (Taylor 1931). In general, muscle groups must perform two major functions: (1) pull on bony levers to move the body, and (2) maintain the body against the pull of gravity in a variety of positions, both moving and stationary. Movement occurs in the body as a result of intricate teamwork among groups of muscles acting in a sequential fashion. Muscle action involves a complex series of sequential events; and muscle function during a given action may change rapidly. As an example, *muscles most involved* in initial movement will act on bony levers to perform a joint motion during one phase of a skill. The same muscle group during a second phase of the same skill, however, may work to *guide* a bony lever a given distance. Toward the last part of the performance it is not uncommon to see the muscles which were originally most involved in moving a joint acting to *stabilize* so another body part may move. Analyzing aggregate muscle actions is challenging, due to such complexity of motion.

The study of muscle function through dissection techniques has been practiced for only about six hundred years. In the earlier stages the joints of the cadavers were moved through their ranges of motion in order to determine muscle actions. This method of determining muscle function has several limitations, because cadaver joint motions bear little resemblance to the motions observed in the joints of the living human being.

Another technique for studying muscle function is to study muscle action by omission. In certain pathologic conditions, such as poliomyelitis, some muscles become paralyzed and others remain normal. Observation of the loss of function at a given joint is an indicator of what the muscle does when it has its neurologic mechanisms intact in the normal individual. The major limitation in studying muscle action by omission is that normal musculature in the damaged area or near the damaged joint will have a tendency to substitute for the loss of function.

Determining the action of a muscle or muscle group by using the sense of touch is known as palpation. The major limitation of this technique is that the only muscles which can be palpated are the superficial muscles located immediately under the surface of the skin. Some of the deeper muscles can be palpated on extremely lean individuals, but most deep muscles, even on people of lean body mass, are too difficult to palpate. Even with this limitation, palpation is recommended as a study technique for the anatomic kinesiology student. This will help the individual to conceptualize the spatial relationship concept and gain a better awareness of muscle contractions. Since each anatomic kinesiology student has a pair of all muscles under study, each person is a potential motion laboratory for palpation, i.e., muscles can be palpated on one's self. However, using the palpation technique with a consenting adult has the infinite advantage of making the study of anatomic kinesiology more meaningful, lively, and sensual!

The most accurate method of studying muscle function is by using electromyographic techniques. *The electromyograph gives a direct electronic readout (via graph or oscilloscope) of the amount and degree of muscle-action potentials occurring during the contraction of a muscle.* These muscle-action potentials are received by electrodes either placed on the skin or implanted with needles in the muscle fibers. Both of these electrode techniques have limitations and tend to be impractical at times, especially when one is trying to study an actual ballistic performance.

Skin electrodes have a tendency at times to record many movement artifacts. These are unwanted recordings of electrical activity from the surrounding area instead of being limited to the muscle under study; consequently, it can be difficult in a complex movement analysis to be certain that the electromyographic data are accurate and valid. It should be noted, however, that there is very little problem with this technique when analyzing simple joint motions in a clinic or laboratory situation.

Needle electrodes can be more accurate, but they do introduce trauma and psychologic factors which tend to inhibit the performer or human subject. There are not many performers, for example, who would serve tennis balls as hard as possible with needle electrodes implanted in their pectoralis major muscles! This simple problem of performing while wired to a machine is also a limitation. However, electromyographic analysis employed in the laboratory situation to study motion problems is the best scientific method for determining the functions of muscles.

Spatial relationship concept

The understanding of muscle function can be enhanced by thoroughly comprehending the spatial relationship concept. The essence of this concept lies in knowing the literal location or spatial relationship of each muscle-tendon to the center of the joint(s) it crosses. If this is known for each muscle, it becomes much easier to classify and identify muscles for their common, aggregate motion function at each joint. *The spatial relationship concept is the most important set of ideas to help the student gain an initial understanding of aggregate muscle action.*

The spatial relationship concept is based upon a synthesis of factual background material from six related areas. These basic facts, when synthesized, will help the student of anatomic kinesiology to understand the spatial relationship concept. This, in turn, will enable the student to deduce the functions of most muscles, either independently or in their common aggregate fashion, to produce motion.

First, the material presented in Chapter Two related to skeletal landmarks and articulations must be known thoroughly. The exact locations of bone landmarks and relationships to surrounding anatomic parts are essential to the subsequent understanding of the position or route a muscle-tendon may take as it attaches to the skeletal landmark or passes over the articulation. For example, the tibial tuberosity is an important anatomic landmark shown in figures 2.10 and 5.1. It is located on the anterior, superior aspect of the tibia inferior to the center of the knee joint. It is an important landmark for the quadricep femoris tendon, because that is where concentric contraction force is applied to extend the knee against resistance. If one does not know the exact location of the tibial tuberosity and its relationship to the knee, it would be impossible to comprehend the functions of the muscles which attach there. The same is true in regard to all of the other important anatomic structures described in Chapter Two.

Second, it is important to have a functional grasp of the planes of motion. The axes of rotation and planes at each joint should be conceptualized. This knowledge, plus knowing the locations of specific bony landmarks, helps one to approximate the centers of joints as accurately as possible.

Third, the motions possible through the planes at each joint must be known. Associated with this knowledge is awareness of the structure of each joint. As an example, one would not expect lateral plane abductions and adductions of the elbow joint simply due to its bone structure (fig. 2.25).

Fourth, the line of pull for each muscle or muscle group must be known. The line of pull of a muscle is from its proximal to distal attachment. This material is covered in Chapters Six–Eight. The *exact* positions of the tendon into the proximal and distal attachment points must be known in order to understand muscle function. As an example, if one thought the ischial tuberosities (figure 2.12) were anterior and superior on the pelvic girdle, it would be impossible to understand "hamstring" muscle group function because those muscles all attach there proximally. (The ischial tuberosities are posterior and inferior on the pelvic girdle.) The muscle line of pull must be known to understand leverage and force application due to muscle contractions.

Fifth, along with the line of pull of the muscle, one needs to define the exact position of the tendon to the center of the joint(s) it crosses. *This is the most important factor within the spatial relationship concept in terms of determining muscle function.* With the exception of the joints within the feet, tendons can be described as passing the center of the joint anteriorly, posteriorly, laterally or medially. For the interphalangeal and metatarsophalangeal joints of the feet, the terms superior and inferior are more appropriate than anterior and posterior. One would describe the biceps femoris tendon in Figure 5.1 as having a posterior/lateral spatial relationship to the center of the knee joint. The quadriceps femoris tendon has an anterior spatial relationship to the knee joint's axis of rotation. These spatial relationships are highly significant in terms of the motion functions of these muscles.

Finally, to fully comprehend the spatial relationship concept and motion at joints, the reader must understand internal force applications at the muscle-tendon attachments. *Internal force is a result of isotonic and isometric (static) contractions of muscles.* The differences between concentric and eccentric (isotonic) contractions are presented in this chapter.

Figure 5.1 is presented as an example to show the spatial relationships of all the muscle-tendons which cross the knee joint. The following are some basic considerations related to the spatial relationship concept applied to this joint:

1. *Important skeletal landmarks:* Tibia, fibula, tibial tuberosity, medial and lateral condyles of the tibia, fibula head
2. *Planes of motion:* Anteroposterior and transverse
3. *Motions possible:* Flexion and extension; medial rotation and lateral rotation when the knee is flexed
4. *Lines of pull:* The quadriceps femoris group is from the anterior, inferior iliac spine (rectus femoris) and superior femur (vastii) proximally to the tibial tuberosity distally. The ''hamstrings'' (semitendinosus, semimembranosus, and biceps femoris) arise on the ischial tuberosities proximally. The biceps femoris attaches distally on the head of the fibula. The semimembranosus attaches distally on the posterior and superior aspect of the medial condyle of the tibia, and the semitendinosus attaches distally on the medial aspect of the shaft of the tibia inferior to the medial condyle. The sartorius has a line of pull from the anterior, superior iliac spine to the same location distally as cited for the semitendinosus. The gracilis has the same distal attachment area as the sartorius and semitendinosus, but its proximal attachment is inferior on the symphysis pubis. The small popliteus goes diagonally from the lateral condyle of the femur to the posterior and medial aspect of the tibia. The gastrocnemius attaches proximally to the posterior, inferior femur condyles, and goes to the posterior calcaneus distally via the Achilles Tendon.

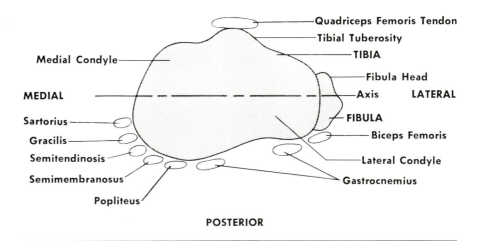

Figure 5.1. Spatial relationships of the right knee joint musculature—cross sectional superior view.

5. *Spatial relationship and function:* For purposes of this example, assume that each of these muscle groups undergo *concentric contraction.* With reference to figure 5.1, the muscles located *anterior* to the joint would cause the knee to extend against resistance. The muscles with a *posterior* spatial relationship to the axis of rotation would flex the knee against resistance. With the knee flexed, the *lateral* muscle (biceps femoris) would be capable of laterally rotating the knee joint. Conversly, the five muscles with a *medial* spatial relationship would be the muscles most involved for medial rotation of the knee joint.

Several of the large knee muscles and their tendons can be palpated. It is recommended that the reader extend the knee while seated and palpate the concentrically contracting quadriceps femoris muscle group with their *anterior spatial relationship* to the joint. Following that, stand with the weight on the left foot and flex the right knee, palpate the medial and lateral tendons of the muscles posterior to the knee. Their functions related to the *posterior spatial relationship* will become obvious. While seated with the knee flexed, laterally rotate the knee while holding the biceps femoris tendon near its distal attachment lateral on the fibula head. The importance of the *lateral spatial relationship* should be noted. The large medial and posterior tendons of the semimembranosus and semitendinosus muscles should be palpated during medial rotation of the knee. Their *medial spatial relationships* to the knee joint provide them with the leverage position to rotate the knee medially when it is flexed.

It should be noted that a drawing of a joint such as figure 5.1 can serve only as a *guide* for study purposes. The exact location or spatial relationship of a tendon as it passes a joint is dependent upon the precise point where the transverse section is made. As an example, the tendons (or part of the muscle) of the semimembranosus and semitendinosus do change their relationship to each other as they go to their distal attachments. This cannot be shown in an illustration; therefore, a drawing such as figure 5.1 is merely a guide showing general spatial relationships—not a precise anatomic diagram.

The reader must ultimately study the bones, skeletal landmarks, proximal and distal muscle attachment points, spatial relationships, and contracting muscles on both a fully articulated skeleton and a consenting adult in order to comprehend joint motions. Rote memory is essential during the early stages of learning anatomic terminology and structures. However, if kinesiology is to become a functional "working tool" for the physical educator, the subject matter must be learned, utilized, and understood to the point of thorough comprehension if it is to be retained. *Comprehension goes beyond memorization!*

Relying upon the study of muscle function by using the spatial relationship concept places the emphasis on logical deduction and conceptualization rather than rote memory. If the reader works at this approach to the study of anatomic kinesiology, better retention of the subject matter and subsequent application of kinesiologic theory in practice is infinitely more likely. Obviously, this has positive implications for the improvement of performance.

**Muscle
action
terminology**

•

Several new terms to describe muscle actions are introduced here. *The main objective in the use of these terms is to better communicate important concepts of anatomic kinesiology.* Some of the traditional muscle action terms tend to be misleading and confusing. The new terms are presented *with their synonyms* from traditional scientific terminology, because the reader must be cognizant of both.

Muscles MOST involved

Muscles which cause or control joint motion through a specified plane of motion are referred to in this book as *muscles MOST involved* (MMI) (Wallis and Logan 1964). The muscles most involved have a spatial relationship with each joint they cross. As a consequence, their lines of pull lie within or parallel to the plane of motion through which the body part will ultimately travel when contraction occurs within the MMI.

The term *muscles most involved* is descriptive of muscle function, and it can easily be integrated into the physical educator's regular vocabulary. As an example, when explaining the "biceps curl" exercise to a secondary school physical education class, one can state: "The muscles most involved in this exercise are located in the front of your upper arm; they are the biceps brachii, brachialis, and brachioradialis." The term fits easily into a common usage context, and that type of anatomic information can be communicated to high school students without any difficulty *if* the physical educator presents the ideas in a logical and progressive sequence.

As can be noted above, an emphasis is placed on the word *most* within the term *muscles most involved.* The reason for this lies in the fact that this term *(MMI)* is *delimited* to include only those muscles involved in causing or controlling joint motion which have the best strength, size, and/or leverage potential. Several muscles are involved in producing any joint motion, but not all muscles are *most* involved. For example, by virtue of their size, strength, and leverage advantages, the MMI for plantar flexion at the ankle joint are the gastrocnemius and soleus. There are five other muscles with a posterior spatial relationship to the ankle joint which contribute force for plantar flexion, but they are not defined as MMI, because they do not meet the aforementioned criteria. These assisting muscles are also described, however, in the appropriate sections of this book.

MMI is used at any time a muscle group causes or controls a joint motion. It was noted that the MMI for elbow flexion are the biceps brachii, brachialis, and brachioradialis during a "biceps curl" exercise. This would denote a concentric contraction, because the elbow is being *flexed against gravity* plus the resistances of the weight of the arm and barbell. If the elbow is extended *slowly* back to the anatomic position from extreme flexion, the MMI for this elbow *extension with gravity* are the eccentrically contracting biceps brachii, brachialis, and brachioradialis. These are the muscles most involved for controlling the speed and extent of motion within the extending elbow.

Our reader is encouraged to read other kinesiology textbooks and to keep abreast of kinesiology literature. Therefore, it is important to know that the most common synonyms for "muscles most involved" are the terms *agonists* and *prime movers*. These are functional terms, but they are not as descriptive as MMI. And, they are not as easy to integrate into common usage to describe muscle functions. One of the main objectives of teaching is to communicate ideas to students in an understandable context. Physical educators know that to teach a given skill to a class it may have to be verbalized and demonstrated in several different ways before learning or true communication occurs. Therefore, it is a good idea to learn how to phrase and rephrase an idea which an individual has learned or is learning; this facilitates comprehension of the subject matter.

Contralateral muscles

The term *contralateral* as used in this book means *opposite side. Contralateral muscles are the muscles located on the opposite side of the joint from the muscles most involved for causing or controlling joint motion.* While the muscles most involved are contracting, the contralateral muscles are being reciprocally innervated and relieved of some tension to allow the MMI to move the joint through the desired range of motion. The extent of the "tension release" is dependent upon the joint velocity and tension desired for skill execution.

This type of cooperative interaction between the muscle groups is what results in functional, sequential muscle action and skilled movement. There must be *teamwork* between the muscles most involved and their contralateral muscles. This connotation of teamwork is lacking in the term *antagonists,* which is the synonym for *contralateral muscles.* Antagonistic muscle action connotes that those muscles are *working against* the agonists or muscles most involved for a joint motion. The opposite, of course, is true, because the contralateral muscle group *cooperates with* the muscles most involved to produce the desired motion. In the "biceps curl" example, the muscles most involved for elbow flexion against resistance have an anterior spatial relationship to the elbow joint. Therefore, the contralateral muscle has a posterior spatial relationship to the same joint. *The term contralateral indicates location once the MMI have been determined.*

The functions of the contralateral muscles often vary, depending upon the skills being performed. Two major functions are: (1) the control of the speed of motion within the muscles most involved and, (2) protection of the joint.

Guiding muscles

The main function of guiding muscles is to rule out undesired motions. Guiding muscles is a descriptive term which connotes the function of these muscles, i.e., they guide a limb or body part through the desired plane of motion providing the necessary force and counterforce to eliminate extraneous motion. Synonyms in the literature for *guiding muscles* are *synergistic action, helping synergy,* and *true synergy.* These are excellent terms, but they do not communicate the concept of the function of these muscles.

Guiding muscles are located parallel to the plane of motion through which the limb or body part will move. Most joints have several different motion capabilities. When a desired motion through a specific plane of motion is performed, the guiding muscles provide a balance of pull on either side of the plane of motion. Therefore, the muscles most involved are allowed to perform as directed volitionally by the central nervous system. This does not rule out the possibility that guiding muscles may also be directly involved in a portion of the volitional movement. As an example, several motions can be performed at the hip joint through four planes of motion, but it is possible to move through one plane of motion at a time. This requires teamwork between and among various muscle groups. When hip flexion is desired through the anteroposterior plane of motion, this exact movement would be impossible if there were not muscles other than the muscles most involved for hip flexion to guide the total action. The abductors and adductors of the hip work in a teamwork fashion with the hip flexors to rule out undesired rotary actions which might occur at the hip joint during flexion.

The hip flexors (MMI) against resistance have an anterior spatial relationship to the hip joint; therefore, the contralateral muscles are located posteriorly. The guiding muscles, in this example, have medial and lateral spatial relationships to the hip joint, i.e., they lie parallel to the anteroposterior plane of motion. They provide a force on one side of the plane and an equal counterforce on the opposite side to rule out transverse, diagonal and lateral plane motions.

Stabilizing muscles

Stabilizing muscles surrounding a joint or body part contract to fixate the area in order to enable another limb or body segment to exert force and move. The terms *stabilizers* and *fixators* are synonyms, and they are used commonly in anatomic kinesiology literature.

Stabilizing muscles undergo varying degrees of static contraction when they fixate a joint or body part. Figure 5.2 shows an isometric abdominal strengthening exercise which serves as an example of static contraction and stabilizing

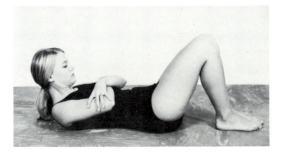

Figure 5.2. Isometric abdominal strengthening exercise. Stabilization of the lumbar-thoracic spine (Jan Stevenson). From Logan, *Adapted Physical Education*.

muscles. The key joint motion in this exercise is cervical spine flexion against gravity. In order for the muscles most involved to move the cervical spine through the flexion range of motion, there must be a stabilized point at which to exert force. In this example, the muscles surrounding the lumbar-thoracic spine are serving as stabilizing muscles by keeping these areas of the spinal column and pelvis in a nonmoving or stable state. The contracting force is exerted against these nonmoving areas. Flexion of the cervical spine tends to add to the resistance; therefore, the abdominal muscles increase their level of static contraction as the head is flexed. This can be palpated, and the contraction gives some residual strengthening benefit to the stabilizing muscles.

Stablized body segments are important for sequential joint motion. As an example, for some upper and lower limb motions, the lumbar-thoracic spine must be stabilized. This is seen during the "jumping jack" exercise where the shoulder and hip joints are abducted and adducted through the lateral plane of motion. The muscles on the anterior, posterior, medial and lateral aspects of the lumbar-thoracic spine are statically contracting to hold that segment stable so the limbs will have a point at which to exert force. This type of force-counterforce situation is an ongoing process in the human body during motion.

When muscles undergo isotonic contraction, they exert equal force on the proximal and distal attachments, i.e., there is force to pull the muscle attachments toward each other. This is particularly observable in a joint such as the elbow. The part that moves is entirely dependent upon the relative stability of the two attachments and the objective of the motion (volitional control). Usually, there will be momentary static contraction by stabilizers at the proximal end of a limb muscle. This allows the force of the muscle contraction to be exerted on the bony landmark (lever) at the distal attachment. This type of stability literally occurs in statically contracting muscles within microseconds. Whereas, stabilized body segments, such as shown in figure 5.2, can be maintained in a static or nonmoving state for relatively long periods of time. Finally, the degree of stabilizing force during muscle contraction can range from mild to extreme. One does not have to contract maximally all muscles surrounding a joint to stabilize it.

The effect of gravity and weight should also be considered in regard to joint stability. A joint can be placed in a stabilized status in a weight bearing situation with minimal or no static contraction by the muscles surrounding the joint. The reader should try standing in a balanced state with his or her weight being borne by the left leg only. Flex the right hip joint forty-five degrees, keep the right knee joint extended, and hold that position for twenty seconds. The left knee is stable, due primarily to the weight bearing situation if equilibrium is maintained. The right knee is stabilized in the extended position, due to the static contraction of muscles surrounding the joint.

Dynamic stabilization

As described above, stabilization is regarded in a nonmoving context by most kinesiologists. This type of stabilization is observed in many performances such as calisthenic exercises, weight training, and weight lifting. However, this type of nonmoving stabilization is the exception rather than the rule in most sport or movement activities. Stabilization must be regarded as a relative concept, because movement to a greater or lesser degree is always taking place within joints considered to be stabilized. Owing to this factor, a different approach to stabilization was introduced by Logan and McKinney in 1970 as moving or *dynamic stabilization*. This appears paradoxical since the terms *dynamic* and *stabilizer* have opposite meanings. This is one of many paradoxes seen in muscle functions. This one is called the *Lomac Paradox*.

A consideration of dynamic stabilization is essential in the understanding of the timing aspect of sequential movements. Dynamic stabilization occurs within stabilizing muscle groups during a sport skill, in instantaneous and fleeting bursts of muscle contractions. There are three major functions of dynamic stabilization. These may occur independently of each other or in an interrelated fashion during the performance of sport skills. These functions are: (1) to maintain the position of the body against gravity, other external forces, and internal force generated by muscle contractions; (2) to prevent trauma within joints due to elongation or compression of the joint structure; or (3) to provide a base from which the original force desired to perform a sport skill can be initiated and transferred from one body segment to another body part in the desired direction or sequence of the skill.

One way to gain an understanding of the concept of dynamic stabilization is to compare it to nonmoving stabilization. For example, the overhead press is a performance skill required in the sport of weight lifting. The athlete is required to bring the weight to his shoulders and then press the barbell over his head by flexing the shoulder joints and extending the elbows. In order for these forces to be exerted vertically, there must be nonmoving stabilization within the musculature surrounding the lumbar-thoracic spine and pelvic girdle, as well as the hip, knee, and ankle joints. Assuming a maximum weight load being moved vertically, the level of static contraction in the stabilizing muscles would be great. If it were not, the upper limbs would not have a point at which to exert enough force to complete a good lift. There would be a strong combination of weight bearing and static contraction stability in this sport example.

What would happen to a distance runner in a 10,000 meter run, as an example, if he or she tried to simulate the same type of lumbar-thoracic spine muscle stability as seen in the execution of an overhead press by a weight lifter? Myologically and physiologically, the results would be disasterous! The runner would not be able to perform, because that extent of stabilization is not needed during the locomotor performance. But there is a need for stabilization to some degree within the pelvic girdle, lumbar-thoracic spine, and shoulder girdle of the runner because of the forces and counterforces between the runner and the earth as well as the moving limbs and trunk. The three body segments (pelvic girdle, lumbar-thoracic spine, and shoulder girdle) are moving under tension. They are providing critical concurrent motions with the hip and shoulder joint motions so the runner can perform in a skilled manner. The *moving tension* within these body segments also means that they are providing *dynamic stability* so the upper and lower limbs will have points at which to exert force.

Dynamic stability is provided by the contraction tension within both the muscles most involved and the contralateral muscles, for movements within segments such as the lumbar spine, pelvic and shoulder girdles. To continue with the runner as an example, running involves concurrent lateral and transverse pelvic girdle rotations with hip joint flexions and extensions. Those four motions must be intricately synchronized for the runner to be skilled. Compared to the hip joint motions, the pelvic segment has a low velocity. Therefore, it can be stated that the lateral and transverse pelvic girdle motions are of the slow tension variety, even for a sprinter. This means that the muscles most involved in these pelvic rotations, plus their contralateral muscles, are both under considerable contractile tension. As a result, both sets of muscles are the dynamic stabilizers for the pelvic girdle during locomotor skills.

Finally, one must also remember that in the process of running, some stabilizing force is being contributed to the pelvic girdle by the momentary stability to the proximal attachments of the hip flexors and extensors. They are located anteriorly and posteriorly on the pelvic girdle.

For most skilled performances dynamic stability is essential within the pelvic girdle, lumbar-thoracic spine, and shoulder girdle. It allows these segments to be optimally stable without impeding motion elsewhere or disrupting physiologic functions. Motions under tension concurrently within those segments are necessary and complement the movements of upper and lower limbs.

Muscle contraction

The specific function of a muscle is to contract and develop tension or internal force. Movement occurs due to changes in tension within muscle groups acting on the bony levers and articulations of the skeletal system.

How does a muscle group contract? A muscle tends to pull from its proximal and distal attachments toward its center. For movement to occur within a joint at either end of the muscle group contracting, one end or attachment of the muscle group must be stabilized momentarily. The range through which a muscle can change its length is known as its amplitude.

There are two general classifications of muscle contraction: (1) isometric and (2) isotonic. Isometric contraction is static contraction, that is, tension is developed within the muscles, but no change in length occurs. As a result, no motion occurs within the joints or body segment involved. Muscle groups surrounding a body segment often undergo static contraction to stabilize the area so isotonically contracting muscles will have a place at which to exert force and cause effective movement.

Isotonic contraction involves both shortening and lengthening of muscle fibers under varying degrees of tension. Concentric contraction takes place when the muscle fibers are shortened, and eccentric contraction occurs when the muscle tissue undergoes lengthening under tension. It is very important to understand the differences between these two types of isotonic contractions. The determination of which muscles are actually most involved in activating and controlling joint motion at all times during a performance of a skill is dependent upon knowing the differences between concentric and eccentric contractions.

Concentric contracton

When innervation to the muscle causes the fibers to shorten, this is known as concentric contraction. *The effect of this type of contraction is to CAUSE MOTION at a joint AGAINST GRAVITY and other resistive external forces.*

Figures 5.3 and 5.4 provide a common example of concentric contraction within a muscle group (the abdominals). The critical joint motion in figure 5.4 is *lumbar flexion* through the cardinal anteroposterior plane of motion. This motion at the lumbar spine has been performed *against gravity.* Therefore, the muscles most involved for *causing* this motion have been contracted *concentrically.* Knowing the motions possible within the lumbar spine, one can deduce that the muscles most involved for lumbar flexion against gravity have an *anterior spatial relationship* to the joints within the lumbar spine. This, furthermore, can be verified by palpation. The pelvic girdle in this example has been dynamically stabilized by the tension developed during contraction of the muscles most involved and the contralateral muscles for anterior pelvic girdle rotation. The pelvis must rotate anteriorly concurrent with lumbar flexion.

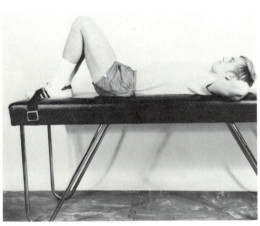

Figure 5.3.

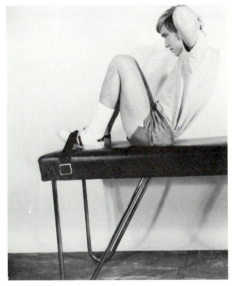

Figure 5.4.

Figure 5.3. Flexed-knee sit-up—start. From Logan, *Adapted Physical Education.*

Figure 5.4. Flexed-knee sit-up—finish. Concentric contraction of the abdominals resulting in lumbar flexion. From Logan, *Adapted Physical Education.*

This dynamic stabilization is necessary, because the concentrically contracting abdominals need a stable point at which to exert force so the motion can be completed by bringing the thoracic-rib cage forward through the anteroposterior plane of motion.

Eccentric contraction

Eccentric contraction of muscle fibers maintains tension during the lengthening process, and this is very important for skilled performance. In addition, this contraction protects joint structure and other body tissues. *The most common effect of eccentric contraction is to CONTROL MOTION at a joint moving WITH GRAVITY.*

The reader should compare and contrast figures 5.5 and 5.6 with figures 5.3 and 5.4. In both sets of figures an exercise has been performed which

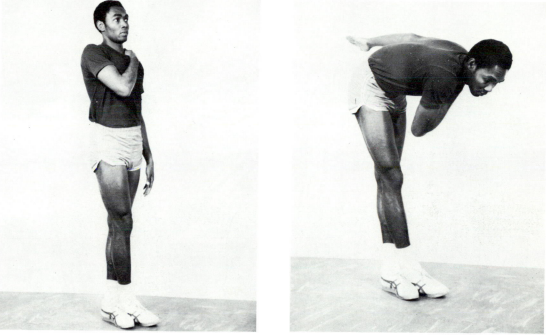

Figure 5.5.

Figure 5.6.

Figure 5.5. Hamstring stretch—start (Billig). From Logan, *Adapted Physical Education.*

Figure 5.6. Hamstring stretch—finish. Eccentric contraction of the erector spinae controlling lumbar flexion. From Logan, *Adapted Physical Education.*

involves lumbar flexion. Although lumbar flexion is a major joint motion in both exercises, the muscles most involved for causing or controlling lumbar flexion in these two examples are entirely different. The lumbar flexion shown in figure 5.6 has been performed through approximately 90 degrees *with gravity*. This means that the muscles most involved for *controlling* the extent and velocity of this lumbar flexion have been contracted *eccentrically*. Knowing the motions possible, and the structure of the lumbar spine, it is not difficult to deduce that the muscles most involved for lumbar flexion with gravity have a *posterior spatial relationship* to the lumbar spine. It is the erector spinae muscle group located posteriorly, *not the abdominals,* which are the muscles most involved in controlling the extent and velocity of lumbar flexion which occurs between figures 5.5 and 5.6. Body position is an important factor to consider while undertaking myologic analyses.

It must be noted that not all motions with gravity require eccentric contraction. If control of the moving body part is desired through its range of motion, the eccentric tension will be maintained. However, it is rather obvious that the whole body, a limb, or the trunk can move through space with gravity, and gravity can be the only moving, external force. Some skills are planned with this in mind, and some performances conclude disasterously when gravitational force gains control.

Reversal of muscle function concept

One should never assume that a joint motion is always caused or controlled by the same muscle group. To make this assumption would be to overlook the differences between concentric and eccentric contractions, as well as the effect of gravity and body positioning, either in terms of bases of support or nonsupported positions in air. Determination of muscle function must depend upon the prevailing situation at each moment during the analysis of any performance.

Traditionally, anatomy and kinesiology textbooks describe muscle functions in terms of their concentric contraction capabilities only. Such descriptions are only myologically correct half of the time! They are correct when the motion is against gravity, but incorrect when the body part is moved with assistance from gravity. *A muscle group which is traditionally described in anatomy and kinesiology textbooks as performing a given function, can contract to control the exactly opposite motion.* This is the essence of the *reversal of muscle function concept.* As an example of this, the muscles with a posterior spatial relationship to the ankle joint *cause plantar flexion* when they *contract concentrically* and move the ankle joint *against gravity.* If *dorsiflexion* of the ankle must be *controlled* slowly through the anteroposterior plane of motion *with gravity,* that motion is the result of *eccentric contraction* by the same group of muscles with a posterior spatial relationship to the ankle joint.

Most anatomy and kinesiology references indicate that the prime movers for knee flexion are the semitendinosus, semimembranosus, and biceps femoris (hamstrings). These muscles are assisted by the gracilis, popliteus, gastrocnemius, and sartorius. This is true *if* resistance must be overcome, but there are situations where these muscles *would not* be the muscles most involved in controlling the extent of knee flexion. Such a case occurs when performing 90-degree knee flexion from a standing position. The effect of the force of gravity must be considered, because the mass of the body is being lowered primarily by gravitational pull. Consequently, the muscles most involved in controlling the extent or degree of knee flexion would be the quadriceps femoris muscle group on the anterior aspect of the thigh. The quadriceps femoris muscle group is actually controlling the degree of knee flexion as well as the velocity by contracting eccentrically. This is not the traditional function listed for the quadriceps femoris muscle group. (Anatomy books simply list this group as knee extensors.) They are receiving cooperative action by the hamstrings on the opposite side of the thigh. Therefore, in this example, one observes a *reversal of traditional muscle function* by the two major muscle groups surrounding the knee joint.

Another example will help illustrate the effect of gravity upon the muscles most involved for a given joint action. In the knee example (above) it was noted that the body was being lowered in the direction of gravitational pull during knee flexion. What would happen to the muscle groups involved if the knee were flexed against gravity? With the individual standing on the right foot only, he is asked to flex the left knee through its full range of motion. Which muscles would be most involved for knee flexion? The answer is the "hamstring" muscle group, because they are moving the knee through a range of flexion *against* resistance caused by the pull of gravity and weight of the lower leg. The muscles on the opposite or anterior side of the thigh, the quadriceps femoris muscle group, are being reciprocally innervated to allow the concentric contraction of the hamstrings to move the knee joint through the desired amount of flexion. In this example, the hamstrings are performing their traditional function of flexing the knee against resistance. Obviously, they are also capable of controlling the extent and velocity of knee extension while contracting eccentrically.

Figure 5.7 shows two highly skilled American football players in action. The tailback (42) is following his fullback or blocking back (36) in this situation. Both knees of the blocking back (36) are being flexed, but there are distinct myologic differences between the muscles most involved for controlling and causing those knee flexions. His right knee is being flexed *with gravity,* and the muscles most involved are the eccentrically contracting quadriceps femoris muscle group on the anterior aspect of the knee. The left knee is being flexed *against gravity,* and the muscles most involved are the concentrically contracting "hamstring" muscle group with a posterior spatial relationship to the knee joint.

Muscle length-force ratio

The force exerted by a muscle is proportional to its length. This principle is reciprocally related to flexibility of joints and eccentric contraction. One can potentially exert a greater force during concentric contraction of a muscle group if the ranges of the motions possible at the joint are better than average. (For mean ranges of motions of joints, the reader is referred to Chapter 4.) Eccentric contraction controlling joint motion with the gravitational field places muscles in a stretched state under tension.

The muscle length-force ratio is also related to the force-time relationship principle from biomechanics. That principle states that the total effect of force on the motion of a body is the product of the magnitude of force and time over which it operates. An increased range of motion in a joint can lead to the potential of greater internal force being generated by the muscle groups most involved for producing a motion, and this also allows for that force to be exerted over a greater time span. The interrelationships between these principles of anatomic kinesiology and biomechanics are important for most skilled performances, especially those of a ballistic nature.

The blocking back (36) in figure 5.7 has the responsibility of exerting extreme force during the act of blocking against an opponent in order for the tailback (42) to gain yardage. He is in the process of *preparing* to do this in figure 5.7, by lowering his center of mass through a series of flexions at the knees, hips and lumbar-thoracic spine. These motions are with gravity, and this stretches the muscle groups eccentrically controlling these flexions, and they are placed under considerable tension.

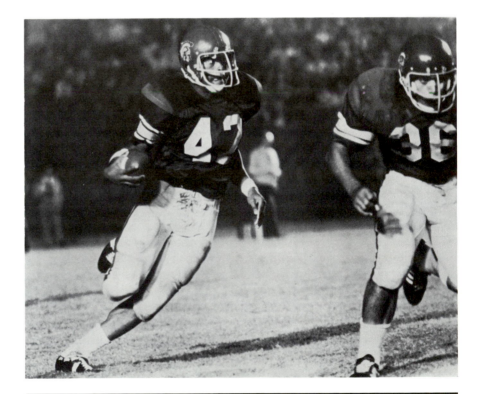

Figure 5.7. Ricky Bell (42), USC tailback, follows his blocking back, Mosi Tatupu (36). Tatupu's left knee is flexed against gravity, and his right knee is being flexed with gravity. Courtesy *USC Athletic News Service.*

The ultimate force will be applied to the opponent by the blocking back through a sequence of *timed extensions* at the ankles, knees, hips, lumbar-thoracic spine, and shoulders primarily. Those extensions would be due to concentric contractions of the muscle groups involved. The total summation of force in this example is greatly enhanced due to the fact that these same muscle groups were placed on *stretch* by being flexed immediately prior to volitionally having them contract concentrically. It is common in sport skills to place critical force producing muscle groups on stretch during the *preparation phase* of the performance as shown in figure 5.7. This preparatory stretching of muscles has important quantitative and qualitative implications for the important *motion phase* of the performance that follows.

In general, muscle groups work in pairs. When a muscle group contracts concentrically on one side of a body part, the muscle group on the opposite, or *contralateral,* side, must lengthen. When the muscle group is lengthening on the contralateral side, it may or may not be under tension. The amount of tension present is dependent upon either the speed of movement of the limb or the amount of resistance overcome during the performance of the skill. If the muscular action must be repeated within the next fraction of a second, there are times when muscle tension cannot be found in either the shortening or lengthening muscle groups on either side of the limb. This is seen in the reciprocal ballistic leg movements of the sprinter. This cooperation among muscle groups is due to *reciprocal innervation* (Sherrington 1955).

Sequential muscle action

During a slow movement, innervation produces tension within the muscle. This tends to be continuous within the muscle group contracting concentrically. In the lengthening contralateral muscle group, there is a relatively small amount of innervation and concurrent tension occurring, provided the slow-moving limb is not overcoming a resistance. When a muscle is lengthened, the stretch receptors within the muscles tend to be stimulated. When concentric contraction occurs within one muscle group on one side of the limb, there is an automatic neural action occurring to dampen the stretch reflex within the muscle group on the contralateral side of a limb. This is known as *inhibition.* When a muscle group is contracting slowly in a concentric fashion against a heavy resistance, the muscle group on the contralateral side of the limb may be under tension.

When both muscle groups on either side of a joint are under tension performing a joint action at a very slow speed against great resistance, they are performing cocontraction (Levine and Kabat 1952). Two of the major purposes of cocontraction of muscles are: (1) to protect the joint from trauma, and (2) to stabilize joints or body parts.

The innervation sequence of muscle groups differs considerably between slow and fast or *ballistic muscle actions* (Hubbard 1960). Ballistic action is fast movement of a body part or limb through a range of motion, assisted in part or wholly by momentum of that part through the range of motion. Ballistic movements are seen most commonly during alternating or reciprocal movements of the limbs. Movements of the upper and lower limbs in running are examples of sequential ballistic muscle actions. Ballistic movements are also seen in sport skills involving transfer of momentum from one body part to another body part.

A ballistic movement is started by muscle contraction within a muscle group most involved for a moving joint. At the time of concentric contraction within this muscle group, there is concurrent lessening of muscle tension of the contralateral musculature. The concentric contraction starts the body part or limb into motion. When momentum takes over, there is a general cessation of muscle action potentials within the muscles most involved *and* the contralateral musculature. In other words, at this point in time, the limb is moving through its plane of motion without benefit of active contraction in either muscle group. The limb continues to move freely through its range of motion. Prior to reaching the end of the range of movement, innervation occurs within the contralateral musculature to slow the moving body part *and* provide the muscular tension or internal force necessary to move the body part in the opposite direction. The "kick-back action" by the contralateral muscles occurs while the original muscles most involved for the joint action are devoid of tension. The original muscles most involved continue to remain devoid of tension until they are required to perform a "kick-back action" at the other end of the range of motion in a reciprocal or alternating action. Ballistic movement, with its "free-running phase," provides human beings with a high degree of conservation of energy during such activities as walking, running, and participation in a wide variety of sport skills. Without this neuro-muscular mechanism, the individual would be unable to sustain muscular activity for prolonged periods of time as seen, for example, in marathon running.

To illustrate reciprocal ballistic movements, the following example is provided. With the arm flexed to ninety degrees at the shoulder joint, and the humerus medially rotated at the shoulder joint to allow flexion and extension of the elbow through a transverse plane, concentric contraction is initiated in the elbow flexors to provide a fast or ballistic movement of the forearm. Following the initial concentric contraction by the elbow flexors, the forearm moves through its range of motion by the momentum provided from the original burst of muscle contraction. The forearm continues to move rapidly through this range of motion until it is slowed when the action is reversed by the contralateral muscle group, the triceps brachii. The contraction of the elbow extensors occurs *before* the forearm has moved through the complete range of motion for elbow flexion. Once the contraction occurs within the contralateral muscles and elbow extension commences, there is a lessening of tension within the elbow extensors *and* flexors. The elbow continues to move into extension by momentum. Momentum is checked or slowed by the elbow flexors at a point near the end of the extension range of motion. This is done when the elbow flexors contract to slow the motion and "kick" the forearm back into flexion. Once elbow flexion starts again, the above process is repeated. It can be seen that ballistic muscle action serves two purposes: (1) to perform reciprocal or alternating fast joint motions without wasteful energy expenditure, and (2) to protect the integrity of the joint.

All throwing and kicking actions are ballistic in nature, but they are not continuously reciprocal. Ballistic action protects the joints involved at the start and conclusion of the motion. For example, during baseball pitching, force is transferred from the trunk to the shoulder area just prior to diagonal adduction of the upper throwing limb. Timed with this force from the trunk musculature is a forceful muscle contraction by the muscles most involved for diagonal adduction and medial rotation on the pitcher's upper limb. This sets the throwing limb into diagonal adduction. Once diagonal adduction has been started, the muscles most involved become devoid of tension. Momentum, augmented by the downward pull of gravity, moves the upper limb through diagonal adduction at the shoulder joint. This force is then transferred to the extending elbow. Just prior to complete elbow extension, diagonal adduction, and medial rotation of the shoulder joint, the elbow flexors and diagonal abductors contract to negatively accelerate the motion and ultimately stop the action. These very important contractions by the elbow flexors and shoulder joint diagonal abductors serve to protect the pitcher's elbow and shoulder joints (fig. 3.16).

It has been observed that throwing too hard during the early part of the season causes pain in the back of the shoulder. This is the result of unaccustomed stress on unconditioned musculature, mainly the long head of the triceps brachii, which is used to stop the ballistic action of throwing.

As mentioned above, ballistic action conserves energy because there are phases within ballistic movements in which no muscle actions are being performed. A further conservation of energy occurs within the body owing to the action of two-joint muscles. Biarticular, or two-joint, muscles have attachments which cross joints at their proximal and distal ends. Biarticular muscles receive kinetic energy through momentum at one of their joints. This energy is subsequently utilized at the other joint. On the other hand, a one-joint muscle would lose this energy by dissipating it as heat.

There tends to be a mechanical advantage of a biarticular muscle over a uniarticular muscle, especially in the lower limbs. It conserves energy, particularly in biarticular muscles capable of flexing at one joint and extending at their other joint. Generally, the individual tends to flex and extend alternately within the hip, knee, and ankle joints during walking, jogging, and running. *It should be remembered that muscles exert force in relation to their length.* As the muscle shortens, its ability to exert force decreases proportionately. For example, when a basketball player jumps to rebound, the player plantar flexes the ankle and extends the knee and hip joints. The biarticular muscle involved in the action at the ankle and knee joints is the gastrocnemius. During plantar flexion and subsequent knee extension, the gastrocnemius tends to maintain a constant length. For example, *flexion at one joint and extension at the second joint by a biarticular muscle results in a constant length. This allows it to exert a greater force throughout the action than if it were shortened at one end only.*

Other important biarticular muscles within the lower limb are the semitendinosus, semimembranosus, biceps femoris, rectus femoris, sartorius, and gracilis. When biarticular muscles are functioning on opposite sides of a limb, a greater force potential is present than when one-joint muscles perform the same function. In general, biarticular muscles work in an aggregate fashion with a strong uniarticular muscle at either end entering into the motion.

Neurologic considerations

The central nervous system has several levels that determine neuromuscular activity (fig. 5.8). These levels are the cerebral cortex, basal ganglia, cerebellum, brain stem, and spinal cord. Each of these areas has unique functions related to motion, and all have integrative functions with other parts of the central nervous system as well as other systems within the human organism (Ayres, 1961). The neurophysiology of exercise and detailed neuroanatomy are not usually considered to be integral parts of the introductory undergraduate course in anatomic kinesiology. Therefore, the greatly simplified neurologic concepts and functions presented in this section are included primarily to remind the reader that a very sophisticated relationship does exist between the central nervous and muscular systems in regard to motion. This relationship is so important that the term *muscular activity* is really a misnomer. To be accurate, the term *neuromuscular activity* should be utilized when describing human performances in exercise, sport, and dance.

Due to the complexity of neurophysiologic research, the functions and interrelationships of the central nervous system are not understood with absolute certainty by scientists. The literature in this area indicates that considerable disagreement exists among the experts, when describing functions of the various brain areas. This should be kept in mind while reading about the functions generalized for the various central nervous system levels below. For a greater awareness of this area, the references listed at the end of this chapter by Ayers, Eccles, Evarts, Gardner and Granit are recommended reading.

The *cortex* is the highest level for integration of neuromuscular activity, and is the area where volitional or willed movements are planned and initiated. Also, the cortex is the area where movement patterns can be inhibited. It must be remembered that the brain does not isolate individual muscles. *Volitional movements are interpreted at the cortical level as aggregate muscle actions or patterns.* Another important function of the cortex is the interpretation of sensory stimuli coming into the body via the various sensory organs. This very important function of interpretation of external and internal sensory stimuli, done in conjunction with the basal ganglia, helps determine the appropriate volitional motions necessary to perform, based upon the sensory input.

The *basal ganglia* are masses of gray matter within the cerebrum. Using a computer analogy, they serve as "storage banks for data." Working in conjunction with the cerebral cortex, the basal ganglia can initiate voluntary *learned* movements. When movements or skills have been learned to that point at which conscious thought is no longer needed, the basal ganglia will initiate movement patterns. The basal ganglia also provide a foundation for various postures and muscle tone. It is from this function that cortically-directed movement can occur. The basal ganglia provide a balancing force for excitatory and inhibitory influences of the brain. There is control of the amount and intensity of the number of neurons working during muscle contractions. Another vital function of the basal ganglia is to control rhythmic movements. Virtually all sport skills and movement patterns have a rhythmic aspect.

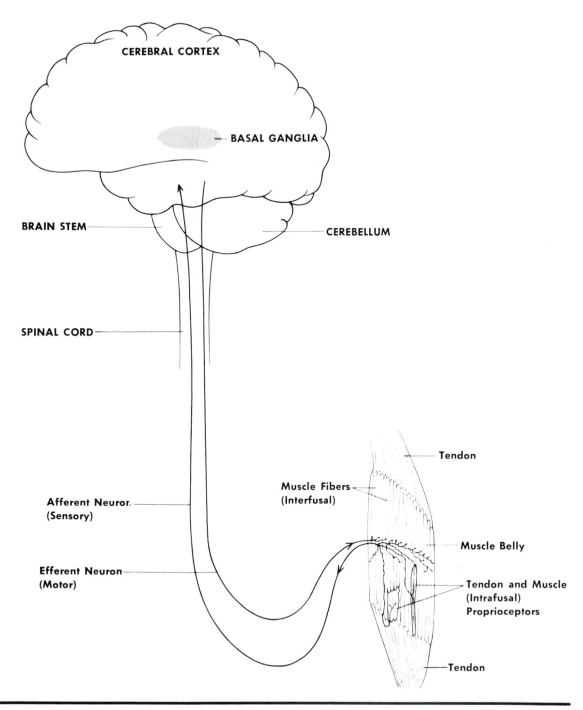

CEREBRAL CORTEX

BASAL GANGLIA

BRAIN STEM

CEREBELLUM

SPINAL CORD

Tendon

Muscle Fibers
(Interfusal)

Afferent Neuron
(Sensory)

Muscle Belly

Efferent Neuron
(Motor)

Tendon and Muscle
(Intrafusal)
Proprioceptors

Tendon

Figure 5.8. Levels of the central nervous system which determine neuromuscular activity. The various central nervous system levels are in uppercase letters.

The *cerebellum* is the major integrator of sensory impulses in the brain. It integrates impulses from all sensory receptors and helps to modulate motor activity initiated elsewhere within the central nervous system. The cerebellum can be thought of as the "control center of the computer." The cerebellum is one area of the body which helps to control equilibrium. Along with this function it serves a related purpose, in that it also controls minute errors in relation to time and distance in movement. Although it controls these factors and acts as an integrator of all sensory stimuli, the cerebellum cannot initiate movements.

The *brain stem* integrates all central nervous system activity through excitation and inhibition of desired neuromuscular functions. Another major function of the brain stem is to control the postural tone of antigravity musculature. It must be remembered that well-conditioned antigravity muscles serve as the "foundation" for skilled performances. This concept will be discussed in chapter 9. The brain stem is also vital because it activates the cerebrum, which serves to help the individual maintain a wakeful state. The cerebrum also helps maintain an attention span, or concentration period, on a task for relatively long periods of time. These factors are all vital to attain satisfactory performance.

The *spinal cord* is simply a common pathway for all neuromechanisms related to the central nervous system. It integrates the various simple and complex spinal reflexes. In addition, it also integrates cortical and basal ganglia activity with the various classifications of spinal reflexes.

Voluntary muscle contractions are the result of a complex relationship between the muscular and central nervous systems. Muscular movement patterns are initiated at various levels within the central nervous system. The quality of movement is, in part, dependent upon the neurologic information fed back from proprioceptors within muscles and joints to the higher brain centers. This information returning to the central nervous system from the periphery includes "data" concerning tension of muscle fibers, tension on tendons, joint angles, and position of the body part being moved. This is analogous to computer systems now in use involving electronic servomechanisms. Thus, volitional movement is autoregulatory.

One of the major purposes of physical conditioning is to assist the athlete in refinement of the neuromuscular integrative functions related to sensory information "fed into" the central nervous system. This information is coming from the eyes, ears, nose, skin, joints, and muscles. The proprioceptors located within muscles, and particularly within joints, are of vital importance to skilled performance. A few examples of these important muscle and joint proprioceptors are the intrafusal fibers or muscle spindles, Golgi tendon organs, and Pacinian corpuscles. These proprioceptors literally inform the central nervous system regarding the degree of tension within the contracting muscle, and the amount of motion occurring within the joints of the body during movements.

Adams, Adrian. "Effect of Exercise Upon Ligament Strength." *Research Quarterly* 37 (May 1966) :163-67.

Ayers, A. Jean. "Levels of Central Integration of Sensorimotor Function." Unpublished report. Los Angeles: University of Southern California, 1961.

Basmajian, John V. "Electromyography of Two-Joint Muscles." *Anatomical Record* 129 (November 1957) :371-80.

Eccles, John C. *The Understanding of the Brain.* (Second Edition) New York: McGraw-Hill Book Company, 1977.

Elftman H. "The Action of Muscles in the Body." *Biological Symposium* 3 (1941) :191-210.

Evarts, Edward V. (ed.). *Central Processing of Sensory Input Leading to Motor Output.* Cambridge: The MIT Press, 1974.

Gardner, Ernest. *Fundamentals of Neurology.* (Fifth Edition) Philadelphia: W. B. Saunders Company, 1968.

Granit, Ragnar, The Purposive Brain. Cambridge: The MIT Press, 1977.

Hinson, Marilyn N., Smith, William C., and Funk, Sandy. "Isokinetics: A Clarification," *Research Quarterly,* 50 (March, 1979), 30-35.

Hubbard, Alfred W. "Homokinetics: Muscular Function in Human Movement." *Science and Medicine of Exercise and Sports,* edited by Warren R. Johnson. New York: Harper & Row, Publishers, 1960.

Levine, M. G., and Kabat, H. "Cocontraction and Reciprocal Innervation in Voluntary Movement in Man." *Science* 116 (1952) :115-18.

Monod, H., and Scherrer, J. "The Work Capacity of a Synergic Muscular Group." *Ergonomics* 8 (July 1965) :329-38.

Razumora, L. L., and Frank, G. M. "An X-Ray Study of the Structure of Muscle Using Different Methods of Fixation." *Biophysics* 6 (1961) :15-19.

Sherrington, Sir Charles. *Man on His Nature.* Garden City: Doubleday & Company, 1955.

Talag, Trinidad S. "Residual Muscular Soreness as Influenced by Concentric, Eccentric, and Static Contractions." *Research Quarterly* 43 (1973) :458-69.

Taylor, James, ed. Selected *Writings of John Hughlings Jackson,* vol 1. London: Hodder & Stoughton, Ltd., 1931.

Wallis, Earl, and Logan, Gene A. *Figure Improvement and Body Conditioning Through Exercise.* Englewood Cliffs, N. J.: Prentice-Hall, 1964.

Selected references

6

Lower Limb Motions

The following discussion is delimited primarily to the extrinsic muscles of the foot. Extrinsic muscles have their proximal attachments outside the foot on the tibia, fibula, or femur. The distal attachments of the extrinsic foot muscles are on bones within the foot; therefore, these muscles cause or control all motions at the ankle and are involved in other foot articulation motions.

The intrinsic muscles of the foot are muscles located entirely within the foot. They are shown in figures 6.1 and 6.2. These muscles work with some extrinsic muscles to produce motions within the interphalangeal, metatarsophalangeal, and tarsometatarsal joints. Most of these intrinsic muscles of the foot are appropriately named to describe their motion functions. For example, the adductor hallucis is shown in figure 6.1. The term *hallucis* refers to the great toe. This small muscle adducts or moves the great toe toward the second toe. The abductor digiti minimi shown in figure 6.2 causes movement of the little or fifth toe (small digit) away from the fourth toe. Thus, the reader can determine function in some of the muscles by the way they are named.

**Transverse tarsal
and subtalar
joint motions**

The subtalar joint involves the articulation between the talus and calcaneus inferior to the talus, as the name implies. The transverse tarsal joint involves articulations between the talus and navicular bones medially as well as the articulation between the calcaneus and cuboid bones laterally (fig. 6.3). The two major motions possible within these joints are inversion and eversion.

Within the subtalar and midtarsal joint areas, some investigators have indicated that a slight amount of abduction and adduction can occur. In these motions, the distal portion of the foot moves laterally and medially. The potential for these motions leads to the motions of *pronation* and *supination* within the foot. Pronation is always a combination of abduction and eversion. Likewise, supination is due to adduction and inversion. The structure of the articulations involved at the tarsal level (figure 6.3) dictates that these special motions always occur together. The emphasis in this text is placed on the major motions of inversion and eversion involving the transverse tarsal and subtalar joints.

Inversion

The soles of the feet are moved medially when inversion occurs. This is a movement problem for many individuals performing locomotor activities such as walking, jogging, and running. Inversion is a particular problem for a potential track athlete, because unusual stresses are placed on the noncontractile tissue (ligaments and tendons) surrounding the transverse tarsal, subtalar, and ankle joints. This can lead to trauma of these tissues as well as the contractile tissue,

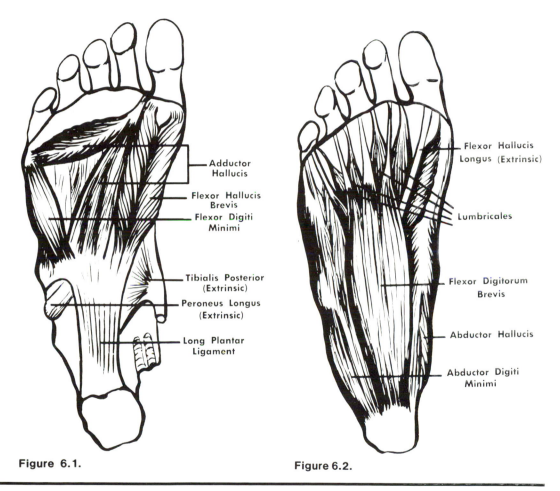

Adductor
Hallucis

Flexor Hallucis
Brevis

Flexor Digiti
Minimi

Tibialis Posterior
(Extrinsic)

Peroneus Longus
(Extrinsic)

Long Plantar
Ligament

Flexor Hallucis
Longus (Extrinsic)

Lumbricales

Flexor Digitorum
Brevis

Abductor Hallucis

Abductor Digiti
Minimi

Figure 6.1.   **Figure 6.2.**

Figure 6.1. Intrinsic muscles of foot (deep)—inferior view. From Logan, *Adapted Physical Education.*

Figure 6.2. Intrinsic muscles of foot (superficial)—inferior view. From Logan, *Adapted Physical Education.*

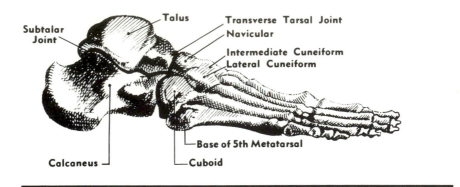

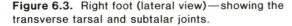

Figure 6.3. Right foot (lateral view)—showing the transverse tarsal and subtalar joints.

and the runner who inverts on each stride is biomechanically less effective than one who does not have this motion problem. It is the responsibility of the physical educator to ameliorate this situation in students through drills and exercises if at all possible. The "toe-in" position of the foot should be eliminated, because that situation must be present to some degree for inversion to occur through a full range of motion.

The muscles most involved for causing inversion through concentric contraction are the tibialis anterior and the tibialis posterior (fig. 6.4). These muscles have a medial spatial relationship to the transverse tarsal and subtalar joints, and possess the best leverage advantage to act as inverters. However, additional inversion force is provided by three other muscles with medial spatial relationships to the transverse tarsal and subtalar joints. These are the flexor hallucis longus, extensor hallucis longus, and the flexor digitorum longus.

The reader will note in figure 6.4 that the *muscles most involved* for inversion appear in uppercase letters. This procedure of placing MMI in uppercase letters is followed in all muscle function figures throughout the text for the convenience of the reader.

The guiding action during inversion is done by the three muscles which pass behind the medial malleolus. These are the tibialis posterior, flexor hallucis longus, and flexor digitorum longus. These muscles are also posterior to the plane of motion. The anterior set of guiding muscles during inversion consists of the extensor hallucis longus and tibialis anterior, that is, they lie anterior to the plane of motion. When inversion occurs against resistance, these five muscles work as a group in performing the motion. They also guide the action through the transverse plane of motion simultaneously.

There is a force-counterforce situation established during contraction on either side of the medial malleolus and the plane of motion. The guiding muscles rule out their other potential motion functions and guide the foot through inversion.

Figure 6.5 shows the surface effect of inversion against resistance. The large tendon of the tibialis anterior muscle is very prominent on the anterior and medial aspect of the foot during inversion, and it can be palpated.

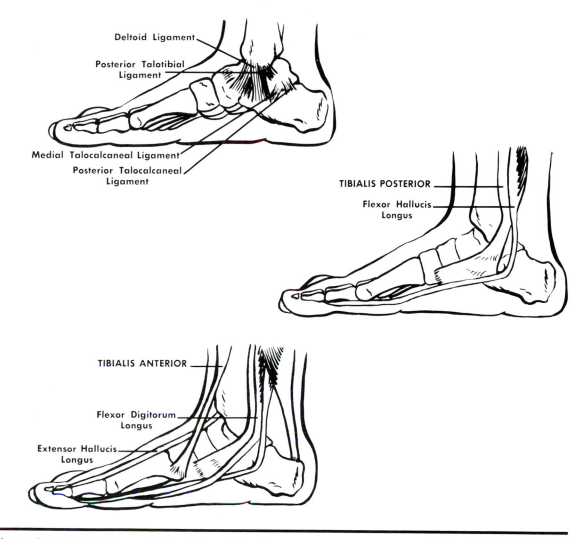

Deltoid Ligament

Posterior Talotibial
Ligament

Medial Talocalcaneal Ligament

Posterior Talocalcaneal
Ligament

TIBIALIS POSTERIOR

Flexor Hallucis
Longus

TIBIALIS ANTERIOR

Flexor Digitorum
Longus

Extensor Hallucis
Longus

Figure 6.4. Medial views of the ankle and foot showing the medial spatial relationships of the inverters. The muscles most involved appear in uppercase letters. From Logan, *Adapted Physical Education*.

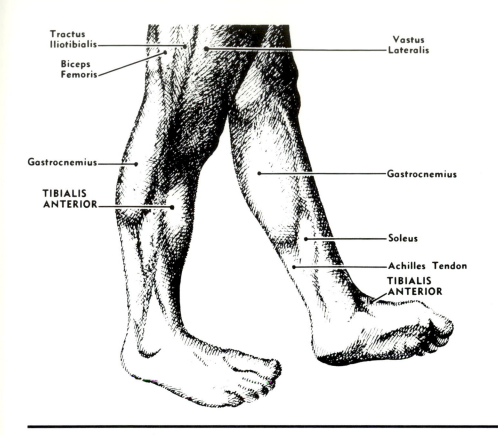

Tractus Iliotibialis

Biceps Femoris

Gastrocnemius

TIBIALIS ANTERIOR

Vastus Lateralis

Gastrocnemius

Soleus

Achilles Tendon

TIBIALIS ANTERIOR

Figure 6.5. Inversion. (Muscles most involved appear in uppercase letters.)

Figure 6.6 shows an excellent golfer's follow-through after he hit a wood shot. It should be noted that his left foot is "toed-in" and inversion has occurred at the subtalar and transverse tarsal joints. These motions were most likely produced more as a residual effect of the external forces involving the total ballistic motion of the golf shot rather than exclusively from concentric contractions involving the left tibialis anterior and tibialis posterior muscles. External forces due to such things as momentum and gravity can cause or contribute to joint motion. This basic fact must be kept in mind when undertaking noncinematographic and basic cinematographic analyses of performers.

Eversion

The soles of the feet are moved laterally during eversion, that is, when eversion occurs through its full range of motion, the individual would be standing or walking on the medial aspect of the foot. Like inversion, this type of foot movement is considered undesirable during locomotor activities.

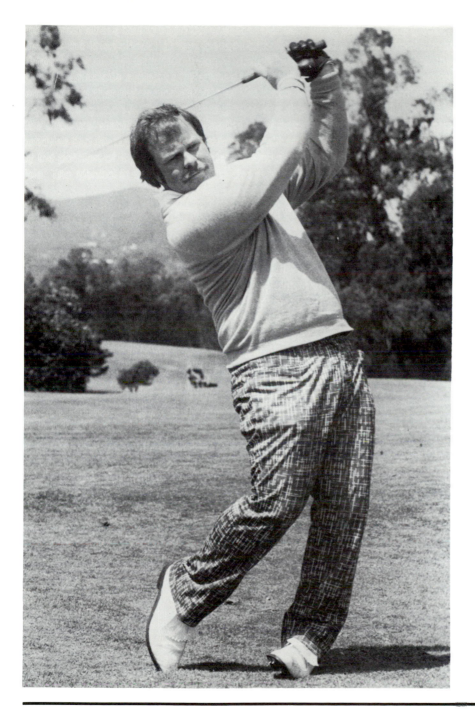

Figure 6.6. Craig Stadler's follow-through on this golf drive includes inversion of his left transverse tarsal and subtalar joints. Courtesy *USC Athletic News Service*.

The "toe-out" position of the foot tends to be accompanied by eversion. This motion pattern places unusual stress on the noncontractile tissue in the immediate area, and this leads to trauma. "Toeing-out" plus eversion during most running is ineffective, because of the undesirability of directing forces away from the intended linear direction of the body. Furthermore, these motions take an additional time fraction for their execution on each stride. That, combined with equal and opposite compensatory motion, tends to be counterproductive for obtaining maximal linear velocity by the runner. As a result, eversion, like inversion, should be considered as a motion to be minimized during most locomotor activities.

The muscles most involved for eversion against resistance are the extensor digitorum longus, peroneus tertius, peroneus longus, and peroneus brevis. These muscles have excellent leverage to produce eversion, and their spatial relationship to the transverse tarsal and subtalar joints is lateral (fig. 6.7). None of the proximal attachments of the everters or inverters has a spatial relationship to the knee joint. Their lines of pull start inferior to the knee joint (as delineated in figure 6.10).

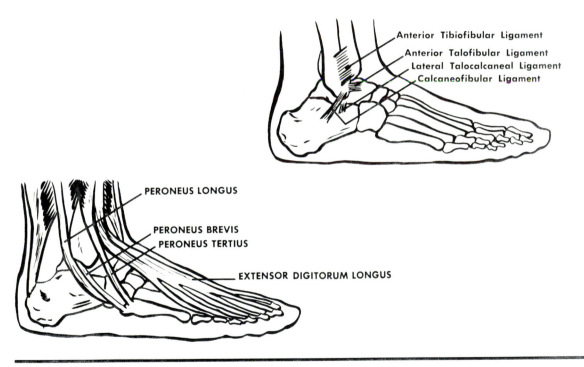

Figure 6.7. Lateral views of the ankle and foot showing the lateral spatial relationships of the everters. The muscles most involved appear in uppercase letters. From Logan, *Adapted Physical Education.*

The four muscles most involved in the producing of eversion against resistance also act as the guiding muscles for the desired amount of eversion. The extensor digitorum longus and peroneus tertius tendons are anterior to the lateral malleolus, and the peroneus longus and peroneus brevis tendons "ride" posterior to the lateral malleolus and have their distal attachments anterior and inferior to it; consequently, the force exerted by these two pairs of muscles against resistance tends to guide the foot as the four muscles combined move it into an everted position against resistance.

Figures 6.8 and 6.9 show the superficial effects of muscles contracting concentrically to produce eversion. While these lateral muscles are contracting to produce eversion, the contralateral muscles on the medial side of the foot (fig. 6.4) are being reciprocally innervated. This allows the everters to move the foot through the volitionally determined range-of-motion desired.

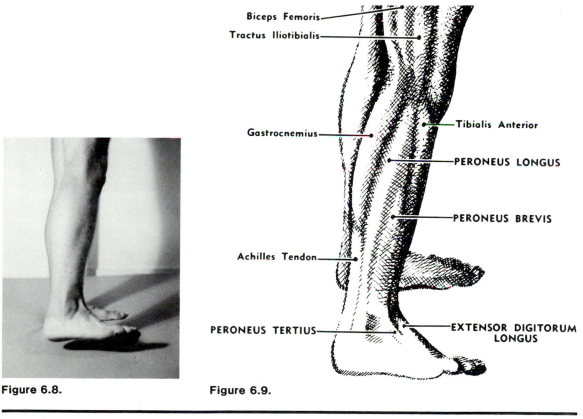

Figure 6.8.

Figure 6.9.

Figure 6.8. Eversion—right foot.

Figure 6.9. Eversion. (Muscles most involved appear in uppercase letters.)

MUSCLES*	PROXIMAL ATTACHMENT	DISTAL ATTACHMENT

I. Transverse Tarsal and Subtalar Joint Musculature

A. Inverters

1. TIBIALIS ANTERIOR	Lateral condyle of the tibia and upper two-thirds of the lateral aspect of the tibia	Medial aspect of the medial cuneiform and base of the first metatarsal
2. TIBIALIS POSTERIOR	Lateral portion of the posterior aspect of the tibia and from the upper two-thirds of the medial aspect of the fibula	Navicular tuberosity with fiber connections to the three cuneiforms, cuboid, and bases of Metatarsals II, III, and IV
3. Extensor hallucis longus	Mid one-half of the anterior aspect of the fibula	Distal phalanx of the great toe (dorsal surface)
4. Flexor hallucis longus	Lower two-thirds of the posterior aspect of the fibula	Distal phalanx of the great toe (plantar surface)
5. Flexor digitorum longus	Posterior surface of the tibia; tendon passes posterior to the medial malleolus and divides into four tendons	Bases of the distal phalanges of the four lesser toes

B. Everters

1. EXTENSOR DIGITORUM LONGUS	Lateral condyle of the tibia; upper three-fourths of the anterior aspect of fibula and divides into four tendons	Dorsal aspect of the four lesser toes
2. PERONEUS TERTIUS	Lower one-third of the anterior fibula	Base of the fifth metatarsal (dorsal surface)
3. PERONEUS LONGUS	Superior, lateral fibula and lateral condyle of tibia	Base of Metatarsal I and lateral aspect of medial cuneiform
4. PERONEUS BREVIS	Lower two-thirds lateral fibula	Tuberosity of Metatarsal V

*The *muscles most involved* for a motion while *contracting concentrically* are listed in uppercase letters. If there are additional muscles contributing concentric contraction force for the same motion, they are listed in lowercase letters. This procedure is followed throughout the book for all muscle line of pull figures.

Figure 6.10. Inverter and everter lines of pull.

The motions of the ankle joint are *dorsiflexion and plantar flexion*. A slight amount of rotation may be possible within the ankle joint, but it is relatively insignificant when related to total ankle movement. It must be remembered that eversion and inversion *do not* take place at the ankle joint. They occur within the transverse tarsal and subtalar joints.

The two major purposes of the foot are weight bearing and locomotion. When executing a kinesiologic analysis of a sport performance, these must be taken into consideration because of their interrelationship. Morton has indicated that body weight should be evenly distributed between the forward weight-bearing aspect of the foot and the heel (Morton 1935). For example, a 120-pound person would bear 60 pounds of weight on each foot. Thirty pounds of weight would be borne on the calcaneus of each foot and 30 pounds distributed on the metatarsal heads of each foot. The weight borne on the metatarsal heads is further subdivided as follows: the lateral four heads have 5 pounds each, and the remaining 10 pounds are distributed under the head of the first metatarsal. Deviations from this normal weight-bearing position in the upright stance will cause changes in bone and muscle relationships. This will result in undesirable locomotion patterns. It is obvious that weight bearing in various sport skills varies widely. The ability to shift and bear weight properly is one characteristic of a highly skilled performer.

The ankle joint (fig. 6.11) is a relatively stable joint owing to its bony arrangement and the support provided by surrounding muscles and ligaments. Stability in this context relates to joint structure and not to muscle function. The so-called instability of the ankle, which results in many athletic injuries, actually occurs at the subtalar and transverse tarsal joints. The malleoli of the tibia and fibula fit firmly over the talus. A series of ligaments help to support the ankle joint on all sides. The most lateral ligament is the calcaneofibular, and the most medial ligament is the deltoid ligament (fig. 6.4). These are often referred to as the collateral ligaments of the ankle. The deltoid ligament in particular has great tensile strength. This is necessary because of its dual function of providing ligamentous support for the ankle and longitudinal arch. The deltoid ligament is so strong that it may pull the bony attachment loose from the tibia before it will tear. Other ligaments support the ankle anteriorly and posteriorly.

The muscles at the ankle joint, as in all major joints of the body, are the most important joint stabilizers. The ligaments help to stabilize joints, but their major function is to prevent further movement within the range of motion at the joint's extreme limit. Muscular support of the ankle is strongest posteriorly. The lateral and medial muscular support is relatively weaker than the anterior muscular support. These spatial relationships can be observed in figure 6.12. *Structural stability of a joint must not be confused with stability due to muscle contraction.*

Dorsiflexion

Movement of the dorsal (top) surface of the foot toward the tibia is dorsiflexion. This motion is of utmost importance, for example, to the traditional placekicker in American football. The degree of dorsiflexion in the ankle of the kicking limb

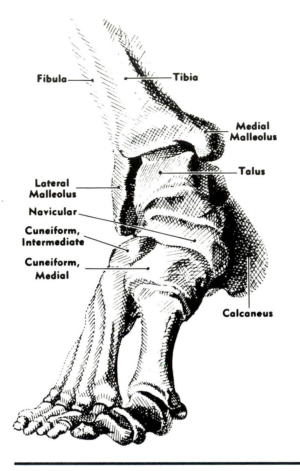

Fibula

Tibia

Medial Malleolus

Talus

Lateral Malleolus

Navicular

Cuneiform, Intermediate

Cuneiform, Medial

Calcaneus

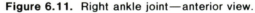

Figure 6.11. Right ankle joint—anterior view.

is one factor which will determine the trajectory of the ball on the kickoff, field goal attempt, or kicking for a point after touchdown. Too much dorsiflexion prior to impact with the football below its center of gravity would result in a high trajectory and less horizontal distance. This would not be desired, for example, on a long field goal attempt.

The muscles most involved for producing dorsiflexion against resistance have anterior spatial relationships to the ankle joint. These dorsiflexors are the tibialis anterior (fig. 6.13), peroneus tertius (figs. 6.7, 6.9, and 6.13), and the extensor digitorum longus (fig. 6.13). Due to its anterior spatial relationship to the ankle joint, the smaller extensor hallucis longus also contributes force to produce dorsiflexion, but it is not an MMI.

The guiding muscles for dorsiflexion against resistance are the tibialis anterior and peroneus tertius. These muscles are located anterior to the ankle joint, but they are positioned medial and lateral to each other. This means their

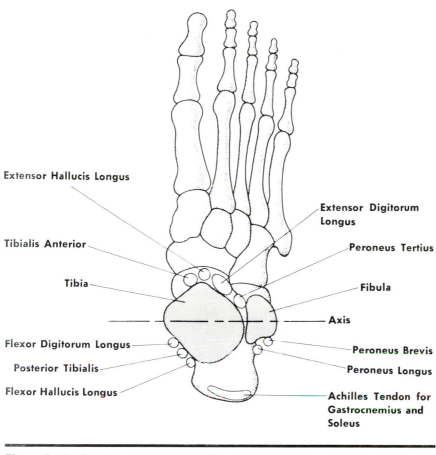

Extensor Hallucis Longus

Extensor Digitorum Longus

Tibialis Anterior

Peroneus Tertius

Tibia

Fibula

Axis

Flexor Digitorum Longus

Peroneus Brevis

Posterior Tibialis

Peroneus Longus

Flexor Hallucis Longus

Achilles Tendon for Gastrocnemius and Soleus

Figure 6.12. Spatial relationships of the extrinsic tendons of the ankle and foot—cross sectional, superior view of the right ankle.

contractile forces lie parallel to the anteroposterior plane of motion traversed by the foot during dorsiflexion. The force-counterforce produced by these muscles for dorsiflexion helps to rule out their undesired motion potential for inversion and eversion respectively.

All four muscles involved in dorsiflexion are superficial and can be palpated. Figure 6.14 shows the general location of the tibialis anterior and extensor digitorum longus. As indicated above, the large tendon of the tibialis anterior can be palpated on the anterior, medial aspect of the foot. The extensor digitorum longus tendon is easy to feel, because it divides into four tendons enroute to its distal attachments on the distal aspects of the lesser toes. The extensor hallucis longus tendon can be palpated beneath the skin on the dorsal aspect of the great toe. The peroneus tertius is anterior to the lateral malleolus.

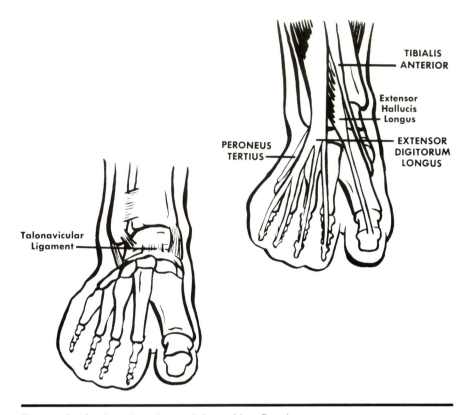

TIBIALIS
ANTERIOR

Extensor
Hallucis
Longus

EXTENSOR
DIGITORUM
LONGUS

PERONEUS
TERTIUS

Talonavicular
Ligament

Figure 6.13. Anterior view—right ankle. Dorsiflexor muscles most involved are shown in upper-case letters. From Logan, *Adapted Physical Education.*

The dorsiflexors against resistance have an anterior spatial relationship to the axis of rotation of the ankle joint, as shown in figure 6.12. These same muscles are the muscles most involved for controlling slow tension plantar flexion by contracting eccentrically. As an example, slow plantar flexion while the body is inverted with the feet as the base of support would indicate eccentric control by the tibialis anterior, extensor digitorum longus, peroneus tertius, and extensor hallucis longus. This could be done with the feet in a harness attached to a horizontal bar. The total body would be hanging in an inverted position, and the ankle joints would be *moved slowly* from the midposition to 45 degrees of plantar flexion. Obviously, the external force of gravity could contribute all the force needed for plantar flexion in this example. But moving slowly through the 45 degrees with gravity means that the muscles most involved for controlling this motion and protecting the ankle joints have an anterior spatial relationship to the joint.

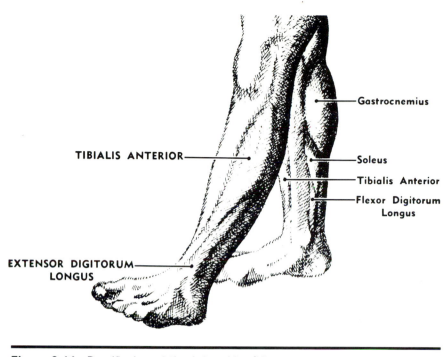

Gastrocnemius

TIBIALIS ANTERIOR

Soleus

Tibialis Anterior

Flexor Digitorum Longus

EXTENSOR DIGITORUM LONGUS

Figure 6.14. Dorsiflexion of the left ankle. (Muscles most involved appear in uppercase letters.) The right ankle is stabilized in a weight bearing position.

Plantar flexion

The bottom or sole of the foot is called the plantar surface. When the plantar surface is moved away from the anterior tibia and fibula, this extension of the ankle joint is paradoxically called plantar flexion.

Plantar flexions of the ankle joint are important to the performance of all locomotor activities. The ballet dancer who works on pointe most certainly must condition the muscles most involved for plantar flexion. A good vertical lift in high jumping is dependent, in part, upon forceful plantar flexion in the ankle joint of the "take-off leg" through as much range of motion as possible while the foot maintains contact with the earth. There are many skills where plantar flexions are important to the performance outcome.

Plantar flexion against resistance is performed by a group of seven muscles which have a posterior spatial relationship to the axis of the ankle joint. However, the muscles most involved for plantar flexion against resistance are the gastrocnemius and soleus. These muscles are large, have excellent leverage, and their line of pull is directly in the anteroposterior plane at the ankle joint. The remaining plantar flexors are the peroneus longus, peroneus brevis, flexor digitorum longus, flexor hallucis longus, and tibialis posterior (fig. 6.15).

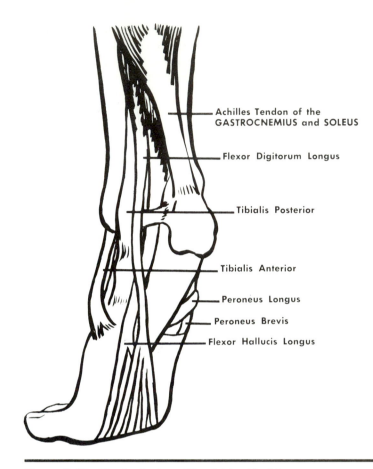

Achilles Tendon of the
GASTROCNEMIUS and SOLEUS

Flexor Digitorum Longus

Tibialis Posterior

Tibialis Anterior

Peroneus Longus

Peroneus Brevis

Flexor Hallucis Longus

Figure 6.15. Plantar flexion of the right ankle. Muscles producing this motion have posterior spatial relationships to the ankle. Muscles most involved are in uppercase letters. From Logan, *Adapted Physical Education.*

     All guiding muscles for plantar flexion through the anteroposterior plane of motion at the ankle joint work in a pulley fashion by utilizing the malleoli (fig. 6.16). On the lateral side, the peroneus longus and peroneus brevis utilize the lateral malleolus of the fibula as a pulley. Their tendons ride in a groove immediately posterior to the lateral malleolus as they move downward toward their distal attachments. On the medial side of the ankle, two guiding muscles—the flexor digitorum longus and tibialis posterior—function in a similar manner. Their tendons pass posterior to the medial malleolus via grooves enroute to their distal attachments. The tendon of the third medial guiding muscle for plantar flexion, the flexor hallucis longus, rides under the sustentaculum tali from the medial side of the calcaneus enroute to its distal attachment on the distal end of the great toe. The sustentaculum tali, like the medial and lateral malleoli, serves as pulleys for the flexor hallucis longus tendons. A critical observation of the spatial relationship and lines of pull of the guiding muscles for dorsiflexion and plantar flexion reveals that these muscles also function as inverters and everters of the subtalar and transverse tarsal joints. This is due to the fact that they are multiarticular muscles which cross those joints. *Generally, if a muscle crosses a joint, it will act at that joint.*

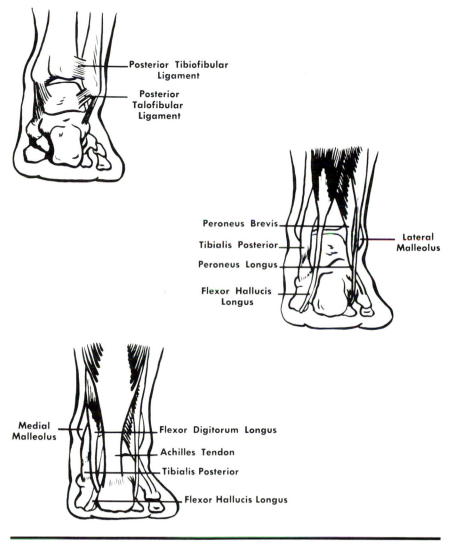

Figure 6.16. Posterior view of right ankle. Guiding muscles for plantar flexion are posterior to both malleoli. From Logan, *Adapted Physical Education.*

The term *triceps surae* is often used to describe the gastrocnemius and soleus muscles as one group. The prefix "tri" indicates that there are three basic structures to be considered. Confusion often exists regarding this point because there are only two muscles involved. The suffix "ceps" gives the answer to this problem. The term "ceps" means "heads." Thus, the term *triceps* refers to three muscle heads. In this case, there are three muscle heads in the two muscles. The gastrocnemius has two heads which attach proximally on the posterior aspect of the femoral condyles. The proximal head of the soleus attaches on the upper and posterior aspects of the tibia and fibula. The distal attachment for the triceps surae group is on the posterior surface of the calcaneus via the Achilles tendon. There is one other muscle which is sometimes missing in this area of the lower limb. It is called the plantaris. When present, the plantaris has its proximal attachment on the lateral aspect of the linea aspera of the femur and its distal attachment is via a long tendon to the posterior and medial aspect of the calcaneus. Since the plantaris is vestigial in man, it will not be discussed further.

Figure 6.17 shows the superficial configuration of the muscles most involved for plantar flexion as they undergo concentric contraction during a "heel raise" exercise. These large muscles can be palpated. The gastrocnemius is

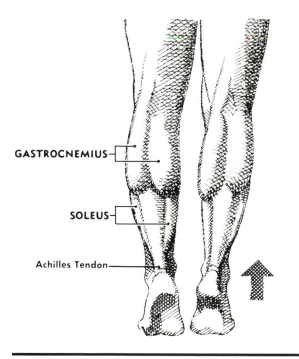

Figure 6.17. Plantar flexion against resistance by the triceps surae. (Muscles most involved appear in uppercase letters.)

the most superficial. During the exercise seen in figure 6.17 the contralateral muscles have spatial relationships anterior to the ankle joint. If the performer *lowers* the body and any other resistance *slowly*, there will be considerable tension in muscle groups on the anterior and posterior sides of the ankle joint. This *dorsiflexion with gravity,* however, is being controlled by the eccentrically contracting gastrocnemius and soleus muscles. The cooperating contralateral muscles are anterior to the joint. This is an example of reversal of muscle function by muscle groups.

The lines of pull for the dorsiflexors and plantar flexors are outlined in figure 6.18.

The basketball player executing the short jump shot in figure 6.19 has plantar flexed both ankle joints through approximately forty-five degrees of motion for each ankle. These motions are an integral component of her summation of force to move vertically and execute the shot. Major internal forces are also derived from concentric contractions of the knee, hip and lumbar-thoracic spine extensors which add to her summation of forces. The plantar flexions of the ankles are the last motions in the sequence, and those motions apply the force to the stable floor.

Metatarso-phalangeal and interphalangeal joint motions

Four extrinsic muscles of the foot are involved in flexion and extension at the metatarsophalangeal joints and interphalangeal joints. The flexors are the flexor digitorum longus and flexor hallucis longus. The extensors are the extensor digitorum longus and extensor hallucis longus. These muscles work in a team-work fashion with the intrinsic muscles of the foot to perform flexion and extension. The muscles which abduct and adduct the toes are located entirely within the foot, i.e., they are intrinsic muscles of the foot (figs. 6.1 and 6.2).

Since shoes are worn for many sport activities, the importance of toe motions are easily overlooked. The flexions and abductions in particular are extremely important for maintaining body equilibrium, increasing resistance, or for added force application. As one example, interphalangeal joint flexion and extension are definitely used and help during the racing start in swimming (fig. 6.20).

Since these muscles are multiarticular, they also have motion functions at the subtalar and transverse tarsal joints as well as the ankle joint. Their lines of pull are discussed in figures 6.10 and 6.18.

Knee joint motions

The motions possible at the knee joint are flexion, extension, medial rotation, and lateral rotation. The rotary action possible in the knee is only seen after flexion has occurred. Rotary movements are not observed at the normal knee joint when it is fully extended. If there seems to be rotation of the extended knee, a close examination will probably reveal that rotation is occurring at the hip joint.

The bones involved at the knee joint are the tibia, posterior aspect of the patella, and the femur (fig. 6.21). The fibula is not a part of the knee joint structure.

MUSCLES	PROXIMAL ATTACHMENT	DISTAL ATTACHMENT
I. Ankle (Talocrural) Joint Musculature		
A. Dorsiflexors		
1. TIBIALIS ANTERIOR	Lateral condyle of the tibia and upper two-thirds of the lateral aspect of the tibia	Medial aspect of the medial cuneiform and base of the first metatarsal
2. EXTENSOR DIGITORUM LONGUS	Lateral condyle of the tibia; upper three-fourths of the anterior aspect of fibula and divides into four tendons	Dorsal aspect of the four lesser toes
3. PERONEUS TERTIUS	Lower one-third of the anterior fibula	Base of the fifth metatarsal (dorsal surface)
4. Extensor hallucis longus	Mid one-half of the anterior aspect of the fibula	Distal phalanx of the great toe (dorsal surface)
B. Plantar Flexors		
1. GASTROC-NEMIUS	Two heads attached to the medial and lateral condyles of the femur posteriorly	Achilles tendon to the calcaneus
2. SOLEUS	Upper one-third of the posterior tibia and fibula	Achilles tendon to the calcaneus
3. Peroneus longus	Superior, lateral fibula and lateral condyle of tibia	Base of Matatarsal I and lateral aspect of medial cuneiform
4. Peroneus brevis	Lower two-thirds lateral fibula	Tuberosity of Metatarsal V
5. Flexor digitorum longus	Posterior surface of the tibia; tendon passes posterior to the medial malleolus and divides into four tendons	Bases of the distal phalanges of the four lesser toes
6. Flexor hallucis longus	Lower two-thirds of the posterior aspect of the fibula	Distal phalanx of the great toe (plantar surface)
7. Tibialis posterior	Lateral portion of the posterior aspect of the tibia and from the upper two-thirds of the medial aspect of the fibula	Navicular tuberosity with fiber connections to the three cuneiforms, cuboid, and bases of Metatarsals II, III, and IV

Figure 6.18. Ankle joint musculature. The muscles most involved for the motions against resistance are in uppercase letters. Muscles supplying supplemental force during concentric contraction are in lowercase letters.

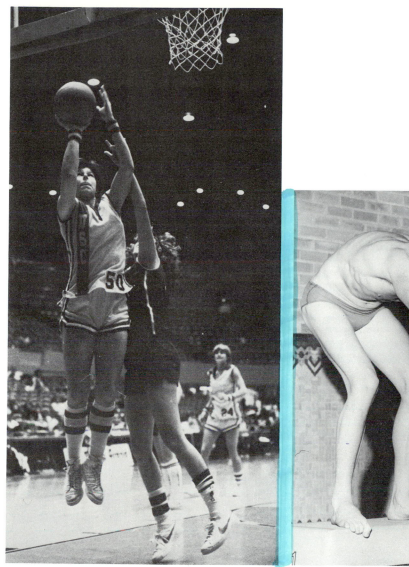

Figure 6.19.

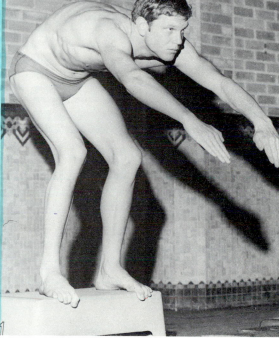

Figure 6.20.

Figure 6.19. Anna Maria Lopez (50), USC basketball player, has plantar flexed both ankles against
gravity to help provide some of the vertical force
necessary to execute a short jump shot. Courtesy
USC Athletic News Service (Michael R. Harriel).

Figure 6.20. Interphalangeal joint flexions of the
toes used during the racing start in swimming by
Jim McConica, USC swimmer. From Northrip, Logan,
and McKinney, *Introduction to Biomechanics Analysis of Sport.*

The knee is constructed to move most efficiently through the anteroposterior plane of motion. When the knees are used in such activities as walking, jogging, sprinting, and running straight or on smooth surfaces, there are a limited number of potential hazards to damage the knee. There are many times, however, when the knee undergoes extreme stresses owing to the medial and lateral pivoting requirements of sport. The knee must function effectively under the extreme stress of sport competition to provide both mobility and stability for the performer. Injuries often occur when the knee is placed in unnatural positions

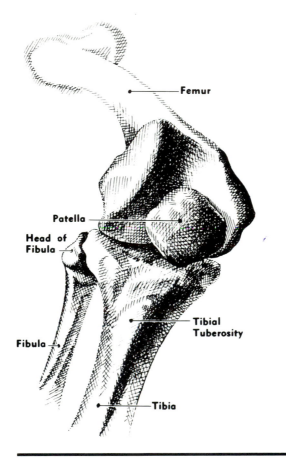

Figure 6.21. Bone structure of the flexed right knee—anterior view.

under great stress during sport competition. Consequently, the supporting structures of the knee should always be well conditioned to reduce the probability of injury.

Ligamentous support of the knee is relatively good; however, it must be remembered that the major stability of the knee joint is derived from muscle groups acting upon it. These muscle groups are shown in figure 6.22. Relatively little structural stability is provided by the bony articulation between the femoral condyles and the superior surface of the tibia, although bony stability is enhanced by the position of the medial and lateral menisci on the superior surface of the tibia. The menisci in this case tend to deepen the articulation (fig. 6.23).

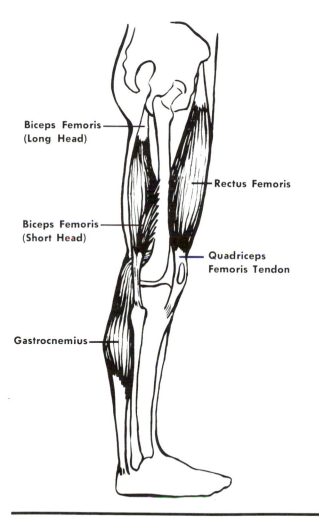

Biceps Femoris (Long Head)

Rectus Femoris

Biceps Femoris (Short Head)

Quadriceps Femoris Tendon

Gastrocnemius

Figure 6.22. Diagrammatic representation of some of the knee stabilizing musculature. From Logan, *Adapted Physical Education.*

There are two major pairs of ligaments which add to the structural stability of the knee. These are the medial and lateral collateral ligaments which have a stabilizing effect in the lateral plane, and the anterior and posterior cruciate ligaments which add anteroposterior stability to the knee joint (fig. 6.23). The medial collateral ligament attaches the femur to the tibia. It also is attached to the medial meniscus. The lateral collateral ligament attaches the femur to the fibula but does not attach to the lateral meniscus. Both collateral ligaments lie slightly posterior to the lateral axis of the knee joint; therefore, they become taut when the knee is moved into complete extension. Conversely, the medial and lateral collateral ligaments become slack when the knee is flexed. *This slackness of the collateral ligaments allows the knee to be rotated medially or laterally when the knee is flexed.*

The cruciate ligaments are named because of their position of attachment on the superior head of the tibia. The term *cruciate* (from *crux*—to cross) implies that these two ligaments cross anteriorly and posteriorly within the septum of the knee joint. The anterior cruciate attaches to the tibia on its anterior-superior surface. It crosses through the knee joint from the medial side diagonally to its lateral attachment on the femur. The posterior cruciate attaches on the posterior-superior aspect of the tibia. It crosses diagonally and medially to its attachment on the femur. The cross-configuration of the cruciates adds structural stability

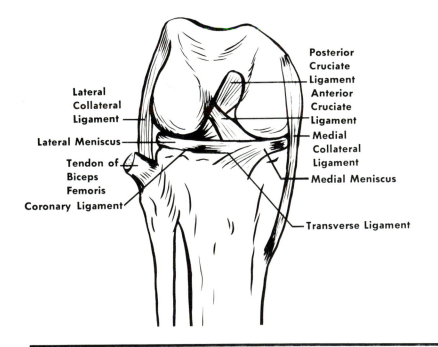

Figure 6.23. Right knee flexed—anterior view showing the cartilage and ligaments of the knee. From Logan, *Adapted Physical Education.*

to the knee joint when it is extended. In addition, the anterior cruciate prevents anterior movement of the tibia when the knee is flexed, and the posterior cruciate prevents posterior movement of the tibia while the knee is flexed. Other ligaments, including the capsular ligaments, provide additional stability for the knee joint.

The patellar ligament is misnamed. The patella is a sesamoid bone; that is, it is a bone located within the quadriceps femoris tendon. Its posterior aspect articulates with the femur during flexion and extension of the knee joint. The structure usually identified as the patellar ligament is actually a continuation of the quadriceps femoris tendon attaching to the tibial tuberosity. Early anatomists assumed that the patellar ligament was actually attached to the patella and connected that bone with the tibia. Were this the case, it would meet the definition of a ligament because it would attach bone to bone. In effect, however, it attaches muscle to bone because of its continuation with the quadriceps femoris tendon.

The menisci are held to the superior aspect of the tibia by the coronary ligaments. These ligaments are located on the periphery of each meniscus, and they are composed of tissue from the joint capsule. The Ligament of Wrisberg is another knee ligament with a direct association to a meniscus. This ligament is attached posterior to the lateral meniscus, and it attaches proximally to the medial condyle of the tibia. The transverse ligament, when present, is located anteriorly. It connects the two menisci.

The oblique popliteal ligament provides considerable structural support posteriorly for the knee. It attaches laterally on the posterior aspect of the lateral condyle of the femur and proceeds diagonally to the medial, posterior head of the tibia. Some of the popliteal space surface posterior and superior to the center of the knee joint is covered by this ligament.

The structural support of the knee by its ligaments is excellent. The laterally placed iliotibial tract also adds to this stable structure. For "normal" locomotor functions through the anteroposterior plane, one would expect minimal knee problems. But the forces generated in sport through that plane, plus the transverse plane of motion, cause tremendous stress on these structures.

The major stability for the knee joint comes from the muscles. The anterior stabilization of the knee joint is provided by the quadriceps femoris muscle group consisting of the rectus femoris, vastus medialis, vastus intermedius, and vastus lateralis. They converge into a fanshaped tendon with its apex at the tibial tuberosity (fig. 6.22). This fan shape is important because it allows for more efficient use of the potential forces of the vastus medialis and vastus lateralis. Any other arrangement of the tendon would dissipate the internal forces generated by these muscles. It is rather interesting to observe that the middle fibers of the quadriceps femoris tendon are thicker than the lateral and medial fibers. The reason for this lies in the fact that this area of the tendon has tremendous forces exerted upon it by the rectus femoris *and* vastus intermedius muscles. Consequently, greater tensile strength of the tendon at this point is desired. These are the main muscles exerting force directly through the anteroposterior plane of motion for knee extension.

A high level of strength within the quadriceps femoris muscle group is important in preventing knee injury; consequently, weight-training programs should include resistance exercises for knee extension and flexion. Upon the initiation of a weight-training program, rapid gains in strength can be expected within the quadriceps femoris muscle group because most individuals have a relatively low level of strength within this muscle group. The potential strength is great in relation to other muscles owing to the fact that the bipedal stance requires relatively little effort by the quadriceps muscle group in activities of daily living. The quadrupedal position probably demanded a muscle group the size of the quadriceps for locomotor purposes.

Posterior stabilization of the knee joint is due to actions of the gastrocnemius popliteus, semitendinosus, semimembranosus, and biceps femoris muscles. Although the hamstring muscles—the semitendinosus, semimembranosus, and biceps femoris—are attached to the medial and lateral sides of the joint, they must be considered posterior muscles. The tendons of the hamstrings lie posterior to the axis of the joint. The hamstring muscles supply lateral and medial support as well as posterior support when the knee is extended. The gastrocnemius, discussed above, is also a posterior stabilizing muscle for the knee joint. Its proximal attachments are on the posterior aspects of the femoral condyles. These posterior attachments add to the stability of the knee when it is in extension. A companion muscle which functions with the gastrocnemius is the popliteus. The primary stability function for the popliteus is to prevent hyperextension of the knee.

Most of the lateral stability of the knee is derived secondarily from forces exerted by anterior and posterior muscle groups. Therefore, much stress and strain is placed on the medial and lateral collateral ligaments. This is one reason these ligaments are often injured in sport activities. Some lateral stability of the knee is given by the tractus iliotibialis, actually a lateral expansion or thickening of the fascia covering the entire thigh. It is thickened laterally to withstand the force exerted upon it at the level of the hip joint by the tensor fasciae latae and gluteus maximus muscles. In a rather remote fashion, the gluteus maximus and tensor fasciae latae add to the lateral stability of the knee also. At the same time they maintain tension on the fascia surrounding the musculature of the total thigh. On the medial side of the knee, the gracilis and sartorius are in a position to maintain minimal stability of the knee joint when it is extended.

Figure 6.24 shows the spatial relationships of all the muscles surrounding the knee. This is a cross section of the right knee joint, viewing the tibia and fibula from above without the femur in place. It is important to know these spatial relationships in terms of both the preceding material related to joint stability and the following discussion of muscle function. It should be noted that all muscles in figure 6.24 have a posterior spatial relationship to the axis of the knee joint, except the quadriceps femoris muscle group. It is also important to note the specific locations of the hamstrings. The biceps femoris lies posterior and lateral to the joint, and the semimembranosus and semitendinosus are posterior and medial. These spatial relationships to the joint and their lines of pull from the ischial tuberosity to these distal attachments determine their functions.

ANTERIOR

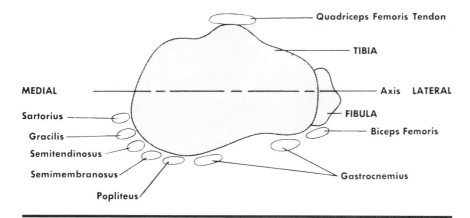

Quadriceps Femoris Tendon

TIBIA

MEDIAL ——————————— — — — — — — — — — — ———————— Axis LATERAL

Sartorius

Gracilis

Semitendinosus

Semimembranosus

Popliteus

FIBULA

Biceps Femoris

Gastrocnemius

Figure 6.24. Spatial relationships of knee joint muscles—superior view, right knee.

Extension

The four muscles most involved for knee extension against resistance are within the quadriceps femoris muscle group: rectus femoris, vastus medialis, vastus intermedius, and vastus lateralis. These four muscles have an anterior spatial relationship to the knee joint. Therefore, when they contract concentrically in a weight-training exercise as shown in figure 6.25, the internal force of the contraction is focused on the tibial tuberosity and the proximal attachments of these four muscles are stabilized. The weight load is moved as the knee joints extend. The contralateral muscles are reciprocally innervated, and they are located posterior to the knee joint.

In general the three vasti muscles envelope the femur anteriorly. The vastus medialis and vastus lateralis are the only two vasti muscles which can be palpated. The vastus intermedius lies between the vastus medialis and vastus lateralis; however, the rectus femoris is superficial to the vastus intermedius. It is the rectus femoris muscle lying between the vastus lateralis and vastus medialis which is palpable on the anterior aspect of the thigh. The vasti muscles are uniarticular with their function at the knee joint only. The rectus femoris is a biarticular muscle with movement functions at knee and hip joints.

The lines of pull of the rectus femoris and vastus intermedius muscles are directly within the anteroposterior plane of motion for knee extension. The line of pull of the vastus lateralis is from lateral to medial, and the line of pull of the vastus medialis is from medial to lateral. As a result, they serve a dual role as the muscles most involved for knee extension as well as providing a minimal guiding function during knee extension. The major guiding muscles during knee extension, however, are the hamstring muscles. In this instance the contralateral

Lower limb motions   139

muscles also serve as guiding muscles. The semimembranosus and semitendinosus muscles lie medial to the anteroposterior plane of motion, and the biceps femoris is lateral to that plane. The force-counterforce developed between these muscles parallel to the plane of motion during knee extension by the quadriceps rules out their undesired rotary capabilities through the transverse plane.

Flexion

Knee flexion occurs when the tibia and fibula are brought closer to the femur posteriorly. The average range of motion for knee flexion is 130 degrees. The range of motion for each individual is determined by the status of the knee ligaments and other noncontractile tissue surrounding the knee plus the size of the muscles located on the posterior aspect of the femur. Figure 6.26 shows a right knee joint which has been flexed through 90 degrees of its range of motion. All joint ranges of motion may be plotted in this manner, utilizing videotape or film. This can be done manually or by means of any of several types of electronic film analyzers available to record and compute joint motion data.

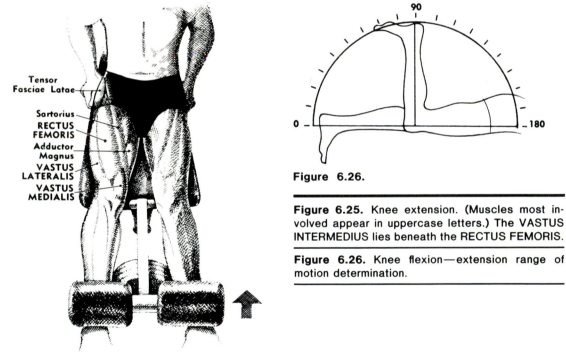

Tensor Fasciae Latae

Sartorius
RECTUS FEMORIS
Adductor Magnus
VASTUS LATERALIS
VASTUS MEDIALIS

Figure 6.25.

Figure 6.26.

Figure 6.25. Knee extension. (Muscles most involved appear in uppercase letters.) The VASTUS INTERMEDIUS lies beneath the RECTUS FEMORIS.

Figure 6.26. Knee flexion—extension range of motion determination.

Knee flexion against resistance is performed by the muscles with spatial relationships posterior to the knee joint as shown in figure 6.24. The one exception to this is the function of the popliteus. It is not considered as a flexor due to its line of pull; however, it plays an important role in flexion by rotating the knee to "unlock" it from complete extension so the flexors can move the joint.

The muscles most involved for knee flexion are the semitendinosus, semimembranosus, and biceps femoris. The sartorius, gracilis and gastrocnemius work with the "hamstrings" to perform knee flexion against resistance; however, their force contribution is relatively small. They simply do not have the size or leverage advantage of the "hamstrings."

Figure 6.27 shows a weight-training exercise involving knee flexion against resistance. Each of the MMI can be palpated during this type of work. It should be noted that rotations of the knee would be undesirable during such an activity. The equal force-counterforce exerted by the biceps femoris laterally and the semitendinosus and semimembranosus medially rule out these rotations; therefore, these muscles serve as guiding muscles as well as MMI. Their distal attachments lie parallel to the anteroposterior plane of motion through which the limb is moving. The contralateral muscles are anterior to the joint in this example.

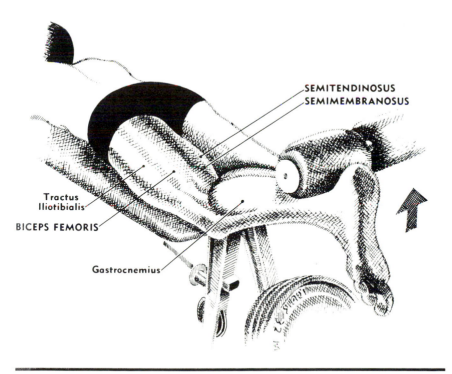

Figure 6.27. Knee flexion. (Muscles most involved appear in uppercase letters.)

Weight training and calisthenic exercises should be performed slowly to take full advantage of both concentric and eccentric contractions and to protect the joints. If the knee flexion exercise as shown in figure 6.27 is performed in this manner, the knee flexors on the posterior aspect of the knee will be worked during the flexion process as noted. And, *if the knee is extended slowly,* these same muscles will be most involved for controlling the speed of extension by means of eccentric contraction. Thus, the "hamstring" muscle group is worked during flexion *and* extension. This would not be the case if the weights were just dropped and the knee joint extended rapidly. The prime moving force in that situation would be gravity.

The knee is a joint which must be protected during calisthenic and weight training programs. It can be traumatized if flexed through its full range of motion in bilateral and unilateral weight bearing situations with the feet or one foot as the base of support. Therefore, exercises such as "deep knee bends" and "duck waddles" are contraindicated from a sport medicine standpoint. Those exercises have the potential of traumatizing the noncontractile tissue of the knee joint, i.e., there is a high probability of ligamentous and/or cartilage damage to the knees of students subjected to "deep knee bends" and "duck waddles."

Exercise of the knee for flexion can be done safely by having the performer assume the prone position as shown in figure 6.27. The submaximal weight load for strength development, as one example, would be significantly lower than the total body weight of the individual doing the exercise. This reduces the stress on the knee, especially if the knee is only allowed to flex through ninety degrees of its range of motion.

If knee flexion-extension is performed in the standing (bilateral weight bearing) position, the knees can be safely flexed to ninety-degrees. To avoid going beyond that point during a weight training exercise, as an example, it is a good idea to place a chair behind the performer. The performer would flex the knees to the point that the gluteus maximus muscles touched the chair. At that point, the knees would be moved into extension by the concentrically contracting quadriceps femoris muscle group. The quadriceps are also the muscles most involved for slowly controlling knee flexion eccentrically in this example.

Figure 6.28 shows an excellent multisport athlete overcoming inertia as he moves out of the blocks during a sprint start in track. The musculature of the knee is very important in terms of the contributions of the contractions of these muscle groups to the overall summation of force to execute the skill. In figure 6.28, the quadriceps are extending the right knee concentrically so force can be applied against the earth. This angular motion within the knee plus angular motions at the other joints contribute the forces necessary to move the total body of the sprinter linearly. The left knee is being flexed against gravity by the concentrically contracting "hamstrings" posterior to the knee while the quadriceps are reciprocally innervated in their contralateral position. The left rectus femoris is plainly visible in a contracted state, because it is contributing force for the left hip flexion. It is a biarticular muscle with anterior spatial relationships to the knee and hip joints.

Medial rotation

Rotation of the knee is only possible when the knee is flexed. The muscles most involved for medial rotation are the semitendinosus, semimembranosus, and popliteus. The sartorius and gracilis also contribute to medial rotation. These five muscles have their distal attachments on the medial aspect of the tibial

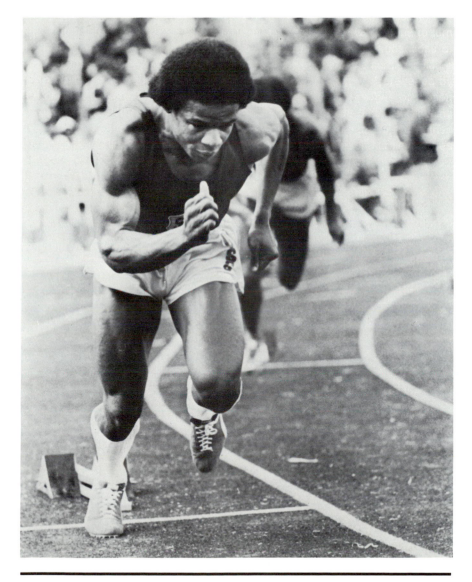

Figure 6.28. Charles White, USC sprinter, demonstrates the necessity for forceful knee extensions and flexions during the sprint start. Courtesy of *USC Athletic News Service.*

condyle. Consequently, when the knee is moved into flexion, their pull during concentric contraction moves the knee into medial rotation unless the force is counteracted by the contralateral muscle, the biceps femoris.

Lateral rotation

The biceps femoris has its distal attachment on the head of the fibula and lateral condyle of the tibia; as a result, when it contracts concentrically against resistance while the knee is being flexed, it is the muscle most involved to rotate the knee laterally, unless its force is counteracted by the five medial rotators of the knee. The lines of pull for all knee joint musculature are presented in figure 6.29.

Hip joint motions   Motions possible at the hip joint include flexion, extension, adduction, abduction, diagonal abduction, diagonal adduction, medial and lateral rotation, and circumduction. Although the hip joint is supported anteriorly by a large amount of connective tissue, there is a wide range and variety of movement within this joint. The hip joint is a very stable structure because of its bone and ligamentous arrangement as well as its muscular support. It is a multiaxial joint.

The bony stability results from the relationship between the deep, cuplike acetabulum of the pelvis and the head of the femur. The femoral head is actually received within the acetabulum area. This type of bony articulation is needed because the hip joint must bear considerable weight in the bipedal stance (fig. 6.30).

Ligamentous support is mainly anterior to the hip joint. Primarily responsible for hip joint stability is the iliofemoral ligament. This ligament is commonly called the "Y" ligament. The pubofemoral ligament provides additional support. The iliofemoral ligament is one of the strongest ligaments in the body and limits extension of the hip. There is no analogous structure for preventing hip flexion. One other ligamentous structure which provides a limited amount of structural stability at the hip joint is the teres ligament. This ligament connects the head of the femur to the concave surface of the acetabulum.

Although there is considerable bony and ligamentous support to maintain structural stability of the hip joint, the major stabilizing force is provided by the muscles surrounding the hip joint. Posterior stabilization of the hip joint comes from the semitendinosus, semimembranosus, biceps femoris, and gluteus maximus. Anterior stabilization, from a muscular standpoint, is provided mainly by the iliopsoas and rectus femoris muscles. However, the iliofemoral ligament provides a great amount of anterior stabilization with the hip extended. Lateral stabilization is due primarily to the interaction of the gluteus medius, gluteus minimus, and tensor fasciae latae muscles, with some help from the gluteus maximus. The muscles have a tendency to counteract the gravitational pull downward. There is an analogy between the actions of these four muscles and the three parts of the deltoid muscle at the shoulder joint. Without these muscles the pelvis would tend to drop on the opposite side during unilateral weight bearing.

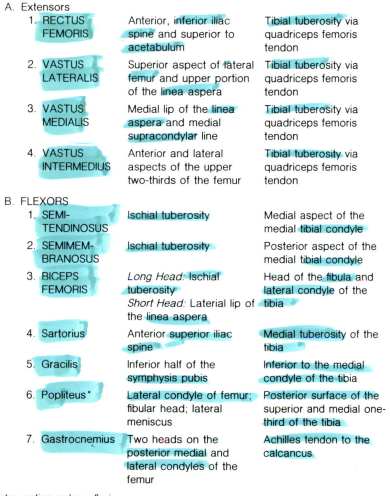

MUSCLES	PROXIMAL ATTACHMENT	DISTAL ATTACHMENT
I. Knee Joint Musculature		
A. Extensors		
1. RECTUS FEMORIS	Anterior, inferior iliac spine and superior to acetabulum	Tibial tuberosity via quadriceps femoris tendon
2. VASTUS LATERALIS	Superior aspect of lateral femur and upper portion of the linea aspera	Tibial tuberosity via quadriceps femoris tendon
3. VASTUS MEDIALIS	Medial lip of the linea aspera and medial supracondylar line	Tibial tuberosity via quadriceps femoris tendon
4. VASTUS INTERMEDIUS	Anterior and lateral aspects of the upper two-thirds of the femur	Tibial tuberosity via quadriceps femoris tendon
B. FLEXORS		
1. SEMI-TENDINOSUS	Ischial tuberosity	Medial aspect of the medial tibial condyle
2. SEMIMEM-BRANOSUS	Ischial tuberosity	Posterior aspect of the medial tibial condyle
3. BICEPS FEMORIS	*Long Head:* Ischial tuberosity *Short Head:* Lateral lip of the linea aspera	Head of the fibula and lateral condyle of the tibia
4. Sartorius	Anterior superior iliac spine	Medial tuberosity of the tibia
5. Gracilis	Inferior half of the symphysis pubis	Inferior to the medial condyle of the tibia
6. Popliteus*	Lateral condyle of femur; fibular head; lateral meniscus	Posterior surface of the superior and medial one-third of the tibia
7. Gastrocnemius	Two heads on the posterior medial and lateral condyles of the femur	Achilles tendon to the calcancus

*Initiates motion so knee flexion can occur

Figure 6.29. Knee joint musculature. The muscles most involved for the motions are in uppercase letters. Muscles supplying supplemental force during concentric contraction are in lowercase letters.

Figure 6.29. Continued.

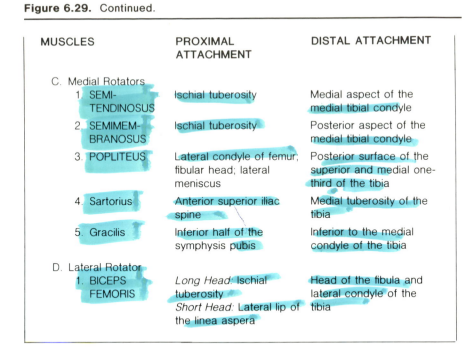

MUSCLES	PROXIMAL ATTACHMENT	DISTAL ATTACHMENT
C. Medial Rotators		
1. SEMI-TENDINOSUS	Ischial tuberosity	Medial aspect of the medial tibial condyle
2. SEMIMEM-BRANOSUS	Ischial tuberosity	Posterior aspect of the medial tibial condyle
3. POPLITEUS	Lateral condyle of femur; fibular head; lateral meniscus	Posterior surface of the superior and medial one-third of the tibia
4. Sartorius	Anterior superior iliac spine	Medial tuberosity of the tibia
5. Gracilis	Inferior half of the symphysis pubis	Inferior to the medial condyle of the tibia
D. Lateral Rotator		
1. BICEPS FEMORIS	*Long Head:* Ischial tuberosity *Short Head:* Lateral lip of the linea aspera	Head of the fibula and lateral condyle of the tibia

The lateral stabilizers are called upon to act at their highest level in a unilateral weight-bearing position. The relationship between the femur and the pelvis is architecturally a cantilever construction. The concentric contraction of the gluteus medius in the unilateral weight-bearing position has a tendency to draw the crest of the ilium down toward the femur on the same side which, in turn, causes lateral pelvic girdle rotation on the opposite side. This is a basic concept which must be understood in virtually all sport skills. For example, this action is seen during running. When the foot strikes the ground and becomes the weight-bearing limb, the lateral stabilizers of the hip on that side must hold the pelvis in position so the opposite limb, the non-weight-bearing limb, can go through the so-called "free-swinging" phase of running. During this phase, all body weight is borne by the hip joint on the weight-bearing side. At this time, the major function of unilateral weight-bearing is assumed by the gluteus minimus, gluteus medius, tensor fasciae latae, and gluteus maximus muscles. Analyses of running and sprinting performances by athletes should be thought of as a sequential and alternating series of unilateral weight-bearing movements.

Medial stabilization of the hip joint by muscles is the direct result of the adductor muscle group: adductor longus, adductor brevis, and adductor magnus muscles. These muscles are assisted in this stabilization function by the gracilis and pectineus muscles.

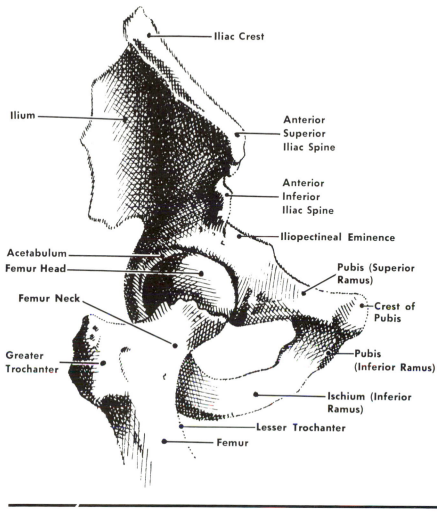

Figure 6.30. Right hip joint.

- Iliac Crest
- Ilium
- Anterior Superior Iliac Spine
- Anterior Inferior Iliac Spine
- Iliopectineal Eminence
- Acetabulum
- Femur Head
- Pubis (Superior Ramus)
- Femur Neck
- Crest of Pubis
- Greater Trochanter
- Pubis (Inferior Ramus)
- Ischium (Inferior Ramus)
- Lesser Trochanter
- Femur

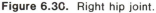

Flexion

Hip joint flexion occurs when there is reduction of the angle between the femur and pelvic girdle. Due to "hamstring tension," a greater range of motion for hip flexion occurs with the knee flexed instead of extended (fig. 6.31). This is an anteroposterior plane motion. The last or "hurdle step" by the springboard diver, for example, is one of the most important phases of diving. This movement, which incorporates hip flexion, determines the amount of board deflection for the final kinetic energy transfer to the body from the board. In addition, this hip flexion helps to determine the trajectory of the dive. Hip flexion range of motion is increased by the diver by concurrently flexing the knee. Hip flexion is an important motion in many skills, but it is especially important in any skill where the mass of the body is being moved vertically.

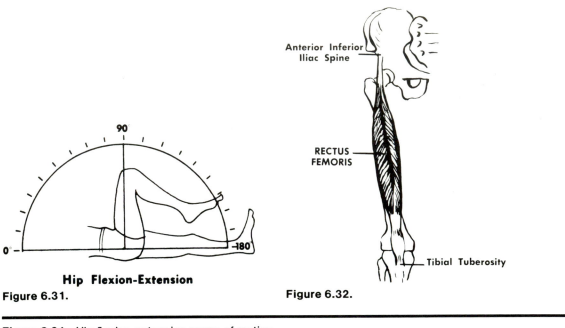

Hip Flexion-Extension

Figure 6.31.

Figure 6.32.

Figure 6.31. Hip flexion-extension range of motion determination.

Figure 6.32. Spatial relationships of the rectus femoris to the right knee and hip joints. From Logan, *Adapted Physical Education.*

The muscles most involved for hip flexion against resistance have anterior spatial relationships to the hip joint. The MMI are the psoas, iliacus, rectus femoris, and pectineus. As indicated, the rectus femoris is a biarticular muscle which extends the knee and flexes the hip joint. The spatial relationships of this muscle to both joints is shown in figure 6.32.

Figure 6.33 shows the remaining hip flexor MMI in uppercase letters and the adductor MMI in lowercase letters. The inguinal ligament is also shown. This ligament provides a type of pulley arrangement to maintain functional positioning of the hip flexors. *All muscles shown in figure 6.33 are located on both sides.* They are separated here to more easily show their relative positions. Of the adductors shown, the gracilis is the only biarticular muscle which has a function at the knee joint.

The term *iliopsoas* appears in figure 6.33. Functionally, the iliacus and psoas muscles have the same line of pull from the iliac fossa to the lesser trochanter of the femur; therefore, the two muscles are considered as one muscle, the iliopsoas, at the hip joint. The psoas, of course, has an independent function at the lumbar spine.

There is some disagreement among kinesiologists regarding the other muscles which contribute to hip flexion besides the iliopsoas, pectineus and rectus femoris.

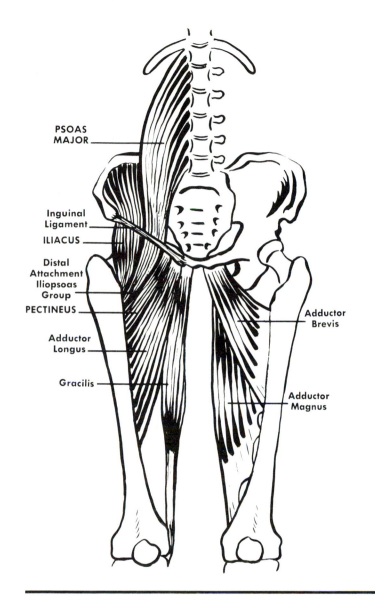

PSOAS
MAJOR

Inguinal
Ligament

ILIACUS

Distal
Attachment
Iliopsoas
Group

PECTINEUS

Adductor
Longus

Gracilis

Adductor
Brevis

Adductor
Magnus

Figure 6.33. Right hip flexor MMI (in uppercase letters)—and adductors. From Logan, *Adapted Physical Education.*

By virtue of their anterior spatial relationships to the hip joint, the sartorius and tensor fasciae latae are involved in hip flexion. Some research investigators have indicated that the anterior fibers of the gluteus medius and minimus, gracilis, adductor longus, and adductor brevis are involved in hip flexion. There is no agreement regarding the role of the adductor magnus. It is believed by the authors that the force contribution of these muscles to hip flexion, if any, is minimal. Some electromyographic action in these muscles during hip flexion and pendular action of the lower limb is to be expected, because of their important guiding (synergistic) function concurrent with flexion.

Of the muscles most involved for hip flexion against resistance, the rectus femoris is the only one readily accessible for palpation. Figure 6.34 shows hip flexion of the right hip joint against resistance provided by an Exer-Genie Exerciser. The concentrically contracting rectus femoris is very prominent superficially in this type of exercise.

Since hip flexion is an anteroposterior plane motion and the MMI against resistance are located anteriorly, the contralateral muscles have spatial relationships posterior to the joint. The guiding muscles, therefore, are located medial

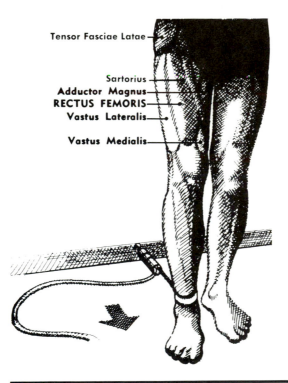

Tensor Fasciae Latae

Sartorius
Adductor Magnus
RECTUS FEMORIS
Vastus Lateralis

Vastus Medialis

Figure 6.34. Hip flexion. (Muscles most involved appear in uppercase letters.)

and lateral or parallel to the anteroposterior plane of motion at the hip joint. The medial guiders are the sartorius, gracilis, adductor longus, adductor brevis, and upper fibers of the adductor magnus. Laterally, the guiding muscles are the tensor fasciae latae, gluteus minimus, and gluteus medius. The relationships of the tensor fasciae latae and sartorious to the hip are shown in figure 6.35. As was the case for the guiders for knee flexion, the guiding muscles can contribute internal forces which add to the flexion and force-counterforce on either side of the motion plane, which rules out undesired motions through other planes. It must be remembered that the hip joint is a multiaxial joint with numerous motion potentialities.

Extension

The muscles most involved for hip extension have a posterior spatial relationship to the joint. These are the gluteus maximus, long head of the biceps femoris, semitendinosus, and semimembranosus. The gluteus maximus, lower fibers, has the best posterior spatial relationship to the joint for force application on the femur. The hamstring muscles' proximal attachment is the ischial tuberosity, and this is posterior *and* inferior to the hip. This latter characteristic minimizes some

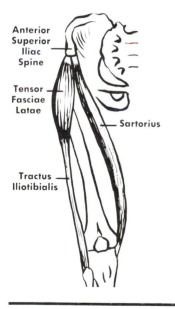

Anterior
Superior
Iliac
Spine

Tensor
Fasciae
Latae

Sartorius

Tractus
Iliotibialis

Figure 6.35. Relationships of the tensor fasciae latae and sartorius muscles to the hip joint. From Logan, *Adapted Physical Education*.

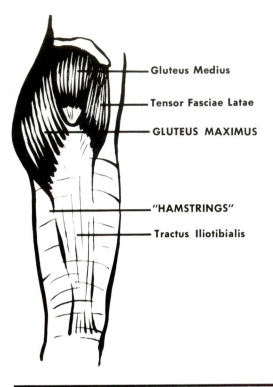

Gluteus Medius

Tensor Fasciae Latae

GLUTEUS MAXIMUS

"HAMSTRINGS"

Tractus Iliotibialis

Figure 6.36. Posterior spatial relationships of the hip extensors to the joint. (Muscles most involved appear in uppercase letters.) From Logan, *Adapted Physical Education.*

of their force potential which can be utilized for hip extension. Figure 6.36 shows the general interrelationships between the gluteus maximus and hamstrings posteriorly, gluteus medius laterally, and the gluteus maximus and tensor fasciae latae laterally.

The guiding muscles for extension have medial and lateral spatial relationships to the hip joint, and they are the same as those guiders listed for hip flexion.

As a ski jumper moves down the hill prior to the jump, there are flexions at the hip joints. This is flexion with gravity; therefore, there is a reversal of the usual function of the muscles most involved. Those muscles posterior to the hip joint are the muscles most involved for controlling the extent of this hip flexion while undergoing eccentric contraction. The gluteus maximus and other posterior muscles are under considerable tension while being stretched. At lift off, the ski jumper forcefully extends the hip joints against gravity. The muscles most involved for this motion are the concentrically contracting gluteus maximus and hamstrings. The stretching or "setting" of these muscles while controlling hip flexion during the moving stance prior to lift off is directly related to the amount of force for hip extension at lift-off. The amount of force available helps determine the angle of take-off and trajectory. Horizontal distance is determined by the parabolic flight pattern, and this helps to determine a portion of the score the jumper receives. Motions and joint angles during the preparatory phase of a sport skill are of considerable importance to the outcome.

The muscles most involved for hip extension are all superficial. A weight-training exercise designed to strengthen and gain muscle endurance in the right gluteus maximus and hamstring muscles is shown in figure 6.37. It is recommended that an exercise of this type be performed by the student, and the muscles should be palpated prior to and during their concentric contractions.

Figure 6.38 shows an excellent offensive American football player starting to accelerate into the open field of the defensive secondary. A portion of the force, which added to his skill, can be seen by the extent of the ranges of motion utilized for hip flexion and extension. The left hip joint has been extended maximally. (There is no hyperextension of the hip.) The left hip extension force as seen in figure 6.38 was generated by concentric contraction of the gluteus

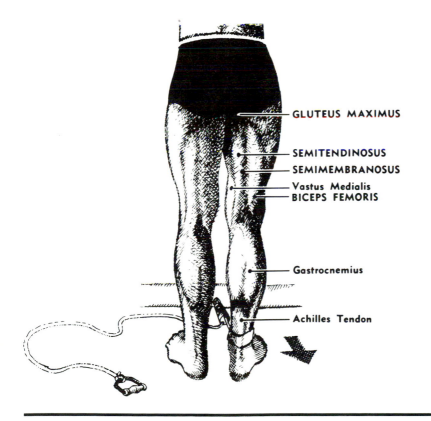

Figure 6.37. Hip extension. (Muscles most involved appear in uppercase letters.)

maximus and other posterior hip muscles as shown in figure 6.37. The summation of forces from the left hip, knee, and ankle muscle contractions contributes to linear motion of the football player through action and reaction with the turf. Concurrently, the right lower limb is being prepared to do the same thing by concentric flexions, at the hip and knee joints. The right lower limb will be thrust against the turf, with the hip and knee joints moving into extension. If continued, these kinds of alternating hip, knee, and ankle joint motions during running have the potential to produce high linear velocity of the body in some runners.

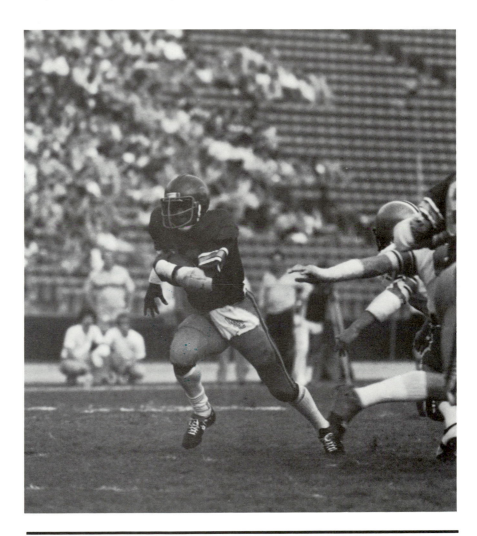

Figure 6.38. Charles White, Heisman Award Winning USC tailback, accelerates into the defensive secondary. Utilization of hip flexion-extension ranges of motion adds to his skill. Courtesy *USC Athletic News Service.*

Abduction

This hip joint motion occurs through the cardinal, lateral plane of motion. The lower limb is moved away from the cardinal anteroposterior plane through a range of motion. Figure 6.39 shows the right hip joint being abducted through approximately thirty-five degrees. The anatomic landmarks and estimated joint centers help determine how many degrees of motion have been negotiated.

Forceful muscle action for abduction is relatively rare in the context of sport and dance performances. The muscle most involved for abduction against resistance is small when compared to many other muscles; however, the leverage advantage of the gluteus medius provides it with considerable potential internal force development. The gluteus medius has a lateral spatial relationship to the hip joint, and lies directly in the lateral plane of motion (figure 6.40).

The remaining gluteal muscles work with the gluteus medius in abduction. The upper fibers of the gluteus maximus and the posterior fibers of the gluteus minimus contribute some contractile force for the motion. The tensor fasciae latae is also involved to some extent in abduction.

Since abduction is a lateral plane motion and the muscle most involved is lateral to the joint, the contralateral muscles have a medial spatial relationship to the joint. This means that the guiding muscles are located anterior and posterior to the joint. The guiders help to rule out medial and lateral rotations during abduction primarily. The anterior guiding muscles for abduction (and adduction) are the iliopsoas, sartorius, rectus femoris, tensor fasciae latae, and gluteus

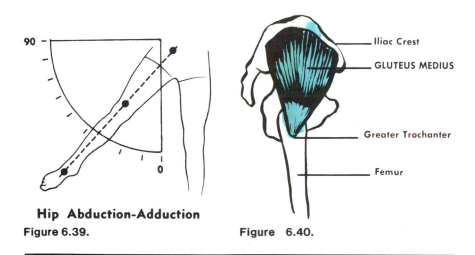

Hip Abduction-Adduction

Figure 6.39.

Iliac Crest

GLUTEUS MEDIUS

Greater Trochanter

Femur

Figure 6.40.

Figure 6.39. Hip abduction-adduction range of motion determination—lateral plane motions.

Figure 6.40. Hip abduction muscle most involved—right hip. From Logan, *Adapted Physical Education.*

---

minimus. Posteriorly, the guiding force is provided by the gluteus maximus, long head of the biceps femoris, semitendinosus, semimembranosus, and the six small lateral rotators of the hip: piriformis, obturator internus, obturator externus, quadratus femoris, gemellus superior, and gemellus inferior. Some of these guiding muscles for abduction and adduction are shown in figure 6.46.

Figure 6.41 shows an exercise for abduction of the right hip joint against resistance. The gluteus medius can be palpated. This type of exercise also demonstrates stabilization and dynamic stabilization. In the lower right limb (fig. 6.41) the muscles surrounding the right ankle and knee joints have contracted statically to *stabilize* these joints. The complete left lower limb is also stabilized, but this is due to the fact that a weight shift has occurred. All of the body weight is borne unilaterally by the left leg and foot. The stabilization in the left lower limb is due primarily to the weight being borne by the supporting bone structures.

For abduction of the right hip joint to occur, the weight must be shifted to the left leg and the pelvic girdle must have a slight amount of right lateral rotation. The latter is needed in order to literally lift the right lower limb. This allows it to turn through its abduction range of motion in pendulum fashion. The lateral rotation of the pelvic girdle is done under considerable tension; therefore, it is described as being dynamically stabilized. It is moving in lateral rotation but

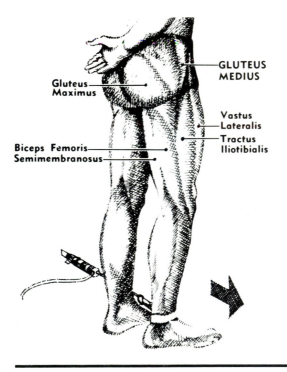

Figure 6.41. Hip abduction. (Muscles most involved appear in uppercase letters.)

stable enough to allow the concentrically contracting gluteus medius and other muscles involved in hip abduction to have a proximal point (pelvic girdle) at which to exert force. If the pelvis were absolutely static or stable, it would be difficult to execute this type of motion smoothly, due to the difficulty of moving from bilateral to unilateral weight-bearing when the feet are equally bearing the body weight. There would have to be some gross motion of the lumbar-thoracic segment to free the hip for abduction if the pelvis could not be rotated laterally.

Adduction

Hip adduction against resistance is performed by the muscles with a medial spatial relationship to the joint. The muscles most involved are the adductor brevis, adductor longus, adductor magnus, and gracilis (figs. 6.33 and 6.42). The lower fibers of the gluteus maximus assist in the adduction process against resistance. The guiding muscles were indicated above as being the same as for those of the abductors.

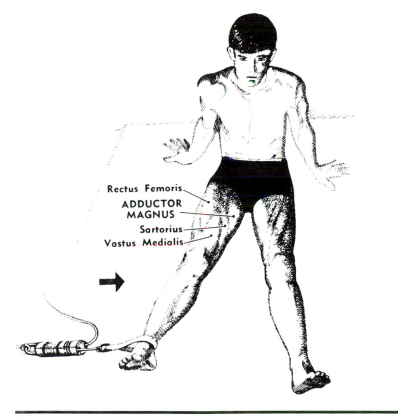

Figure 6.42. Hip adduction. (muscles most in-volved appear in uppercase letters.)

Adduction against resistance in the standing position with the weight borne unilaterally is unusual, unless the individual is attached to wall pulley weights or an exercise device. Adduction in that position can be performed entirely by gravity by releasing the tension in the muscles surrounding the hip joint. If, however, the lower limb is adducted slowly, the muscle most involved for controlling this motion would be the eccentrically contracting gluteus medius on the same side as the adducting hip. In this example there is a reversal of muscle function and the traditional adductors (medial spatial relationship) would serve as contralateral muscles.

Figure 6.42 shows adduction against resistance of the right hip joint in the seated position. This is a functional position to exercise the adductors, because extraneous motions elsewhere in the body are minimized. Consequently, the adductors are isolated and must perform the work through the lateral plane of motion. This, for example, would be a good exercise for swimmers who perform the breaststroke. The adductors are used forcefully in the whip kick against the resistance of the water; therefore, this group of muscles must have excellent strength and muscle endurance.

Diagonal abduction

Due to the enarthrodial structure of the hip joint, it is possible to move the lower limb through a low diagonal plane of motion. Motion at the hip joint through this plane away from the longitudinal axis of the body in the anatomic position is diagonal abduction.

The muscles most involved for diagonal abduction have lateral and posterior spatial relationships to the hip joint. They are the gluteus medius, gluteus maximus, semitendinosus, semimembranosus, long head of the biceps femoris, and the six lateral rotators.

The gluteal muscles involved in diagonal abduction contribute the greatest amount of force for the motion during concentric contraction. They have diagonal lines of pull. Diagonal abduction at the hip is a combination of abduction, extension, and lateral rotation in most instances. Lateral rotation may not be a part of some nonballistic diagonal abductions.

Soccer-style kicking is one skill which utilizes the hip joint diagonal plane motions of diagonal abduction and diagonal adduction. During the preparatory phase of the kick, the kicking limb is diagonally abducted as far as possible to place the diagonal adductors (the contralateral muscles) on stretch. For greater force potential, the hip joint is usually laterally rotated during diagonal abduction prior to a soccer-style kick. Therefore, it is advantageous for a person working on soccer-style kicking skills to increase the range of motion for diagonal abduction as much as possible. The increased flexibility in the hip joint has the potential to increase kicking limb velocity which might have the implication of more points scored.

The guiding muscles for diagonal plane motions at the hip have medial and lateral spatial relationships to the joint primarily. Medially, the three adductor muscles and the gracilis provide some guiding force. Laterally, the tensor fasciae latae, gluteus minimus, and gluteus medius provide a counterforce to rule out undesired motions.

Figure 6.43 shows the start of diagonal abduction against resistance in the right hip joint. The muscles most involved are not identified in this view, because they are lateral (under the swim suit) and posterior to the hip joint.

Hurdling technique (figure 6.44) involves diagonal plane motions at the hip joints in order to clear the hurdles efficiently instead of jumping them. The hurdler must keep his or her center of mass as close to the hurdle as possible. Anteroposterior plane motions used exclusively at the hip joints would tend to turn the hurdler into a "jumper." Diagonal abductions and diagonal adductions of the hip joints allow the skilled hurdler to *run* over the hurdles. The hurdler in figure 6.44 is diagonally adducting her right hip joint. This motion was preceded by diagonal abduction in the same hip. Hurdlers with excellent ranges of motion (flexibility) through the diagonal planes at hip joints are capable of almost touching their buttocks on top of each hurdle during the race. That greatly improves their times, because time is not lost by excessive vertical lift at each hurdle. It takes

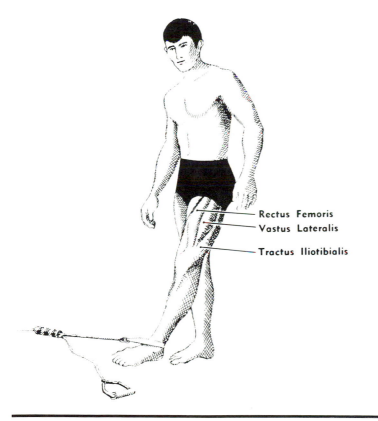

Rectus Femoris
Vastus Lateralis

Tractus Iliotibialis

Figure 6.43. The start of diagonal abduction of the right hip against resistance. (Muscles most involved are not seen in the anterior view.)

time for the center of mass to rise and fall through space. The good hurdler uses diagonal plane motions at the hip to eliminate that negative time factor during a race. This means that there is very little change in the height of the good hurdler's center of mass throughout a complete event such as the 120 yard high hurdle race.

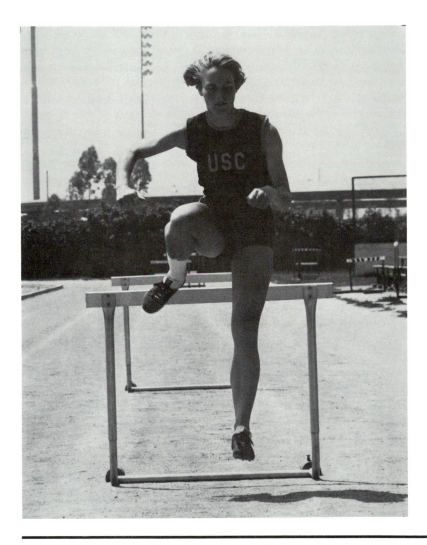

Figure 6.44. Mitzi McMillin, USC hurdler, utilizing diagonal adduction of her right hip joint to clear the hurdle efficiently. Courtesy *USC Athletic News Service.*

Diagonal adduction

The diagonal adductors at the hip joint have anterior and medial spatial relationships to the joint. They are located to pull the lower limb through the diagonal plane of motion toward the midline of the body when they contract concentrically. The muscles most involved for diagonal adduction against resistance are the iliopsoas, rectus femoris, pectineus, adductor brevis, adductor longus, and adductor magnus. Figure 6.45 shows diagonal adduction of the right hip against resistance at a point approximately midway through the potential range of motion.

To continue with the example of the soccer-style kick, the diagonal abduction serves the purpose of placing the muscles most involved for diagonal adduction on stretch. When the muscles most involved for diagonal adduction contract concentrically, this moves the kicking limb from the end of its diagonal abduction range of motion forward into diagonal adduction or the kicking phase.

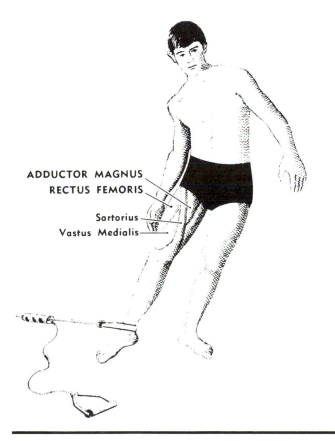

ADDUCTOR MAGNUS
RECTUS FEMORIS
Sartorius
Vastus Medialis

Figure 6.45. Hip diagonal adduction. (Superficial muscles most involved appear in uppercase letters.)

In terms of potential internal force, diagonal adduction is a more powerful motion than hip flexion. It will be noted that diagonal adduction utilizes both the hip flexor *and* adductor muscles. This is one reason why relatively small soccer-style kickers attain great distances in their kicks. This is also one reason that this style of kicking is being adopted by American football place-kickers. These larger men will be able to kick great distances using diagonal adduction once they have mastered the kicking skill. Some American football place-kickers use a toe-kicking style employing hip flexion and knee extension through the antero-posterior plane of motion. In American-style place-kicking a relatively small amount of the foot surface contacts the ball; whereas, in soccer-style kicking a large portion of the medial aspect of the foot comes into contact with the football. This has a tendency to result in greater accuracy as well as greater distance.

Lateral rotation

The spatial relationships of the lateral rotators of the hip are posterior to the joint. The muscles most involved for this motion are the gluteus maximus and six lateral rotators. The gluteus maximus is shown in figure 6.36, and figure 6.46 shows the six lateral rotators.

The gluteus maximus may be palpated during lateral rotation at the hip joint. However, the six lateral rotators are deep and cannot be felt during this motion. Figure 6.47 shows lateral rotation through almost a complete range of motion. This is a problem motion for many people during locomotor activities. The potential strength of the muscles most involved for lateral rotation is great, especially in the gluteus maximus. The medial rotators, on the other hand, are not as powerful. This imbalance of force is one reason individuals, in the absence of tibial torsion, "toe out" as they walk and run. Tibial torsion is an abnormal twisting of the tibia which also can cause a "toe out" type of lower limb motion. This lateral rotation of the hip is an extraneous motion during most locomotor activities and leads to a loss of average linear velocity of the body. As noted previously, the "toe out" problem is further complicated by that fact that eversion of the subtalar and transverse tarsal joints can also be present as an extraneous motion for running, jogging, and walking.

Lateral rotations of the hip joints may be more functional in curvilinear movement of the entire body, as seen in baserunning, and for directional changes during running by a football halfback. Lateral rotation adds to equilibrium in these situations by widening the base of support in unilateral and bilateral weight-bearing positions.

Medial rotation

The muscle most involved for medial rotation of the hip joint against resistance is the gluteus minimus, anterior fibers. This muscle is assisted by the anterior fibers of the gluteus medius and the tensor fasciae latae. Kinesiologists tend to disagree regarding muscles which may or may not contribute to this motion.

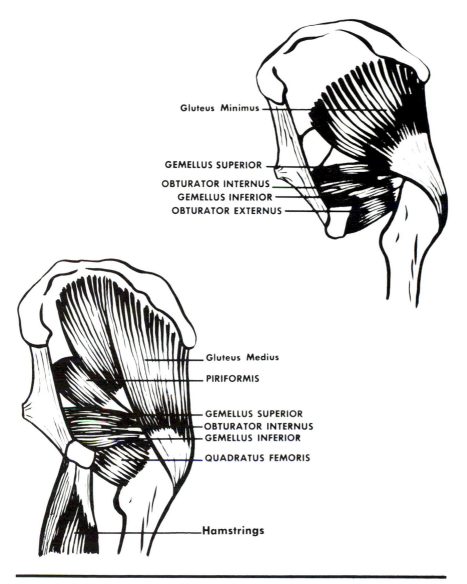

Gluteus Minimus

GEMELLUS SUPERIOR

OBTURATOR INTERNUS

GEMELLUS INFERIOR

OBTURATOR EXTERNUS

Gluteus Medius

PIRIFORMIS

GEMELLUS SUPERIOR

OBTURATOR INTERNUS

GEMELLUS INFERIOR

QUADRATUS FEMORIS

Hamstrings

Figure 6.46. Lateral rotators of the right hip joint. Gluteus maximum is not shown. (Muscles most involved appear in uppercase letters.) From Logan, *Adapted Physical Education.*

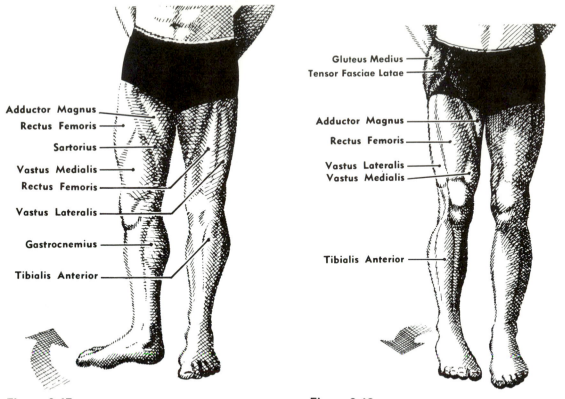

Adductor Magnus
Rectus Femoris
Sartorius
Vastus Medialis
Rectus Femoris
Vastus Lateralis
Gastrocnemius
Tibialis Anterior

Gluteus Medius
Tensor Fasciae Latae
Adductor Magnus
Rectus Femoris
Vastus Lateralis
Vastus Medialis
Tibialis Anterior

Figure 6.47.

Figure 6.48.

Figure 6.47. Hip lateral rotation. (Muscles most involved are not seen in anterior view.)

Figure 6.48. Hip medial rotation.

For ballistic activities involving the lower limbs, it should be noted that the lateral and medial rotations of the femur around its longitudinal axis probably requires very little, if any, generation of internal force to produce the rotations. Considering the bony configuration of the joint and a high limb velocity during diagonal adduction in a kick or punt situation, medial rotation can occur very easily in the follow-through phase without concentric contraction occurring in the medial rotators.

The "toe-in" effect of medial rotation is seen in figure 6.48. If this is a permanent type of condition in an individual, it may not be due to a muscular dysfunction. There could be some torsion or torque in the tibia or femur causing the permanent medial rotation effect. This type of motion through a transverse plane is not desirable despite the myth about the great "pigeon-toed sprinters." Some men and women who are great sprinters may walk with slight hip medial rotations, but when they are twenty meters into a 100-meter dash their hip, knee, and ankle joints are moving through anteroposterior planes.

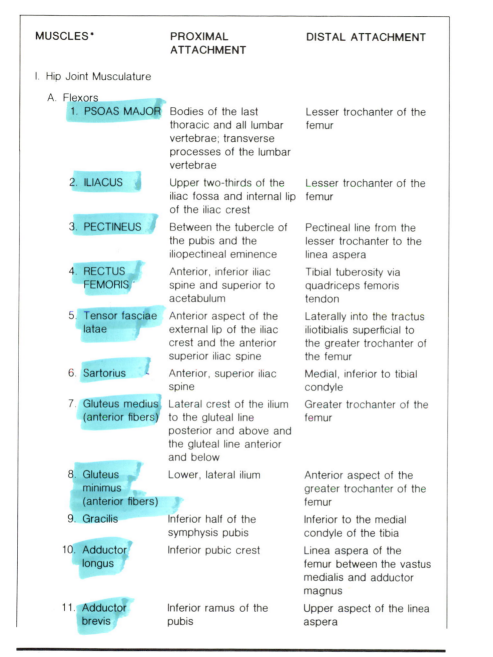

MUSCLES*	PROXIMAL ATTACHMENT	DISTAL ATTACHMENT

I. Hip Joint Musculature

A. Flexors

	MUSCLES*	PROXIMAL ATTACHMENT	DISTAL ATTACHMENT
1.	PSOAS MAJOR	Bodies of the last thoracic and all lumbar vertebrae; transverse processes of the lumbar vertebrae	Lesser trochanter of the femur
2.	ILIACUS	Upper two-thirds of the iliac fossa and internal lip of the iliac crest	Lesser trochanter of the femur
3.	PECTINEUS	Between the tubercle of the pubis and the iliopectineal eminence	Pectineal line from the lesser trochanter to the linea aspera
4.	RECTUS FEMORIS	Anterior, inferior iliac spine and superior to acetabulum	Tibial tuberosity via quadriceps femoris tendon
5.	Tensor fasciae latae	Anterior aspect of the external lip of the iliac crest and the anterior superior iliac spine	Laterally into the tractus iliotibialis superficial to the greater trochanter of the femur
6.	Sartorius	Anterior, superior iliac spine	Medial, inferior to tibial condyle
7.	Gluteus medius (anterior fibers)	Lateral crest of the ilium to the gluteal line posterior and above and the gluteal line anterior and below	Greater trochanter of the femur
8.	Gluteus minimus (anterior fibers)	Lower, lateral ilium	Anterior aspect of the greater trochanter of the femur
9.	Gracilis	Inferior half of the symphysis pubis	Inferior to the medial condyle of the tibia
10.	Adductor longus	Inferior pubic crest	Linea aspera of the femur between the vastus medialis and adductor magnus
11.	Adductor brevis	Inferior ramus of the pubis	Upper aspect of the linea aspera

Figure 6.49. Hip joint musculature. The muscles most involved for the motions against resistance are ahown in uppercase letters. Muscles supplying supplemental force during concentric contraction are in lowercase letters.

Figure 6.49. Continued.

MUSCLES	PROXIMAL ATTACHMENT	DISTAL ATTACHMENT
B. Extensors		
1. GLUTEUS MAXIMUS	Gluteal line posterior of the ilium and a portion of the posterior iliac crest	Upper fibers into the tractus iliotibialis and lower fibers into posterior femur
2. BICEPS FEMORIS (LONG HEAD)	*Long Head:* Ischial tuberosity	Head of the fibula and lateral condyle of the tibia
3. SEMITEN-DINOSUS	Ischial tuberosity	Medial aspect of the medial tibial condyle
4. SEMIMEM-BRANOSUS	Ischial tuberosity	Posterior aspect of the medial tibial condyle
C. Abductors		
1. GLUTEUS MEDIUS	Lateral crest of the ilium to the gluteal line posterior and above and the gluteal line anterior and below	Greater trochanter of the femur
2. Gluteus maximus (upper fibers)	Gluteal line posterior of the ilium and a portion of the posterior iliac crest	Upper fibers into the tractus iliotibialis and lower fibers into posterior femur
3. Gluteus minimus (posterior fibers)	Lower, lateral ilium	Anterior aspect of the greater trochanter of the femur
4. Tensor fasciae latae	Anterior aspect of the external lip of the iliac crest and the anterior superior iliac spine	Laterally into the tractus iliotibialis superficial to the greater trochanter of the femur
D. Adductors		
1. ADDUCTOR BREVIS	Inferior ramus of the pubis	Upper aspect of the linea aspera
2. ADDUCTOR LONGUS	Inferior pubic crest	Linea aspera of the femur between the vastus medialis and adductor magnus
3. ADDUCTOR MAGNUS	Inferior ramus, anterior pubis and inferior ischial tuberosity	Entire linea aspera and the adductor tubercle on the medial condyle of the femur
4. GRACILIS	Inferior half of the symphysis pubis	Inferior to the medial condyle of the tibia
5. Gluteus maximus (lower fibers)	Gluteal line posterior of the ilium and a portion of the posterior iliac crest	Upper fibers into the tractus iliotibialis and lower fibers into posterior femur

Figure 6.49. Continued

MUSCLES	PROXIMAL ATTACHMENT	DISTAL ATTACHMENT
E. Diagonal Abductors		
1. GLUTEUS MEDIUS	Lateral crest of the ilium to the gluteal line posterior and above and the gluteal line anterior and below	Greater trochanter of the femur
2. GLUTEUS MAXIMUS	Gluteal line posterior of the ilium and a portion of the posterior iliac crest	Upper fibers into the tractus iliotibialis and lower fibers into posterior femur
3. SEMITEN-DINOSUS	Ischial tuberosity	Medial aspect of the medial tibial condyle
4. SEMIMEM-BRANOSUS	Ischial tuberosity	Posterior aspect of the medial tibial condyle
5. BICEPS FEMORIS (LONG HEAD)	*Long Head:* Ischial tuberosity	Head of the fibula and lateral condyle of the tibia
6. PIRIFORMIS	Anterior aspect of pelvis	Greater trochanter
7. OBTURATOR INTERNUS	Surrounds obturator foramen	Greater trochanter
8. GEMELLUS SUPERIOR	Outer aspect of the ischial spine	Greater trochanter
9. GEMELLUS INFERIOR	Upper aspect of the ischial tuberosity	Greater trochanter
10. QUADRATUS FEMORIS	External border of the ischial tuberosity	Intertrochanter line of the femur
11. OBTURATOR EXTERNUS	Medial aspect of the obturator foramen, inferior ramus of the pubis and ischial ramus	Trochanter fossa of the femur
F. Diagonal Adductors		
1. ILIOPSOAS	Lumbar vertebrae and iliac fossa	Lesser trochanter of the femur
2. RECTUS FEMORIS	Anterior, inferior iliac spine and superior to acetabulum	Tibial tuberosity via quadriceps femoris tendon
3. PECTINEUS	Between the tubercle of the pubis and the iliopectineal eminence	Pectineal line from the lesser trochanter to the linea aspera
4. ADDUCTOR BREVIS	Inferior ramus of the pubis	Upper aspect of the linea aspera

Figure 6.49. Continued.

MUSCLES	PROXIMAL ATTACHMENT	DISTAL ATTACHMENT
5. ADDUCTOR LONGUS	Inferior pubic crest	Linea aspera of the femur between the vastus medialis and adductor magnus
6. ADDUCTOR MAGNUS	Inferior ramus, anterior pubis and inferior ischial tuberosity	Entire linea aspera and the adductor tubercle on the medial condyle of the femur
G. Lateral Rotators		
1. GLUTEUS MAXIMUS	Gluteal line posterior of the ilium and a portion of the posterior iliac crest	Upper fibers into the tractus iliotibialis and lower fibers into posterior femur
2. SIX LATERAL ROTATORS		
a. PIRI-FORMIS	Anterior aspect of pelvis	Greater trochanter
b. OBTURA-TOR INTERNUS	Surrounds obturator foramen	Greater trochanter
c. GEMELLUS SUPERIOR	Outer aspect of the ischial spine	Greater trochanter
d. GEMEL-LUS IN-FERIOR	Upper aspect of the ischial tuberosity	Greater trochanter
e. QUAD-RATUS FEMORIS	External border of the ischial tuberosity	Intertrochanter line of the femur
f. OBTU-RATOR EXTER-NUS	Medial aspect of the obturator foramen, inferior ramus of the pubis and ischial ramus	Trochanter fossa of the femur
H. Medial Rotators		
1. GLUTEUS MINIMUS (ANTERIOR FIBERS)	Lower, lateral ilium	Anterior aspect of the greater trochanter of the femur
2. Gluteus medius (anterior fibers)	Lateral crest of the ilium to the gluteal line posterior and above and the gluteal line anterior and below	Greater trochanter of the femur
3. Tensor fasciae latae	Anterior aspect of the external lip of the iliac crest and the anterior superior iliac spine	Laterally into the tractus iliotibialis superficial to the greater trochanter of the femur

Allington, Ruth Owne, et al. "Strengthening Techniques of the Quadriceps Muscles: An Electromyographic Evaluation." *Physical Therapy* 46 (November 1966) :1173-76.

Andres, T. L., et al. "Involvement of Selected Quadriceps Muscles During a Knee Extension Exercise." *American Corrective Therapy Journal* 33 (July-August, 1979):111-114.

Basmajian, John V., and Stecko, George. "The Role of Muscles in Arch Support of the Foot." *Journal of Bone and Joint Surgery* 45-A (September 1963) :1184-90.

Bierman, William, and Ralston, H. J. "Electromyographic Study During Passive and Active Flexion and Extension of the Knee of the Normal Human Subject." *Archives of Physical Medicine and Rehabilitation* 46 (January 1965) :71-75.

Bosco, C., et al. "Mechanical Characteristics and Fiber Composition of Human Leg Extensor Muscles." *European Journal of Applied Physiology* 41 (August, 1979) :275-284.

Brewerton, D. A. "The Function of the Vastus Medialis Muscle." *Annals of Physical Medicine* 2 (1955) :164-68.

Cavagna, G. A., and Margaria, R. "Mechanics of Walking." *Journal of Applied Physiology* 21 (January 1966) :271-78.

Damholt, V., et al. "Asymmetry of Plantar Flexion Strength in the Foot." *ACTA Orthopaedica Scandinavica* 49 (April, 1978) :215-219.

Dempster, W. T. "The Range of Motion of Cadaver Joints: The Lower Limb." *University of Michigan Medical Bulletin* 22 (1956) :364-79.

Deutsch, H., et al. "Quadriceps Kinesiology (EMG) with Varying Hip Joint Flexion and Resistance." *Archives of Physical Medicine and Rehabilitation* 59 (May, 1978) :231-236.

Elftman, H. "Forces and Energy Changes in the Leg During Walking." *American Journal of Physiology* 125 (1959) :339-56.

Fugal-Meyer, A. R., et al. "Human Plantar Flexion Strength and Structure." *ACTA Physiologica Scandinavica* 107 (September, 1979) :47-56.

Gollnick, Philip D. "Electrogoniometric Study of Walking on High Heels." *Research Quarterly* 35 (October 1964) :370-78.

Grieve, D. W., and Gear, Ruth J. "The Relationships Between Length and Stride, Step Frequence, Time of Swing and Speed for Walking for Children and Adults." *Ergonomics* 9 (September 1966) :379-99.

Hall, W. L., and Klein, K. K. "The Man, the Knee and the Ligaments." *Medicina Dello Sport* 1 (October 1961) :500-11.

Hallen, L. G., and Lindahl, O. "The Lateral Stability of the Knee Joint." *Acta Orthopaedica Scandinavica* 36 (1965) :179-91.

————. "The 'Screw-Home' Movement in the Knee Joint." *Acta Orthopaedica Scandinavica* 37 (Fasc. 1, 1966) :97-106.

Hooper, A. C. "The Role of the Iliopsoas Muscle in Femoral Rotation." *Irish Medical Journal* 146 (April, 1977) :108-112.

Houtz, S. J., and Walsh, Frank P. "Electromyographic Analysis of the Function of the Muscles Acting on the Ankle During Weight Bearing with Special Reference to the Triceps Surae." *Journal of Bone and Joint Surgery* 41-A (1959) :1469–81.

Inman, Verne T. "Functional Aspects of the Abductor Muscles of the Hip." *Journal of Bone and Joint Surgery* 29 (1947) :607–19.

Jonsson, Bengt, and Steen, Bertil. "Function of the Gracilis Muscle." *Acta Morphologica Neerlando-Scandinavica* 6 (1966) :325–41.

Kaplan, Emanuel B. "The Iliotibial Tract." *Journal of Bone and Joint Surgery* 40-A (1958) :817–32.

Karpovich, Peter V., and Manfredi, Thomas G. "Mechanisms of Rising on the Toes." *Research Quarterly* 42 (1971) :395–404.

Karpovich, Peter V., and Wilklow, Leighton B. "Goniometric Study of the Human Foot in Standing and Walking." *Industrial Medicine and Surgery* 29 (July 1960) :338–47.

Klein, Karl K. "The Deep Squat Exercise as Utilized in Weight Training for Athletics and Its Effect on the Ligaments of the Knee." *Journal of the Association for Physical and Mental Rehabilitation* 15 (January–February 1961) :6–11.

————. "The Knee and the Ligaments." *Journal of Bone and Joint Surgery* 44-A (September 1962) :1191–93.

Knight, K. L., et al. "EMG Comparison of Quadriceps Femoris Activity During Knee Extension and Straight Leg Raises." *American Journal of Physical Medicine* 58 (April, 1979) :57–67.

Kroll, Walt, et al. "Muscle Fiber Type Composition and Knee Extension Isometric Strength Fatigue Patterns in Power and Endurance Trained Males." *Research Quarterly for Exercise and Sport* 51 (May, 1980) :323–333.

Lawrence, Mary S; Meyer, Harriet R.; and Matthews, Nancy L. "Comparative Increase in Muscle Strength in the Quadriceps Femoris by Isometric and Isotonic Exercises and Effects on the Contralateral Muscle." *Journal of the American Physical Therapy Association* 42 (January 1962) :15–20.

Mann, R. A., et al. "The Function of the Toes in Walking, Jogging, and Running." *Clinical Orthopaedics and Related Research* 142 (July–August, 1979) :24–29.

Mathews, Donald; Shaw, Virginia; and Bohnen, Melra. "Hip Flexibility of College Women as Related to Length of Body Segments." *Child Development Abstracts and Bibliography* 32 (June–August 1958) :85.

Mathews, Donald K.; Shaw, Virginia; and Woods, John B. "Hip Flexibility of Elementary School Boys as Related to Body Segments." *Research Quarterly* 30 (October 1959) :297–302.

Meyers, Earle J. "Effect of Selected Exercise Variables on Ligament Stability and Flexibility of the Knee." *Research Quarterly* 42 (1971) :411–22.

Morton, Dudley J. *The Human Foot.* New York: Columbia University Press, 1935.

Murray, M. P., et al. "Function of the Triceps Surae During Gait: Compensatory Mechanisms for Unilateral Loss." *Journal of Bone and Joint Surgery* 60 (June, 1978) :473-476.

O'Connell, A. L. "Electromyographic Study of Certain Leg Muscles During Movements of the Free Foot and During Standing." *American Journal of Physical Medicine* 37 (December 1958) :289-301.

Rarick, L., and Thompson, J. "Roentgenographic Measures of Leg Muscle Size and Ankle Extensor Strength" *Research Quarterly* 27 (October 1956) :321.

Ricci, Benjamin, and Karpovich, Peter V. "Effect of Height of Heel Upon the Foot." *Research Quarterly* 35 (October 1964) :385-88.

Sheffield, F. J., et al. "Electromyographic Study of the Muscles of the Foot in Normal Walking." *American Journal of Physical Medicine* 35 (1956) :223-36.

Stern, Jack T. "Anatomical and Functional Specializations of the Human Gluteus Maximus." *American Journal of Physical Anthropology* 36 (1972) :315-39.

Sutherland, David H. "An Electromyographic Study of the Plantar Flexors of the Ankle in Normal Walking on the Level." *Journal of Bone and Joint Surgery* 48-A (January 1966) :66-71.

Wheatley, M. D., and Johnke, W. D. "Electromyographic Study of the Superficial Thigh and Hip Muscles in Normal Individuals." *Archives of Physical Medicine* 32 (1951) :508-15.

Woodman, R. M., et al. "Testing Hip Extensor Strength when Passive Hip Extension is Restricted." *Physical Therapy* 58 (July, 1978) :882.

7

Pelvic Girdle and Spinal Column Motions

The spinal column consists of seven vertebrae in the cervical (neck) area, twelve in the thoracic region, and five in the lumbar portion of the spine. Movement within and between these twenty-four vertebrae is extensive; however, movement between any two vertebrae is relatively small. The majority of motion occurs at the cervical and lumbar areas of the spine. The thoracic area, including the rib cage, is a relatively stable or fixed portion of the spinal column. In addition to the twenty-four vertebrae in the cercival, thoracic, and lumbar areas, five fixed vertebrae compose the sacrum, the four partially movable vertebrae comprise the coccyx. Thus, the spinal column consists of thirty-three vertebrae (fig. 7.1).

The twelve thoracic vertebrae and the rib cage to which they are attached can be considered as one functional unit. This unit has a limited degree of movement potential, with the exception of rib movement required in breathing. From a kinesiologic standpoint, this unit can be thought of as a constant volumetric structure, because the rib cage, unlike the lungs, does not change its size appreciably during movement.

Functioning with the thoracic spine-rib cage unit to make up what is commonly known as the "trunk" is the pelvic girdle. The pelvic girdle, like the thoracic rib cage area, can also be thought of as a functional unit. These two units of the trunk are joined together by the five lumbar vertebrae. The lumbar vertebrae can be considered a pivotal support structure linking the two units together.

The seven cervical vertebrae function as another pivotal support structure. These vertebrae serve as a connective link between the rib cage and the head. This area, the neck, is moved by muscles connecting the rib cage to the head. The head, like the rib cage, can be thought of as a nonchanging volumetric structure. Thus, it can be seen that in the so-called trunk area there are three nonchanging volumetric units connected by two pivotal support structures. As a result, virtually all movements of the spinal column take place within two supportive areas known as the lumbar and cervical portions of the spine.

For noncinematographic analysis purposes, it is a good idea to focus attention primarily on six separate segments of the body. This analytic procedure is known as *segmental analysis.* The six major segments which need to be analyzed independently are: (1) pelvic girdle, (2) lumbar-thoracic spine, (3) head and cervical spine, (4) shoulder girdle, (5) upper limbs, and (6) lower limbs. The

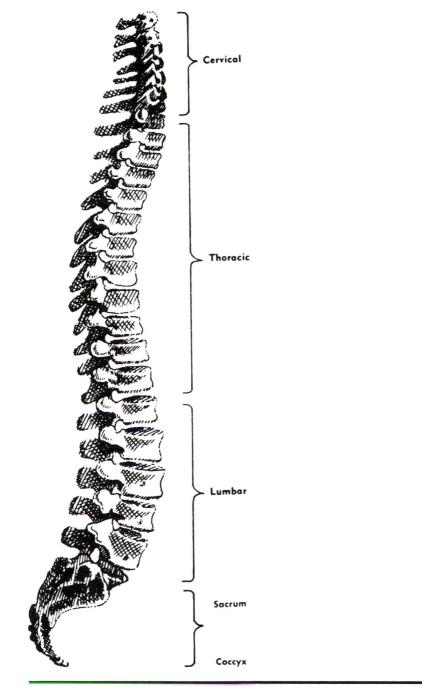

Figure 7.1. Spinal column—lateral view.

pelvic and lumbar-thoracic segments are good points to start a segmental analysis, because the velocities generated in these segments are relatively slow even during a ballistic skill involving the limbs. The motions in these segments often indicate directional tendencies of the total body.

Numerous motions are seen within the various units of the spinal column, and occur between the facets of the vertebrae which lie posterior to the longitudinal axis of the spinal column. Motions possible within the lumbar and cervical spinal column segments are flexion, extension, rotation around the longitudinal axis, and lateral flexion.

Reduction is the return from lateral flexion to the anatomic position. The cervical and lumbar spines can also be circumducted and hyperextended.

In general, the entire spinal column has relatively good ligamentous support given to it by short, strong ligaments connecting individual vertebrae. The most important of these are the anterior longitudinal ligament, posterior longitudinal ligament, and the ligamentum nuchae. The anterior longitudinal ligament is continuous from the occipital bone to the sacrum. It is relatively thin in the cervical region and thick in the thoracic area. The posterior longitudinal ligament is continuous from the occipital bone to the coccygeal region. The ligamentum nuchae is located in the posterior cervical region. It is a continuation of the supraspinous ligament from the seventh cervical vertebra to the occipital region. It is a strong, but thin, fibrous membrane in this area. The supraspinous ligament is actually a continuation of the ligamentum nuchae from the seventh cervical vertebra to the sacrum. The supraspinous ligament and its continuation in the cervical region, the ligamentum nuchae, help to maintain the spinal column in an erect position. In this regard, they function as antigravity ligaments adding to the extension capacity of the antigravity musculature.

The bony support between the articulations of the spinal column is relatively unstable. The main bony support is posterior. The spinous processes, for example, serve as limiting structures for extension and hyperextension of the spine. There also is some bony support in the area of the rib cage. This is provided by the articulation of the ribs with the articular facets of the vertebrae in the thoracic area.

Muscle stability within the spinal area is of vital importance. The muscles connecting the pelvic girdle to the rib cage as well as the muscular connection of the rib cage to the head serve as dynamic stabilizers when required for movements of the upper and lower limbs. Because man has assumed the bipedal, or upright position, the muscles in the lumbar region are required to do less work than they would in a flexed, or quadrupedal, position. Consequently, the strength of these muscles is usually much less than their potential strength level. In addition, the muscles connecting the pelvic girdle to the rib cage are often overlooked in the conditioning process for sport skills involving the use of the limbs. In terms of maximum performance in sports, these two factors must be considered, especially during the conditioning process and when writing exercise prescriptions.

It was noted in Chapter 2 that different muscle attachment terminology can be used for muscles located entirely on the pelvis, lumbar-thoracic spine, and cervical spine areas. The two sets of terms are: (1) superior and inferior attachments and (2) medial and lateral attachments. Superior and inferior attachment terminology can be used for muscles with vertical lines of pull on the trunk. Medial and lateral attachment terminology can be used for those muscles with oblique or horizontal lines of pull.

Some readers may find it easier to conceptualize lines of pull by using the above terms. All muscles in this chapter, *with the exceptions of the internal oblique, external oblique, and transversus abdominis,* can be considered to have superior/inferior lines of pull. The three abdominal muscles cited have lateral/medial lines of pull.

The motions of the pelvis are functionally related to hip and spinal column movements. However, pelvic motions are observable as distinct, albeit slight, motions through the three traditional planes. To enhance communication related to pelvic motions, new terminology was introduced in chapter 4.

Pelvic girdle motions

Aggregate muscle action for pelvic motions change, depending upon what the performer is using as a base of support. The discussion at this point concerns aggregate muscle actions for pelvic motions while the individual is: (1) standing with the weight distributed unilaterally or bilaterally, or (2) using the hands as a base of support while hanging from a piece of apparatus.

Pelvic motions are an integral part of many sport skills when there is a summation of force or velocity from lower to upper limbs. Internal force generated through sequential contractions of the muscles most involved for ankle, knee, and hip joint motions is summated and transferred to the moving pelvic and spinal column of a performer involved in throwing and striking skills as examples.

The perfectly timed and appropriate pelvic rotation must occur to add to and transfer force to the next contracting body segment in the kinetic chain. For throwing, in particular, the pelvic rotations are important to the ultimate outcome. These pelvic rotations are interrelated with spinal column rotations and have a direct bearing on how much force will be transferred to the throwing limb.

The pelvic girdle and lumbar spine segment of the body is a good observation area from which to gain insights regarding such factors as weight shifts, total body movement direction, line of thrust of the center of mass, transfer of forces, and other pertinent factors of motion. The pelvis is a relatively slow-moving area and easily observed during a sport skill. This is particularly true during a ballistic skill in which limbs and other body segments move rapidly. A performer highly skilled in using feint or faked movements to gain an advantage over opponents cannot manipulate the pelvic girdle advantageously. Rotary motions in the thoracic and cervical spine can be used to indicate total body movement in one direction while the performer actually moves in a different direction. As an example, coaches of offensive ends and flanker backs in American football teach a wide variety of these kinds of motions to be used to gain body position advantage while running pass patterns. Conversely, defensive football backfield coaches teach the defensive backs to "key" or watch the pelvic girdle-lumbar area of their opponents. If they watch the pass catcher's head (cervical spine) motions, there is a good chance he will show motion in one direction and go another. However, the same thing cannot be accomplished with pelvic girdle rotations. The center of mass moves with the pelvic girdle; consequently, if a defensive performer watches the pelvis of an opponent, that individual's total body direction will always be a known factor—information that can be used to advantage.

There are six pelvic girdle motions: (1) left transverse rotation, (2) right transverse rotation, (3) anterior rotation, (4) posterior rotation, (5) left lateral rotation, and (6) right lateral rotation. Movements through the anteroposterior and lateral planes of motion are also referred to as "tilts" or "inclinations." Observation of the iliac crests helps to determine the direction of movement of the pelvic girdle (figs. 7.2–7.6).

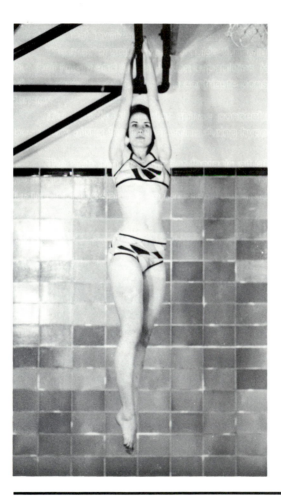

Figure 7.2. Left transverse pelvic rotation (Ruth Miller).

Transverse pelvic rotation

These rotations are a functional part of all locomotor activity: for example—there are slight transverse pelvic rotations on each stride during walking, jogging, and running. These transverse rotations are also important to ballistic skill performance utilizing the upper and lower limbs.

The muscles most involved in left transverse rotation against resistance in a *hanging position* using the hands as the base of support are the left external oblique and right internal oblique muscles (fig. 7.2). The transverse rotation in this hanging position, which would be used frequently by gymnasts, is the result of concentric contraction of *the external oblique muscle on the same side as the rotation working with the internal oblique on the opposite side.* The MMI for right transverse rotation can be determined by using this guideline. External and internal oblique muscles are shown in figure 7.12.

The most common use of transverse pelvic girdle rotation is in unilateral weight-bearing and weight-shifting situations. Functionally, especially in ballistic skills, the transverse pelvic girdle rotation is in one direction concurrent with lumbar-thoracic rotation in the opposite direction.

This can be seen in figure 7.3. The left handed pitcher completed right transverse pelvic rotation during the unilateral weight shift immediately prior to the right leg receiving weight force. The lumbar-thoracic spine is rotated in the opposite direction. These critical pelvis-spine motion relationships completed during the preparation phase of a ballistic skill are very important and will be discussed in more detail in Chapter 10.

The muscles most involved for right transverse pelvic rotation in unilateral weight-shifting situations are the right external oblique, left internal oblique, and left erector spinae muscles. There would also be some internal force supplied by the deep spinal muscles on the right side. The contralateral muscles for this motion are the same muscles on the opposite side of the body. This musculature rotated the pitcher's pelvis as shown in figure 7.3 a fraction of a second before the photograph was taken, i.e., the muscles most involved contracted concentrically to rotate the pelvic girdle right (clockwise) through the transverse plane while the weight was on the left leg. The right transverse pelvic rotation continued until the weight shift to the right leg was completed. The pelvic girdle is dynamically stabilized continually in this type of situation. (The musculature is diagrammed in figures 7.9, 7.10, and 7.12).

When a performer is bearing the body weight equally and bilaterally on both feet, left transverse pelvic rotation occurs with right lumbar-thoracic rotation. The muscles most involved for left transverse pelvic rotation are the left gluteus maximus and right tensor fasciae latae, right gluteus minimus, and the anterior fibers of the right gluteus medius. Some hip-joint rotation might also be noted. Rotation of the pelvis in this context is relatively rare in sport; however, there are some golf shots, as examples, which may employ transverse rotations of the pelvic girdle in a bilateral weight-bearing stance with the knees flexed. *Muscles which attach to the pelvis or sacrum serve to initiate or control pelvic motions.*

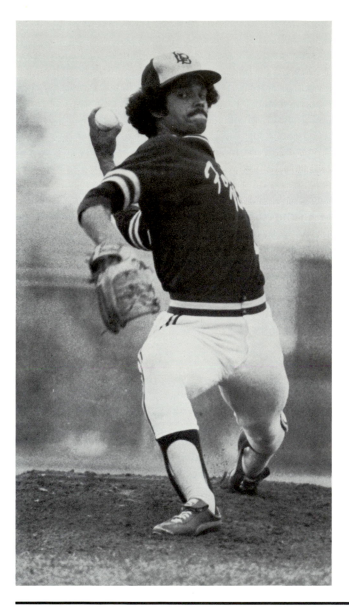

Figure 7.3. Rich Rivera, California State University-Long Beach pitcher, has just completed right
transverse pelvis rotation during the unilateral
weight shift of his preparation phase. The concurrent opposite rotation in the lumbar-thoracic spine
prior to the motion phase adds to his effectiveness.
Photo by Bruce Hazelton. Reprinted with permission
of the Sports Information Bureau, California State
University-Long Beach.

Anterior pelvic rotation

This rotation is observed when the iliac crests move *forward* through the cardinal anteroposterior plane of motion. Such motion is observed, to cite one example, concurrent with complete extension of both hip joints through their anteroposterior ranges of motion. These concurrent hip and pelvic motions give the illusion of hyperextension in the hip joints. A gymnast makes this type of maneuver swinging on the horizontal bar to develop angular velocity. A stripteaser uses a sequential combination of anterior and posterior pelvic rotations in her dance to communicate exotic ideas to the audience. Wrestlers use the same pelvic motions to try to alleviate near-pin situations as they move into the bridge position.

When the performer is using the hands as a base of support in the *hanging position,* the MMI are the erector spinae muscles which attach to the pelvis from the lumbar spine (fig. 7.13). Both halves of the erector spinae must contract with equal intensity for the rotation to be anterior. Unequal force would cause rotations through other planes. Both halves of the rectus abdominis serve as the contralateral muscles (fig. 7.10).

Figure 7.4 shows anterior pelvic girdle rotation in a bilateral weight-bearing position. The extent of the rotation can be observed by comparing the angle of the iliac crest with lines on the background wall. When the individual is in a weight-bearing position, some caution must be given to ascribing muscle action to pelvic movements, because the effect of gravity *and* resistance must be considered. For example, while doing a hip extension exercise by pulling on a heavy wall-pulley device or an Exer-Genie Exerciser from above, the muscles most involved in anterior pelvic rotation, which accompanies hip extension in this case, are the hip flexors. These are the rectus femoris, iliopsoas, and pectineus muscles. The contralateral muscles in anterior pelvic rotation against resistance are the gluteus maximus, semitendinosus, semimembranosus, and biceps femoris. While in the standing position, with the trunk being flexed slowly by the pull of gravity, there is concurrent hip flexion and anterior pelvic rotation. The muscles most involved in this anterior pelvic rotation are the gluteus maximus, semitendinosus, semimembranosus, and long head of the biceps femoris. These muscles are allowing rotation to occur in the pelvic girdle by contracting eccentrically. The muscles contralateral to anterior pelvic rotation in the weight-bearing position are the pectineus, rectus femoris, and iliopsoas.

Posterior pelvic rotation

When the iliac crests move *backward* through the cardinal, anteroposterior plane, posterior pelvic rotation has taken place. This can be seen by comparing figure 7.5 with figure 7.4.

In a situation where the hands are the base of support with the feet off the ground, the muscles most involved for posterior pelvic rotation are the equally contracting rectus abdominis muscles. They literally contract and exert a rotary force component on the superior aspect of the symphysis pubis (fig. 7.10).

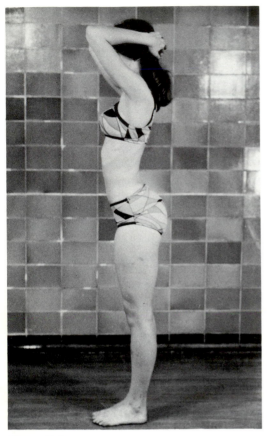

Figure 7.4.

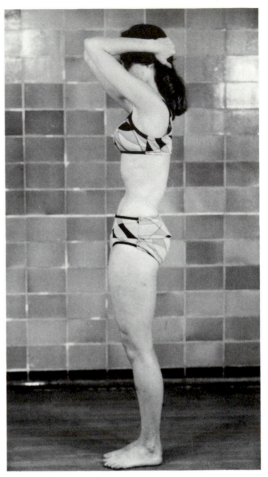

Figure 7.5.

Figure 7.4. Anterior pelvic girdle rotation.

Figure 7.5. Posterior pelvic girdle rotation.

The generation of internal force for posterior pelvic girdle rotation while standing on both feet or lying on the back involve a cooperative action between posterior and anterior musculature. Posteriorly, the muscles most involved are the concentrically and bilaterally contracting gluteus maximus, semitendinosus, semimembranosus, and biceps femoris—long head. Anteriorly, both rectus abdominus muscles contract concentrically. This anterior/posterior force tandum is very effective for posterior pelvic rotation in the supine position.

Lateral pelvic rotation

What appears to be the lifting of the iliac crest on one side is defined as a lateral rotation. Right lateral rotation is shown in figure 7.6.

Like the transverse pelvic girdle rotations, lateral rotations occur both left and right. When the performer is hanging by the hands, the muscles most involved in right lateral pelvic girdle rotation are the erector spinae on the right side and the three abdominal muscles on the right side excluding the transverse abdominis. The contralateral muscles in the right lateral pelvic girdle rotation are the left erector spinae and the left half of the three major abdominal muscles, excluding the transverse abdominis. The quadratus lumborum muscle on the same side as the movement may assist in this rotation.

During locomotor activities, lateral pelvic rotations occur in unilateral weight-bearing situations. There is unilateral weight-bearing on each stride, as an example, during walking, jogging, and running. The pelvis laterally rotates to allow the nonweight-bearing leg to move forward through an anteroposterior plane of motion.

If the pelvic girdle were not rotated laterally on each walking or running stride, the anteroposterior, pendular action of the leg would not be possible. The "lifting effect" of the lateral rotation on the pelvis allows the nonweight-bearing limb to be moved through its range of motion by the hip flexors and extensors.

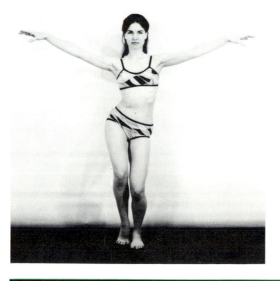

Figure 7.6. Right lateral pelvic girdle rotation (Ruth Miller).

Without this synchronized interaction of motions between the pelvic girdle and hip joints, normal walking, jogging, and running would be described as "shuffling." Obviously, that motion pattern would have many negative ramifications in terms of sport performance.

If the weight is being borne on the left leg, right lateral pelvic rotation is the result of concentric contraction of the left gluteus medius. The right gluteus medius is the muscle most involved for left lateral pelvic rotation when the weight is on the right lower limb. The adductor muscles are the contralateral muscles for lateral pelvic rotations in the unilateral weight-bearing position.

The pole vaulter in figure 7.7 is in a unilateral weight-bearing situation, with the body weight being borne on his left lower limb. There has been right lateral pelvic girdle rotation, and this has allowed the right lower limb to be moved through an anteroposterior plane of motion at the right hip joint. His hip joint is moving into flexion at the point of pole implant and prior to lift off. The pelvic girdle-hip motion combinations at this point are of significant importance to the outcome of pole vaulting performance.

Side-to-side shifting movement of the pelvis is not to be confused with lateral pelvic girdle rotation. The side-to-side shifting movement of the pelvis in the lateral plane is simply a matter of adduction and abduction of the hip joint. The crest of the ilium remains relatively level when abduction and adduction are occurring within this context and weight is distributed over both feet. Variations of this type of motion are seen in various dances. The hula dance is an example. The knees are usually flexed to add to the effect of the hip and pelvic girdle motions. These motions plus lateral and transverse pelvic motions are utilized by the skilled dancer to provide the aesthetic aspects of the dance.

Figure 7.8 provides a summary of the pelvic girdle musculature and the motions for which they are responsible.

Lumbar-thoracic spine motions

An understanding of the spatial relationships of the muscles which move the spinal column is basic to comprehending their functions. Also, to facilitate learning, some of the spinal column muscles with common functions have been placed into groups. For the most part, these muscles are discussed in terms of their function as a group, instead of individually. These muscle groups and the muscles which constitute the group are as follows:

ERECTOR SPINAE (Lumbar)
    Iliocostalis thoracis
    Iliocostalis lumborum
    Longissimus thoracis
    Spinalis thoracis
DEEP POSTERIOR SPINAL GROUP
    Intertransversarii
    Interspinales
    Rotatores
    Multifidus

ERECTOR SPINAE (Cervical)
    Iliocostalis cervicis
    Longissimus cervicis
    Longissimus capitis
    Spinalis cervicis
ABDOMINALS
    Rectus abdominis
    External oblique
    Internal oblique

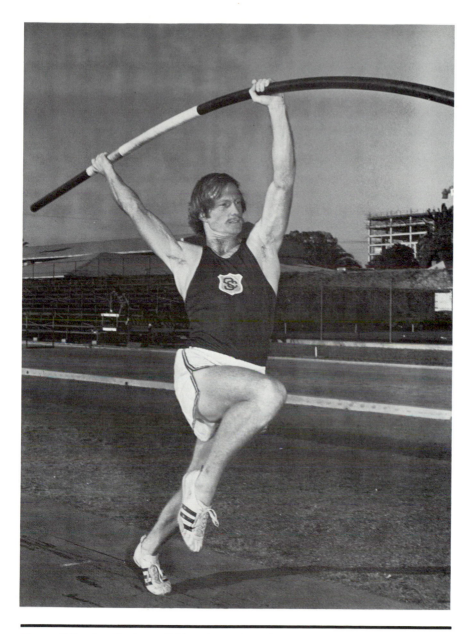

Figure 7.7. Jim Cochran, USC pole vaulter, demonstrates the importance of right lateral pelvic rotation to the anteroposterior, pendular motions of the right hip joint at lift-off in the pole vault. Courtesy *USC Athletic News Service.*

I. Pelvic Girdle Musculature

A. Transverse pelvic rotation—LEFT
   1. Hanging position
      a. LEFT EXTERNAL OBLIQUE
      b. RIGHT INTERNAL OBLIQUE
   2. Unilateral weight bearing
      a. LEFT EXTERNAL OBLIQUE
      b. RIGHT INTERNAL OBLIQUE
      c. RIGHT ERECTOR SPINAE
   3. Bilateral weight bearing
      a. LEFT GLUTEUS MAXIMUS
      b. RIGHT TENSOR FASCIAE LATAE
      c. RIGHT GLUTEUS MINIMUS
      d. RIGHT GLUTEUS MEDIUS (ANTERIOR FIBERS)

B. Anterior pelvic rotation
   1. Hanging position
      a. ERECTOR SPINAE
   2. Bilateral weight bearing
      a. RECTUS FEMORIS
      b. ILIOPSOAS
      c. PECTINEUS

C. Posterior pelvic rotation
   1. Hanging position
      a. RECTUS ABDOMINIS
   2. Bilateral weight bearing
      a. GLUTEUS MAXIMUS
      b. SEMITENDINOSUS
      c. SEMIMEMBRANOSUS
      d. BICEPS FEMORIS (LONG HEAD)
      e. RECTUS ABDOMINIS
   3. Prone position
      a. Same MMI as bilateral

D. Lateral pelvic rotation—RIGHT
   1. Hanging position
      a. RIGHT ERECTOR SPINAE
      b. RIGHT RECTUS ABDOMINIS
      c. RIGHT EXTERNAL OBLIQUE
      d. RIGHT INTERNAL OBLIQUE
      e. Right quadratus lumborum
   2. Unilateral weight bearing
      a. LEFT GLUTEUS MEDIUS

Figure 7.8. Pelvic girdle musculature. The muscles most involved for the motions against resistance are shown in uppercase letters. Muscles supplying supplemental force during concentric contraction are in lowercase letters.

Figure 7.9 shows a transverse section of the spinal column through a lumbar vertebra. The spatial relationships of the abdominals and erector spinae to the spinal column are clearly seen in cross section. Also, the positions of the muscles relative to each other should be noted.

The abdominal muscles are positioned around the lumbar-thoracic spine to perform strong rotary motions and flexions through two planes of motion. A diagrammatic outline of the rectus abdominis muscles is shown in figure 7.10.

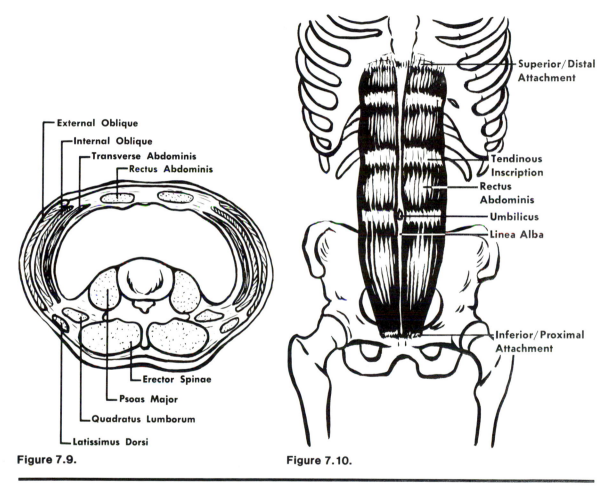

Figure 7.9.

Figure 7.10.

Figure 7.9. Transverse section of the lumbar spine showing spatial relationships of trunk musculature to the spinal column. From Logan, *Adapted Physical Education*.

Figure 7.10. Rectus abdominis muscles—anterior view. From Logan, *Adapted Physical Education*.

As can be seen, these muscles have an anterior spatial relationship to the lumbar-thoracic spine. These are relatively long muscles with a vertical line of pull in the cardinal anteroposterior plane. This position makes them potentially very strong. The length might be detrimental to their strength potential, but the tendinous inscriptions tend to compartmentalize the muscles. This configuration gives the well-trained rectus abdominis muscles considerable strength. A male athlete with a good level of lean body mass (low percentage of body fat) should have rectus abdominis muscles which look much like those in figure 7.10. A photographic example of a teenage boy is shown in figure 7.11. An adult female whose rectus abdominis muscles are very strong may not be able to see tendinous inscriptions. The mature woman has more subcutaneous adipose tissue in this area than the mature male. This is a normal secondary sex characteristic. A man has an unscientific device to tell him when the percentage of body fat is too great. It is called a mirror! If the line that separates the two rectus abdominis muscles (linea alba) and the tendinous inscriptions cannot be seen, the male is most likely too fat for his own well-being, especially as an athlete.

The remaining abdominal muscles are shown in figure 7.12. These are the external oblique, internal oblique, and transverse abdominis. These muscles are in layers as noted in figure 7.9. The internal oblique is the deepest of the abdominal muscles which move the lumbar-thoracic spine. It should be noted that the deeper transverse abdominis does not function to move the lumbar spine. This muscle acts to compress the visceral contents. It helps in the normal elimination functions of the body, and it is a very important muscle during normal childbirth.

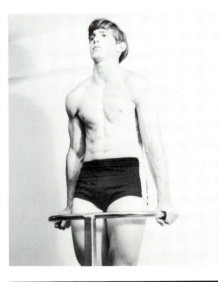

Figure 7.11. Developing abdominal musculature in a 15-year-old athlete with good, lean body mass. (Mike McKinney)

The external oblique fibers lie in a diagonal pattern from lateral to medial. The two pairs of muscles composed of the external oblique of one side and the internal oblique on the same side form the shape of an *X*. This design provides the muscles with the ability to work in conjunction with each other for spinal flexion and functionally with each other for spinal rotation and lateral flexion. This functional relationship means that one set of muscles is shortening while the other set of muscles is lengthening. At any one point in the motion,

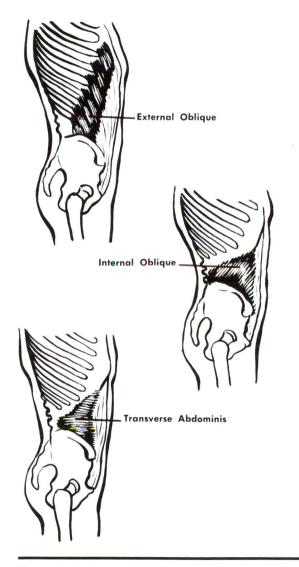

Figure 7.12. Lateral views of the three abdominal muscles with lateral/medial lines of pull. From Logan, *Adapted Physical Education.*

the interaction between shortening and lengthening muscles provides a moving stabilization of the lumbar-thoracic spine. This area of the spinal column is constantly receiving forces from the upper and lower limbs. The lumbar-thoracic spine must be stable enough to provide a counterforce for the other body segments to complete their movements, and it must move to provide compensatory and force-producing motions at the same time. This is *dynamic stabilization* or *The Lomac Paradox,* i.e., the paradox of motion with stability.

Figure 7.13 shows the erector spinae muscle group in a diagrammatic fashion. This muscle group actually has three subdivisions, and the individual muscles which constitute this group are in bilateral pairs throughout each of these subdivisions, from the posterior ilium and sacrum to the mastoid processes. The erector spinae group is considered as a unit for its major functions, extension and hyperextension. These two motions through the anteroposterior plane require equal and bilateral contraction. Other motion capabilities of the erector spinae require unilateral contractions. These functions of the erector spine will be discussed in conjunction with the individual spinal column motions.

Figure 7.13 includes examples of three of the muscles in each of the three erector spinae subdivisions: (1) iliocostalis lumborum, (2) longissimus thoracis, and (3) spinalis cervicis. As stated, these muscles are in bilateral pairs over the posterior length of the spinal column. All of the iliocostalis muscles from inferior to superior are lateral. The longissimus muscle pairs are between the iliocostalis and spinalis muscle pairs. The spinalis muscles within the erector spinae group lie virtually within the cardinal anteroposterior plane of motion.

Flexion

Due to the structure of the lumbar-thoracic spine, the muscles which flex it against resistance must have an anterior spatial relationship to the vertebrae. Therefore, the muscles most involved for lumbar-thoracic flexion against resistance are the rectus abdominis, external oblique, and internal oblique muscles contracting equally and bilaterally. The line of pull of the rectus abdominis muscles lies directly in the cardinal, anteroposterior plane of motion. This gives these muscles good leverage for flexion.

The hook-lying sit-up as shown in figure 7.14 actually involves the abdominals and psoas muscles. This is the case any time the feet are held in place during the lumbar-thoracic flexion by a device or person. The feet must be held while performing sit-ups on a slant board. If they were not, the individual would roll backwards. When the individual is in a supine position with hips and knees flexed and feet flat on the floor unheld, movement of the rib cage toward the pelvis is strictly an abdominal exercise. The psoas and other anterior hip muscles tend to be slackened by the hip and knee flexions; consequently, they do not contribute force for the lumbar-thoracic flexion. The hook-lying sit-up with the feet unheld is, therefore, an abdominal exercise for individuals who have no history of back problems. It *is not* an abdominal exercise automatically good for everyone to perform.

The safest lumbar-thoracic spine flexion exercise is the "curl-up exercise." It is both efficient and safe for developing abdominal strength and/or muscular

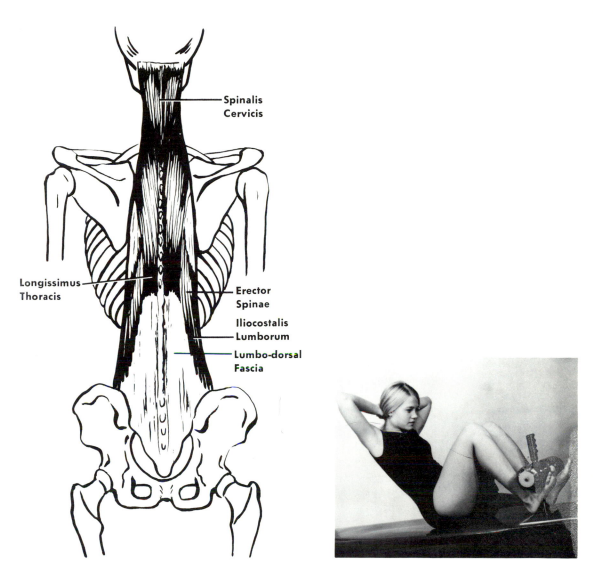

Spinalis
Cervicis

Longissimus
Thoracis

Erector
Spinae

Iliocostalis
Lumborum

Lumbo-dorsal
Fascia

Figure 7.13.

Figure 7.14.

Figure 7.13. Erector spinae muscle group—posterior view. From Logan, *Adapted Physical Education.*

Figure 7.14. Lumbar-thoracic flexion against resistance provided by gravity, body weight, and slant board angle. The abdominals are the MMI, and the psoas assists due to the feet being held (Jan Stevenson). From Logan, *Adapted Physical Education.*

endurance. This exercise is done from the prone position. The hips are flexed slightly to take the hip flexors off stretch. This puts the force factor for the motion on the concentrically contracting abdominals. The cervical spine is flexed and stabilized. The hands are placed on the anterior thighs, and the feet *are not* held. The performer flexes the lumbar-thoracic spine through approximately 45 degrees and returns slowly to the mat. This exercise works the abdominals concentrically during flexion and eccentrically during extension.

The guiding muscles for lumbar-thoracic flexion are both pairs of the internal and external obliques. These muscles have lateral spatial relationships to the vertebrae and have an anterior position as well; consequently, they are capable of rotating the lumbar-thoracic spine (fig. 7.9). When the flexion is through the anteroposterior plane of motion exclusively, the left and right pairs of oblique muscles provide a force-counterforce situation which rules out their rotary capabilities. This type of guiding action is highly desirable during lumbar-thoracic flexion, as seen in the sit-up exercise. Due to potential trauma infliction to the intervertebral discs and other tissue surrounding the vertebrae, it is unwise to include a transverse plane rotation during an anteroposterior sit-up.

The contralateral muscles for lumbar-thoracic flexion against gravity are located posterior to the vertebrae. These are the muscles in the erector spinae muscle group. When the lumbar-thoracic flexion is with gravity as seen in figure 7.15, the erector spinae become the muscles most involved by contracting eccentrically to control the extent and speed of flexion. In this reversal of function, the abdominals become the contralateral muscles.

Lumbar-thoracic flexion can also occur by changing the moving body segments. Figure 7.14 shows lumbar-thoracic flexion with the rib cage moving toward the stabilized pelvic girdle and lower limbs. With a performer in a supine position, the legs can be moved to a position over the head. Flexion has taken place in the lumbar-thoracic spine. The pelvic girdle and lower limbs are the moving body segments (fig. 7.16). Stabilization occurs in the upper thoracic region, cervical spine, shoulders, and upper limbs. *The direction in which a body part moves when contraction occurs depends upon which attachments of the muscles are stabilized at the time.*

Palpation should be used to gain more insight into the function of the superficial lumbar-thoracic flexors. The rectus abdominis and external oblique muscles can be palpated during a sit-up exercise. The effect of their concentric contractions can be felt during the first several degrees of the movement. Once the movement goes beyond forty-five degrees, the resistance is not as great. As the performer extends the spine slowly to return to the mat, palpation will reveal that the abdominals are under considerable eccentric contraction to control the velocity of the extending spine.

Extension

Powerful extension of the lumbar-thoracic spine is an integral motion within many sport skills. As examples, oarsmen and cross-country skiers must have excellent strength and muscle endurance in the muscles most involved for lumbar-thoracic extension. A basketball player rebounding, volleyball player spiking, and football player tackling all use spinal column extension to help summate force for their skills.

From a more functional standpoint, providing internal force to counteract gravity and maintain the upright stance is the responsibility of the extensors of the lumbar-thoracic spine. The magnitude of contraction increases as the center of mass is displaced forward. This is very important, because this area of the human body is susceptible to considerable gravitational stress. The musculature surrounding the lumbar-thoracic spine tends to show degeneration relatively early in the aging process if the flexors and extensors are not kept in a good state of muscular tone through exercise. The "visceral ptosis syndrome" is too common among sedentary individuals. This is a displacement forward of the abdominal wall and the visceral contents due to a lack of strength. Extra stress is placed on the extensor musculature located posteriorly. Lower back pain is commonly associated with this syndrome.

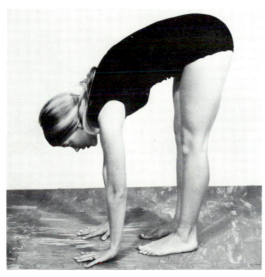

Figure 7.15.

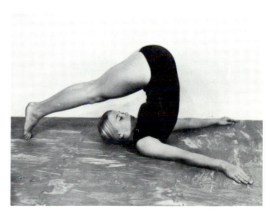

Figure 7.16.

Figure 7.15. Lumbar-thoracic flexion with gravity. The erector spinae as the MMI control the extent and speed of motion (Jan Stevenson). From Logan, *Adapted Physical Education.*

Figure 7.16. Lumbar-thoracic flexion—pelvic girdle moving toward the rib cage (Jan Stevenson). From Logan, *Adapted Physical Education.*

In the upright stance, it must be remembered that the anterior abdominal musculature plays an important role to counteract the potential posteriorward motion of the spine due to gravity or loss of equilibrium. The abdominals in this context control extension in the lumbar-thoracic spine by contracting eccentrically.

Extension of the lumbar-thoracic spine against resistance is the result of bilateral concentric contraction by the pairs of muscles within the erector spinae muscle group. In order to have spinal extension without any rotation, these muscles must contract equally and bilaterally. Individually each muscle in the erector spinae group is not exceptionally large. Collectively, however, this muscle group is large and has considerable strength potential. The deep posterior spinal group and both semispinalis thoracis muscles contribute contractile force for extension. These muscles are very small and do not meet the criteria for being muscles most involved for spinal column extension.

The erector spinae help to guide during lumbar-thoracic extension by ruling out their rotary and lateral flexion capabilities. However, the internal and external oblique muscles on both sides contribute considerable guiding force during extension.

The effects of erector spinae concentric contraction can be observed posteriorly along the lumbar spine during hyperextension. This is seen in figure 7.17.

The high jumper's lumbar-thoracic situation in figure 7.18 is virtually the myologic opposite of the situation seen in figure 7.17. Hyperextension of the lumbar-thoracic spine is being caused against the gravitational field on the slant

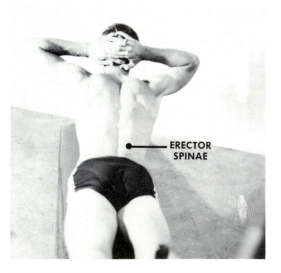

ERECTOR
SPINAE

Figure 7.17. Lumbar-thoracic hyperextension on a slant board. Muscles most involved in uppercase letters.

board. The high jumper, prior to and at the position shown in figure 7.18, must control her lumbar-thoracic extension-hyperextension range of motion as well as the velocity of motion of that body segment. This means that the abdominal muscle group, with its anterior spatial relationship to the spinal column, exerts control in this situation by contracting eccentrically.

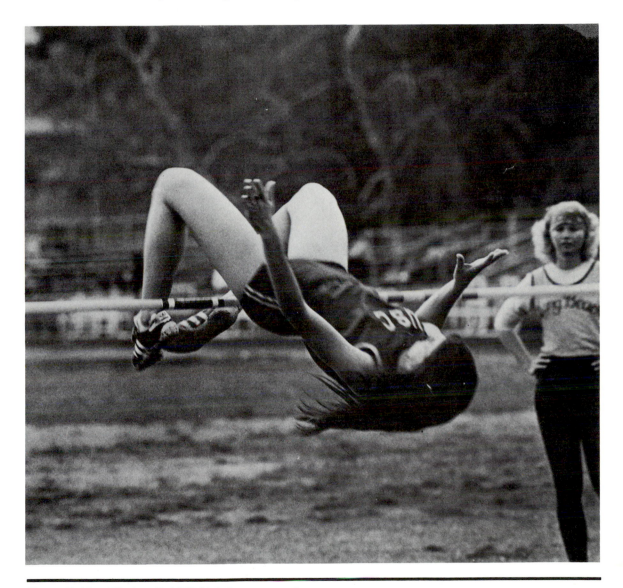

Figure 7.18. Julie Lendl, USC high jumper, must eccentrically control the lumbar-thoracic extension-hyperextension range of motion and velocity to execute a successful jump. Courtesy *USC Athletic News Service.*

Rotations

The structure of the lumbar spine does not allow this area to rotate freely. Most of the spinal rotation observed in the lumbar-thoracic segment actually occurs within the thoracic spine. The rotations are left and right in direction; for example, if the upper part of the spine rotates to the right in relation to the lower part, this would be right lumbar-thoracic rotation (fig. 7.19).

Spinal rotations through the cardinal transverse plane are utilized in numerous sport skills involving throwing and striking movements. The right-handed tennis player during the serve, as one example, utilizes right lumbar-thoracic rotation during the preparatory phase of the skill as the racket limb is being diagonally abducted at the right shoulder. Left lumbar-thoracic rotation will precede diagonal adduction of the right shoulder joint. These are the principal motions which provide the racket with velocity to contact the ball. If the spinal rotations were eliminated as motions in the tennis serve, force application to the ball would be reduced significantly. This is the case in most throwing and striking ballistic skills (fig. 7.3).

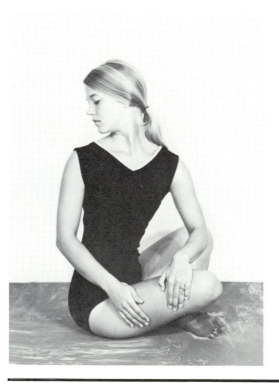

Figure 7.19. Right lumbar-thoracic and cervical spine rotations (Jan Stevenson). From Logan, *Adapted Physical Education.*

The muscles most involved for *right* lumbar-thoracic rotation against re-sistance are the right internal oblique, left external oblique, and right erector spinae muscles. Some force is also provided by the left semispinalis thoracis, left rotatores, and left multifidus muscles. Conversely, the paired muscles on the opposite side (contralateral muscles for right lumbar-thoracic rotation) would be the muscles most involved for rotating the lumbar-thoracic spine to the *left. The internal oblique and erector spinae muscles on the side of the body in the direction of the rotation contribute force along with the external oblique muscle on the opposite side.* The diagonal lines of pull of these muscles to the axis of rotation allow this function.

Some individuals find lumbar-thoracic rotary function of the spinal muscles somewhat abstract to conceptualize. An analogous situation is more readily observable in the cervical spine rotations. Figure 7.19 also shows cervical rotation to the *right.* The *left* sternocleidomastoid is a muscle most involved for *right* cervical rotation, and it is very prominent in the figure. The sternocleidomastoid function at the cervical spine is analogous to the external oblique rotary function at the lumbar-thoracic spine. It is recommended that observations and palpations be made of both sternocleidomastoids while rotating the cervical spine. This may help in understanding the muscle functions of lumbar-thoracic rotations. It must be remembered that the external obliques can also be palpated during motion through the transverse plane.

Lateral flexions

The lumbar-thoracic spine can be moved both left and right through the lateral plane of motion. This can be a distinct motion such as seen in figure 7.20. Lateral flexion to some extent always accompanies rotation, and it occurs on the same side as the rotation. This motion helps place muscle groups on greater stretch to exert more force for subsequent movements.

The muscles most involved for lumbar-thoracic lateral flexion to the left against resistance are the abdominal and erector spinae muscles on the left side

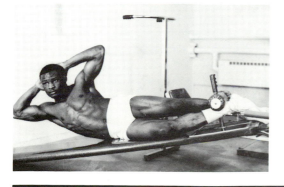

Figure 7.20. Left lateral flexion of the lumbar-tho-racic spine against resistance (Ardie McCoy).

of the body. The effect of the concentric contractions in the left rectus abdominis and left external oblique muscles for left lateral flexion can be observed in figure 7.20. There is a difference in external configuration in these muscles in the figure, as opposed to their reciprocally innervated contralateral counterparts. Internally, the left quadratus lumborum and left semispinalis thoracis also contribute force for left lateral flexion. The contralateral muscles for left lateral flexion would be the muscles most involved for right lateral flexion against resistance.

The guiding force during lateral flexion is provided by equal contraction anteriorly and posteriorly within the muscles most involved. This tends to reduce undesired rotation by these muscles located on either side of the lateral plane of motion.

As is the case in all joint motions, one must myologically analyze on the bases of: (1) gravitational considerations and (2) base of weight bearing support. The reader is asked to compare and contrast the motions of the lumbar-thoracic spines of the performers in figures 7.20 and 7.21. Both have laterally flexed their lumbar-thoracic spines, but that is where the similarity ceases. The exercise performed in figure 7.20 is against the resistances of his body weight and gravity primarily. In the side lying position on a slant board, the muscles most involved, as noted previously, must contract concentrically to produce left lateral flexion. The gymnast on the balance beam in figure 7.21 is using her feet as the base of support while laterally flexing the lumbar-thoracic spine to her left. This means that eccentric control was provided for this motion by the right half of her abdominals and erector spinae primarily. For reduction to occur (return to the anatomic position from lateral flexion), she would concentrically contract those same muscles. If the performer in figure 7.20 eases himself slowly down to the slant board, the muscle control for this would be from the eccentrically contracting left half of his abdominals and erector spinae primarily.

Cervical spine motions

The vertebrae of the cervical spine are much smaller than the lumbar vertebrae. As a result, the head-neck segment of the spine has considerable motion potential. The motions possible are: (1) flexion, (2) extension, (3) hyperextension, (4) lateral flexion, (5) rotation, and (6) circumduction. Owing to the relatively small size of each cervical vertebrae and only moderate ligamentous support in the area, stability of the cervical spine must be maintained by all of the musculature surrounding the neck. This region must receive considerable strength work, for example, by athletes in impact sports such as American football and ice hockey. In any sport where high velocity contacts may be possible between performers, whether advertently or inadvertently, such as English football, field hockey, baseball, or basketball, off-season and in-season weight training programs should include exercises for the cervical spine. This process has some potential for reducing spinal column injuries in this area if the muscles can negate some unusual external forces, e.g., the ''whip-lash'' effect of contact.

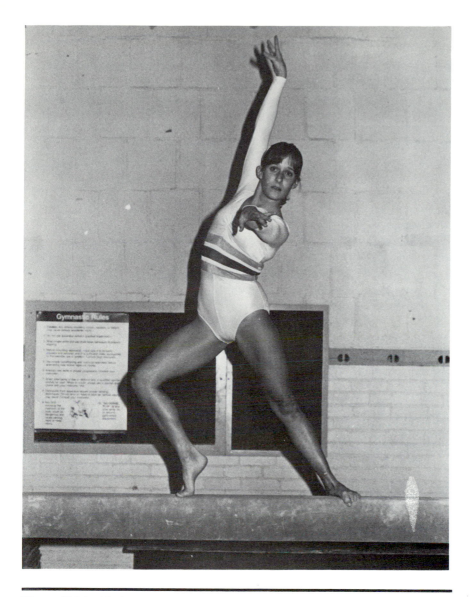

Figure 7.21. Linda Harding, USC gymnast, executes a balance beam maneuver involving lateral lumbar-thoracic flexion with gravity. Courtesy *USC Athletic News Service.*

Flexion

Flexion of the cervical spine against resistance is performed by both sternocleidomastoid muscles (MMI) contracting concentrically. These two muscles have a spatial relationship anterior to the cervical spine. An example of this type of movement performed by the sternocleidomastoids is seen when the individual is lying in the supine position and raises the head from the floor. The head moves toward the rib cage through the anteroposterior plane of motion. When the individual is standing and flexes the cervical spine, gravity is a major moving force. The muscles most involved in controlling this action are the erector spinae muscles contracting eccentrically on the posterior aspect of the cervical spine, i.e., the erector spinae are lengthening to allow the head to move forward slowly. The contralateral muscles for cervical flexion against resistance are the erector spinae muscles in the cervical region. The guiding component for cervical flexion is provided by the equal bilateral pull of the contracting sternocleidomastoid muscles. If one sternocleidomastoid muscle were contracting unilaterally, a rotary component would be introduced into the movement.

It should be noted that the sternocleidomastoid muscles receive some helping force for cervical flexion against resistance, by means of several small muscles. These are the prevertebral, hyoid, and scaleni muscles. However, these smaller muscles do not have either the size or the leverage of the two sternocleidomastoids.

In figure 7.22, the gymnast has flexed his cervical spine. His base of support is the right arm as he maneuvers on the sidehorse. If the cervical flexion occurred rapidly, the external force of gravity would be responsible for the motion. If the motion were performed slowly through the range of motion shown, the muscles most involved would be the eccentrically and bilaterally contracting erector spinae.

Extension

Extension of the cervical spine against resistance occurs as a result of concentric contraction by the erector spinae muscle group within the cervical region. The spatial relationship of the erector spinae to the cervical vertebrae is posterior. Extension through the anteroposterior range of motion is brought about due to the equal bilateral contraction of the erector spinae muscles on both the right and left halves of the body. The contralateral muscles for cervical extension are the sternocleidomastoid muscles on the anterior aspect of the neck. Guiding action is performed by equal tension within the contracting erector spinae on the right and left sides of the spinal column. If the muscles within the erector spinae group were to contract unilaterally, there would be a rotary action occurring within the cervical spine.

Muscles within the deep posterior spinal group, both splenius cervicis, both splenius capitis, both semispinalis cervicis, and both semispinalis capitis muscles also provide some force for spinal extension against resistance.

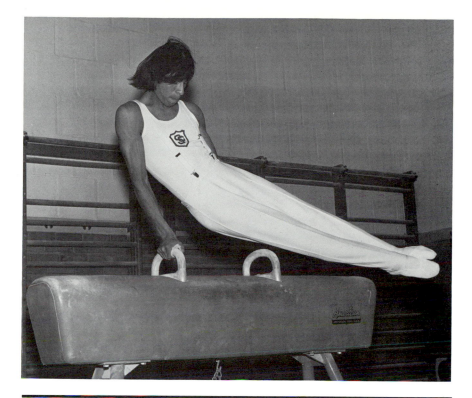

Figure 7.22. Juan Aguilar, USC gymnast, executing a sidehorse skill. The base of support is the right hand. Cervical flexion was either due to the external force of gravity or eccentric contraction of the erector spinae. Courtesy *USC Athletic News Service.*

Figures 7.23 and 7.24 are included in order to compare and contrast cervical extension-hyperextensions against and with gravity. The two excellent volleyball players in figure 7.23 are using their erector spinae to extend-hyperextend their cervical spines. Since there are no rotary components, it can be assumed that equal, bilateral concentric contractions of the erector spinae occurred to move the head-neck (cervical spine) to the position shown. This position of cervical hyperextension is of utmost importance to the volleyball players in order to view such things as ball flight, ball spin, opponent floor positioning, and positions of teammates.

The excellent gymnast on the beam in figure 7.24 has moved her cervical spine into extreme hyperextension with gravity. If this were done slowly, the muscles most involved would be both sternocleidomastoids contracting eccentrically. These muscles can be seen very prominently in figure 7.24. The gymnast is using cervical hyperextension for aesthetic purposes in her routine.

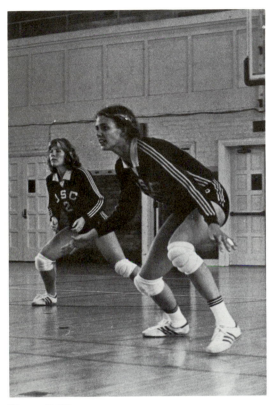

Figure 7.23.

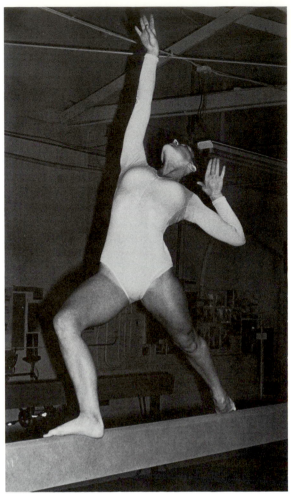

Figure 7.24.

Figure 7.23. Star Clark (13) and Paula Dittmer (2), USC volleyball players, utilize cervical extension-hyperextensions to make critical visual observations during the contest. Courtesy *USC Athletic News Service*. Photo by Michael R. Harriel.

Figure 7.24. Gale Wyckoff, USC gymnast, uses cervical hyperextension with gravity for aesthetic effect during her balance beam routine. Courtesy *USC Athletic News Service*.

Rotations

The cervical spine can be rotated left and right through a transverse plane of motion. These rotations are extremely important for increasing the degrees of the field of vision. If a performer had to rely strictly on peripheral vision with the cervical spine stabilized in the anatomic position, performing would be very awkward. Many extraneous and inefficient motions would have to be made elsewhere in the body to position the head. This would be a performance problem. Anyone who has ever had a "stiff neck" and tried to perform a skill has some firsthand insight into the problem.

Left cervical spine rotation is movement of the face toward the left shoulder. The muscles most involved for this motion against resistance are the right sternocleidomastoid and the left half of the erector spinae muscles. The left splenius capitis and left splenius cervicis muscles also assist in left cervical rotation. Right cervical spine rotation is shown in figure 7.19, the muscles listed above would be the contralateral muscles for right cervical spine rotation. Their contralateral counterparts would be the muscles most involved for right cervical spine rotation. The guiding function for the rotations comes from the forces developed within the muscles most involved. Flexion and extension capabilities are eliminated to bring about the desired rotation.

Lateral flexions

Right and left lateral flexions of the cervical spine occur through the lateral plane of motion. These motions occur with gravity for the most part when the performer is in the bipedal position. Figure 7.25 shows lateral cervical flexion to the left with the right hand and upper limb musculature providing the resistive force. In this situation, the muscles most involved for left lateral flexion of the cervical spine contracting concentrically are the left sternocleidomastoid plus the left half of the erector spinae muscles in the cervical region. The left scalenus anterior, medius, and posterior, left splenius capitis and cervicis, and the left semispinalis cervicis, along with the left levator scapulae, also provide some force for left lateral cervical flexion.

If the cervical spine were allowed to slowly flex laterally to the left *with gravity,* the muscles most involved would be the eccentrically contracting right sternocleidomastoid and the right erector spinae muscles.

The guiding muscles are located anterior and posterior to the cervical spine. The muscles most involved have these spatial relationships as well as being lateral to the cervical spine. Consequently, they rule out their flexion, extension, and rotation components to guide the head through the lateral plane of motion.

Figure 7.26 shows the lines of pull for all the muscles with spatial relationships to the spinal column.

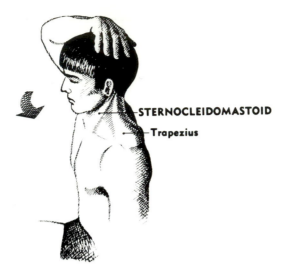

Figure 7.25. Left lateral cervical flexion against resistance. (Superficial muscles most involved appear in uppercase letters.)

MUSCLES	PROXIMAL ATTACHMENT	DISTAL ATTACHMENT
I. Lumbar-Thoracic Spine Musculature		
A. Flexors		
1. RECTUS ABDOMINIS	Pubic crest, superior	Anterior on the cartilages of ribs 5–7 and the xiphoid process
2. EXTERNAL OBLIQUE	Inferior border of the lower eight ribs	Anterior half of the iliac crest, pubic crest, and linea alba
3. INTERNAL OBLIQUE	Anterior two-thirds of the iliac crest, lateral half of the inguinal ligament and lumbodorsal fascia	Cartilage of the lower four ribs of the linea alba
4. Psoas	Twelfth thoracic and all lumbar vertebrae	Lesser trochanter of femur

Figure 7.26. Spinal column musculature. The muscles most involved for the motions against resistance are shown in uppercase letters. Muscles supplying supplemental force during concentric contraction are in lowercase letters.

Figure 7.26. Continued.

MUSCLES	PROXIMAL ATTACHMENT	DISTAL ATTACHMENT
B. Extensors		
1. ERECTOR SPINAE	Thoracolumbar fasciae; posterior lumbar, thoracic and lower cervical vertebrae; posterior ribs	Posterior ribs; posterior cervical and thoracic vertebrae and mastoid processes
2. Deep posterior spinal group	Posterior sacrum and processes of all vertebrae	Spinous and transverse processes and laminae of vertebrae superior to proximal attachments
3. Semispinalis thoracis	Transverse processes of thoracic vertebrae 6–10	Spinous processes of upper four thoracic and lower two cervical vertebrae
C. Rotators		
1. INTERNAL OBLIQUE	Anterior two-thirds of the iliac crest, lateral half of the inguinal ligament and lumbodorsal fascia	Cartilage of the lower four ribs and the linea alba
2. EXTERNAL OBLIQUE	Inferior border of the lower eight ribs	Anterior half of the iliac crest, pubic crest, and linea alba
3. ERECTOR SPINAE	Thoracolumbar fasciae; posterior lumbar, thoracic and lower cervical vertebrae; posterior ribs	Posterior ribs; posterior cervical and thoracic vertebrae and mastoid processes
4. Semispinalis thoracis	Transverse processes of thoracic vertebrae 6–10	Spinous processes of upper four thoracic and lower two cervical vertebrae
5. Deep posterior spinal group	Posterior sacrum and processes of all vertebrae	Spinous and transverse processes and laminae of vertebrae superior to proximal attachments
D. Lateral Flexors		
1. RECTUS ABDOMINIS	Pubic crest, superior	Anterior on the cartilages of ribs 5–7 and the xiphoid process
2. INTERNAL OBLIQUE	Anterior two-thirds of the iliac crest, lateral half of the inguinal ligament and lumbodorsal fascia	Cartilage of the lower four ribs and the linea alba
3. EXTERNAL OBLIQUE	Inferior border of the lower eight ribs	Anterior half of the iliac crest, pubic crest, and linea alba

Figure 7.26. Continued

MUSCLES	PROXIMAL ATTACHMENT	DISTAL ATTACHMENT
4. ERECTOR SPINAE	Thoracolumbar fasciae; posterior lumbar, thoracic and lower cervical vertebrae; posterior ribs	Posterior ribs; posterior cervical and thoracic vertebrae and mastoid processes
5. Semispinalis thoracis	Transverse processes of thoracic vertebrae 6–10	Spinous processes of upper four thoracic and lower two cervical vertebrae
6. Quadratus lumborum	Iliac crest and iliolumbar ligament	Inferior aspect of the twelfth rib and transverse processes of the upper four lumbar vertebrae
II. Cervical Spine Musculature		
A. Flexors		
1. STERNOCLEI DOMASTOID	*Sternum head:* Anterior manubrium	Mastoid process and superior nuchal line
B. Extensors		
1. ERECTOR SPINAE	Thoracolumbar fasciae; posterior lumbar, thoracic and lower cervical vertebrae; posterior ribs	Posterior ribs; posterior cervical and thoracic vertebrae and mastoid processes
2. Deep posterior spinal group	Posterior sacrum and processes of all vertebrae	Spinous and transverse processes and laminae of vertebrae superior to proximal attachments
3. Splenius capitis	Ligamentum nuchae, spinous processes of the seventh cervical and upper three thoracic vertebrae	Mastoid process and occipital bone
4. Semispinalis cervicis	Transverse processes of upper five thoracic vertebrae	Spinous processes of first five cervical vertebrae
5. Semispinalis capitis	Articular processes of 4–6 cervical vertebrae; transverse processes of the seventh cervical and superior six thoracic vertebrae	Occipital area between the superior and inferior nuchal lines

Figure 7.26. Continued.

MUSCLES	PROXIMAL ATTACHMENT	DISTAL ATTACHMENT
C. Rotators		
1. STERNOCLEI-DOMASTOID	*Sternum head:* Anterior manubrium	Mastoid process and superior nuchal line
2. ERECTOR SPINAE	Thoracolumbar fasciae; posterior lumbar, thoracic and lower cervical vertebrae; posterior ribs	Posterior ribs; posterior cervical and thoracic vertebrae and mastoid processes
3. Splenius capitis	Ligamentum nuchae, spinous processes of the seventh cervical and upper three thoracic vertebrae	Mastoid process and occipital bone
4. Splenius cervicis	Spinous processes of thoracic vertebrae 3–6	Transverse processes cervical vertebrae two and three
D. Lateral Flexors		
1. STERNOCLEI-DOMASTOID	*Sternum head:* Anterior manubrium	Mastoid process and superior nuchal line
2. ERECTOR SPINAE	Thoracolumbar fasciae; posterior lumbar, thoracic and lower cervical vertebrae; posterior ribs	Posterior ribs; posterior cervical and thoracic vertebrae and mastoid processes
3. Three Scaleni	First two ribs	Transverse processes of cervical vertebrae
4. Splenius capitis	Ligamentum nuchae, spinous processes of the seventh cervical and upper three thoracic vertebrae	Mastoid process and occipital bone
5. Splenius cervicis	Spinous processes of thoracic vertebrae 3–6	Transverse processes cervical vertebrae two and three
6. Semispinalis cervicis	Transverse processes of upper five thoracic vertebrae	Spinous processes of first five cervical vertebrae
7. Semispinalis capitis	Articular processes of 4–6 cervical vertebrae; transverse processes of the seventh cervical and superior six thoracic vertebrae	Occipital area between the superior lines

Selected references

Benteler, A. M. "Change in Tone of the Spinal Muscles in Man." *Sechnor Physiological Journal of the U.S.S.R.* 47 (1961) :393-98.

Colachis, S. C., Jr., et al. "Movement of the Sacroiliac Joint in the Adult Male: Preliminary Report." *Archives of Physical Medicine and Rehabilitation* 44 (September 1963) :490-98.

Davis, P. R. "Posture of the Trunk During the Lifting of Weights." *British Medical Journal* 5114 (1959) :87-89.

Davis, P. R.; Troup, J. D. G.; and Burnard, J. H. "Movements of the Thoracic and Lumbar Spine When Lifting: A Chronocylophotographic Study." *Journal of Anatomy* 99 (January 1965) :13-26.

Defibaugh, Joseph J. "Measurement of Head Motion, Part I: A Review of Methods of Measuring Joint Motion." *Physical Therapy* 44 (March 1964) :157-63.

————. "Measurement in Head Motion, Part II: An Experimental Study of Head Motion in Adult Males." *Physical Therapy* 44 (March 1964) :163-68.

Ferlic, Donald. "The Range of Motion of the 'Normal' Cervical Spine." *Bulletin of the Johns Hopkins Hospital* 110 (February 1962) :59-65.

Flint, M. M. "Effect of Increasing Back and Abdominal Muscle Strength on Low Back Pain." *Research Quarterly* 29 (May 1958) :160-71.

Frankel, Saul A., and Hirata, Isao. "The Scalenus Anticus Syndrome and Competitive Swimming." *Journal of the American Medical Association* 215 (1971) 1796-98.

Gough, Joseph G., and Koepke, George H. "Electromyographic Determination of Motor Root Levels in Erector Spinae Muscles." *Archives of Physical Medicine and Rehabilitation* 47 (January 1966) :9-11.

Gutin, Bernard, and Lipetz, Stanley. "An Electromyographic Investigation of the Rectus Abdominis in Abdominal Exercises." *Research Quarterly* 42 (1971) :256-63.

Halpren, A. A., et. al. "Sit-up Exercises: An Electromyographic Study." *Clinical Orthapaedics and Related Research* 145 (November-December, 1979):172-178.

Keagy, Robert D.; Brumlick, Joel; and Bergan, John J. "Direct Electromyography of the Psoas Major Muscle in Man." *Journal of Bone and Joint Surgery* 48-A (October 1966) :1377-82.

Kottke, Frederic J., and Mundale, Martin O. "Range of Mobility of the Cervical Spine." *Archives of Physical Medicine and Rehabilitation* 40 (September 1959) :379-82.

La Ban, Myron M., et al. "Electromyographic Study of Function of Iliopsoas Muscle." *Archives of Physical Medicine and Rehabilitation* 46 (October 1965) :676-79.

Michele, Arthur A. *Iliopsoas.* Springfield: Charles C Thomas, Publisher, 1962.

Morris, J. M.; Benner, G.; and Lucas, D. B. "An Electromyographic Study of the Intrinsic Muscles of the Back in Man." *Journal of Anatomy* 96 (October 1962) :509-20.

Nachemson, A. "Electromyographic Studies on the Vertebral Portion of the Psoas Muscle." *Acta Orthopaedica Scandinavica* 37 (Fase. 2 1966) :177-90.

Partridge, Miriam J., and Walters, C. Etta. "Participation of the Abdominal Muscles in Various Movements of the Trunk in Man." *Physical Therapy Review* 39 (December 1959) 791-800.

Rab, G. T. "Muscle Forces in the Posterior Thoracic Spine." *Clinical Orthopaedics and Related Research* 139 (March–April, 1979) :28-32.

Rab, G. T., et. al. "Muscle Force Analysis of the Lumbar Spine." *Orthopedic Clinics of North America* 8 (January, 1977) :193-199.

Raper, A. Jarrell, et al. "Scalene and Sternomastoid Muscle Function." *Journal of Applied Physiology* 21 (1966) :497-502.

Sheffield, F. J. "Electromyographic Study of the Abdominal Muscles in Walking and Other Movements." *American Journal of Physical Medicine* 41 (August 1962) :142-47.

Singh, Mohan, and Ashton, T. Edwin. "Study of Back-lift Strength with Electrogoniometric Analysis of Hip Angle." *Research Quarterly* 41 (1970) :562-68.

Steen, B. "The Function of Certain Neck Muscles in Different Positions of the Head with and without Loading of the Cervical Spine." *Acta Morphologica Neerlando-Scandinavica* 4 (1966) :301-10.

Walters, C. Etta, and Partridge, Miriam J. "Electromyographic Study of the Differential Action of the Abdominal Muscles During Exercises." *American Journal of Physical Medicine* 36 (October 1957) :259-68.

Wilson, Gary L., Capen, Edward K. and Stubbs, Nancy B. "A Fine-Wire Electromyographic Investigation of the Gluteus Minimus and Gluteus Medius Muscles." *Research Quarterly* 47 (December, 1976): 824-828.

8

Shoulder Girdle and Upper Limb Motions

For academic reasons only the shoulder girdle is discussed as an entity separate from the shoulder joint in this chapter. The reader must remember that functionally these two areas are reciprocally related to one another. The motions of the shoulder girdle and shoulder joint cannot be separated when analyzing total shoulder area movements.

There are five muscles of the shoulder girdle with both attachments on the trunk or spinal area. If the reader prefers, the attachments of these muscles can be conceptualized as being either superior/inferior or lateral/medial, instead of the more traditional, proximal/distal type of attachment situation. The muscles with superior/inferior lines of pull are: (1) pectoralis minor, figure 8.5; (2) levator scapulae, figure 8.3; and (3) trapezius, figure 8.2. The muscles which have lateral/medial lines of pull are: (1) serratus anterior, figure 8.3, and (2) the rhomboids, figure 8.3. The attachment points for these muscles are included in figure 8.12.

Shoulder girdle structure

The shoulder girdle is composed of the clavicles and scapulae (fig. 8.1). This is a relatively weak bony arrangement. The clavicle joins the trunk at the sternum forming the sternoclavicular joint, and the acromioclavicular joint is formed by the clavicle articulating with the scapula. The rhomboid muscles complete the girdle posteriorly by attaching the scapulae to the spinal column in the thoracic region.

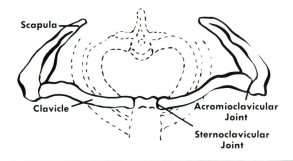

Figure 8.1. Shoulder girdle—superior view. From Logan, *Adapted Physical Education.*

Sternoclavicular joint

The sternoclavicular joint is one of the most freely movable gliding joints in the body. There is considerable motion allowed because this joint has an interarticular disc. The clavicle moves approximately forty degrees during depression and elevation. It also moves approximately forty degrees anteriorly and posteriorly.

From a ligamentous standpoint, the support of the sternoclavicular joint is very strong. There is a fibrocartilage to assist in preventing the upward and medial displacement of the clavicle. This fibrocartilage also absorbs shock received laterally through the acromion process. For example, shock received by a wrestler who is thrown on the "point of his shoulder" is partially absorbed at the sternoclavicular joint. This joint receives further support by anterior and posterior sternoclavicular ligaments. These ligaments, working in conjunction with the costoclavicular ligament, prevent upward and lateral displacement of the clavicle. The interclavicular ligament connects the clavicles. This ligament prevents the clavicles from being displaced laterally.

The subclavius muscle has a type of "ligamentous function" because it supports or stabilizes the clavicle. It has an attachment on the first rib and another attachment on the inferior aspect of the clavicle. Its structural support function for the sternoclavicular joint is very important. It contributes some force when contracting concentrically for depression of the shoulder girdle against resistance. Due to its small mass and relatively poor leverage, it is not considered to be a muscle most involved for shoulder girdle depression. If a woman must have a radical mastectomy, removal of the breast along with a portion of the *upper fibers* of the pectoralis major, due to cancer, the surgeon will make adaptations where the subclavius fibers will serve a substitute role for the removed muscular tissue of the pectoralis major. This is a good example of adaptation and substitution of muscle function.

Surgeons often use normal muscles to assume motion functions of muscles rendered inactive by virtue of disease or trauma. They will change the lines of pull and spatial relationships to joints so normal muscle-tendons can assume motion functions where abnormalities exist. As an example by doing this, a normal flexor can be changed to have an extension function. This procedure is utilized when the quadriceps femoris muscle group at the knee is incapacitated by disease or trauma. The distal attachments of the semitendinosus and biceps femoris are changed to the medial and lateral superior margin of the patella. This change of spatial relationships to the knee joint allows these muscles to extend the knee when they contract concentrically.

Acromioclavicular joint

The acromioclavicular joint is a relatively fixed joint held together by the superior and inferior acromioclavicular ligaments as well as by the coracoclavicular ligament from below. Due to this ligamentous stability of the bony structures, the movements of the shoulder girdle are seen functionally within the sternoclavicular joints. There is very little, if any, muscle support of the acromioclavicular joint because muscles do not cross it.

The trapezius, rhomboid, levator scapulae, serratus anterior, and pectoralis minor are the muscles which cause the shoulder girdle motions. With the exception of the pectoralis minor, these muscles are seen as they attach to the scapulae in figures 8.2 and 8.3. The pectoralis minor is shown in figure 8.5.

Figure 8.2 shows the trapezius. This is a large, superficial muscle which covers the rhomboids. It has several different functions depending upon which fibers are activated. The upper fibers are from the base of the skull to the acromion and lateral scapular spine area. The middle fibers lie in the transverse plane, and the lower fibers exert their pull from the medial aspect of the scapular spine to the thoracic vertebrae. It is a prominent muscle of the back, and the various parts may be palpated during contraction.

It should be noted that the trapezius muscle is often described as being a four part muscle in the literature. As seen in figure 8.2, the upper trapezius includes parts I and II. Part III is the middle trapezius, and part IV is shown as the lower trapezius.

The rhomboid muscles are considered as one muscle in terms of function. This muscle has a diagonal line of pull from the medial border of the scapula to the last cervical and first five thoracic spinous processes. Functionally, the rhomboid interacts with the serratus anterior at the medial border of the scapula.

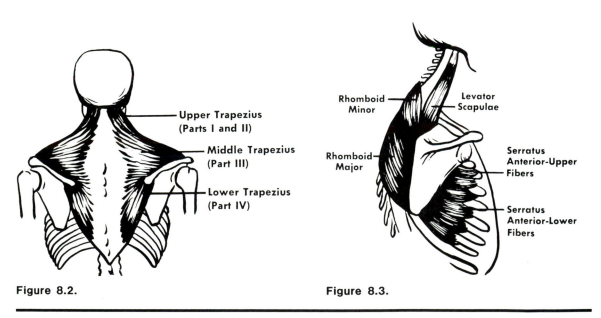

Figure 8.2.

Figure 8.3.

Figure 8.2. The trapezius—posterior view. From Logan, *Adapted Physical Education.*

Figure 8.3. Shoulder girdle musculature—lateral view. From Logan, *Adapted Physical Education.*

The serratus anterior then continues its line of pull diagonally to the lateral aspects of the first eight ribs (fig. 8.3). The levator scapulae is superior to the scapula with a line of pull from the transverse processes of the cervical vertebra to the superior angle of the scapula. The pectoralis minor lies beneath the pectoralis major anteriorly attaching to the coracoid process of the scapula and projecting diagonally downward to attach on the lateral aspects of ribs, three, four, and five.

The spatial relationships of the muscles discussed in the shoulder girdle area are in terms of their positions to the *scapulae* instead of to joints *per se*. This approach to spatial relationship differs from other body areas, due to the fact that the scapula is used as a reference point and moving part instead of a joint.

The motions of the shoulder girdle are abduction, adduction, downward rotation, upward rotation, elevation, and depression. The main purpose of these motions is to maintain the position of the glenoid fossa of the scapula with the head of the humerus during shoulder joint motions.

There must be a constant, functional relationship between the shoulder girdle and shoulder joint motions. The muscles contracting to move the shoulder joints and upper limbs must have stable areas proximally for the limb motions to be functional. Those areas are the shoulder girdle and trunk (spinal column). The glenoid fossa of the scapula must move to accomodate the humeral head during shoulder joint motions. Therefore, the shoulder girdle area must move, and it must also provide enough tension to allow proximal attachments of upper limb muscles with a relatively stable area at which to exert their contractile forces to produce shoulder joint motion. *This moving tension provided by the shoulder girdle muscles concurrent with shoulder joint muscle contraction furnishes dynamic stability.* Stable motion of this type is known as the Lomac Paradox. *The dynamic stability of the shoulder girdle is provided by tension within the muscles most involved for a motion plus their contralateral muscles.*

Abduction

The scapulae move away from the spinous processes during abduction without any rotation. From the anatomic position as the shoulders are protracted, the scapulae are abducted. Scapular abduction is observed during push-up and bench-press exercises, but this abduction follows upward rotation. Due to the fact that ninety degrees of shoulder joint flexion occurs to position the performer to execute the push-up or bench-press, a few degrees of scapular upward rotation must occur concurrent with the shoulder flexion. The scapulae are "set" in the upward rotation position and abducted without further rotation as the body resistance or weights are lifted.

The muscles most involved for scapular adbuction against resistance are the pectoralis minor and upper serratus anterior. The contralateral muscles are the middle fibers of the trapezius and rhomboid muscles. Guiding force for scapular abduction is provided by a balance of power between the concentrically contracting upper and lower fibers of the serratus anterior. This rules out rotation motions of the shoulder girdle.

Adduction

Scapular adduction is the return of the scapulae to the anatomic position from abduction. This occurs with the retraction movement of the shoulder area.

The middle fibers of the trapezius and rhomboids are the muscles most involved for scapular adduction against resistance. With the spine attachments stabilized, these muscles have good leverage advantage and exert force in a medial direction. The muscles most involved guide the motion by ruling out their rotary capabilities. Figure 8.4 shows the trapezius contracting prominently during a weight-training exercise which involves shoulder joint extension and scapular adduction.

Scapular adbuction and adduction can be understood best by study of the relationship between the serratus anterior and rhomboid muscles. These two muscles can be thought of as one myologic unit because they both attach at the vertebral borders of the scapulae. When the serratus anterior contracts concentrically against resistance, the rhomboids must lengthen while the serratus anterior abducts the scapula. These two muscles maintain a close contact with the rib cage throughout this movement. This action holds the scapulae in a relatively close relationship to the rib cage. Because of the semicylindrical shape

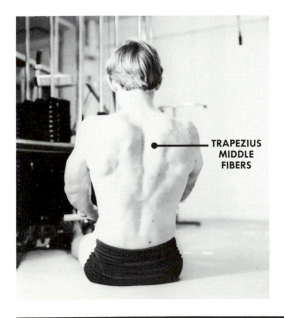

TRAPEZIUS
MIDDLE
FIBERS

Figure 8.4. Scapular adduction concurrent with shoulder joint extension.

of the rib cage, it is obvious that the scapulae describe an arc during abduction and adduction. The myologic unit consisting of the serratus anterior and rhomboids also has a relationship with the internal and external oblique muscles. These four muscles are discussed in chapter 10 in terms of a larger myologic construct known as "the serape effect."

Downward rotation

Downward rotation of the scapula involves teamwork among muscles located anterior and posterior to the rib cage. The glenoid fossa is rotated downward anytime the humerus is moving downward through any plane of motion; for example, if the shoulder joint is being adducted through the lateral plane of motion, the concurrent motion in the shoulder girdle is downward rotation.

The muscles most involved for downward rotation against resistance are the rhomboid and pectoralis minor muscles (fig. 8.5). The main guiding force is derived from contraction of the lower fibers of the rhomboid and the levator scapulae. The contralateral muscles are all parts of the trapezius and lower fibers of the serratus anterior.

Downward rotation of the scapula can be the result of gravitational and other external forces exclusively during high velocity extension, adduction, and diagonal adduction of the shoulder joint. However, if downward rotation of the scapula is performed slowly with these shoulder motions, the eccentric control comes from the trapezius and lower fibers of the serratus anterior.

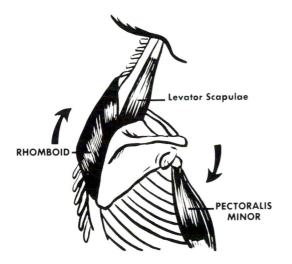

Figure 8.5. Scapular downward rotators. (Muscles most involved appear in uppercase letters.) From Logan, *Adapted Physical Education.*

It must be borne in mind that the muscles involved in downward rotation may need special attention for strength and muscular endurance development. This motion routinely receives considerable gravitational assistance; consequently, performers need exercises which will place the downward rotators in concentric contraction situations. Figures 8.6 and 8.7 show a weight-training exercise designed to work the downward rotators of the shoulder girdle and the shoulder joint adductors against resistance. The muscles most involved for downward rotation are not seen, because they are not superficial muscles.

Upward rotation

Upward rotation of the scapula involves lateral and upward movement of the inferior angle of the scapula and glenoid fossa. It should be noted that during this movement the anteroposterior axis of the scapula is moving laterally as well as upward during upward rotation. This is due primarily to the fact that motion

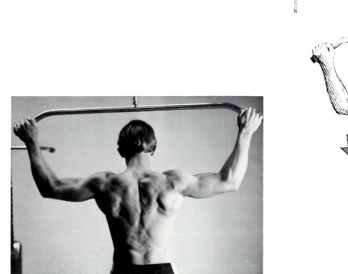

Figure 8.6.

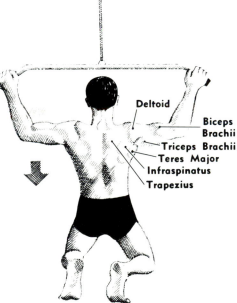

Figure 8.7.

Figure 8.6. Downward rotation of the scapulae—superficial posterior muscles.

Figure 8.7. Downward rotation of the scapulae—concurrent with shoulder joint adduction.

is allowed within the freely movable sternoclavicular joint. The clavicle actually provides a radius for shoulder girdle movement to occur. It also allows lateral and upward displacement of the scapula.

The position of the upper limbs must be taken under consideration when analyzing or determining the muscles most involved for upward rotation. As pointed out previously, upward rotation of the scapula accompanies any upward, lateral, or diagonal motion of the upper limbs at the glenohumeral joint. The muscles most involved for upward rotation of the scapulae differ in relation to shoulder joint abduction and flexion. This is because of the change in position of the scapula relative to the rib cage when the shoulder joint is abducted or flexed. As can be observed by palpation techniques, the scapulae are in a position closer to the spinal column when the shoulder joint is abducted than when the shoulder joint is flexed. The scapulae are moved away from the vertebral column when the upper limbs are flexed at the shoulder joint. When the upper limbs are flexed at the shoulder joint, the function of the trapezius muscle in upward rotation of the scapula is less because the trapezius is placed in a position of leverage disadvantage for functional concentric contraction and subsequent movement of the scapula into upward rotation.

The muscles most involved in upward rotation of the scapula against resistance while the shoulder joint is being abducted or diagonally abducted are all parts of the trapezius and lower fibers of the serratus anterior (fig. 8.8). All parts of the trapezius are active during upward rotation against resistance, but part IV (lower fibers) and part II (inferior portion of the upper fibers) have the best leverage to upwardly rotate the scapula against resistance.

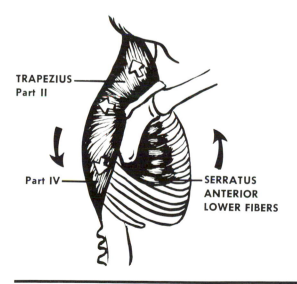

TRAPEZIUS
Part II

Part IV

SERRATUS
ANTERIOR
LOWER FIBERS

Figure 8.8. Upward rotation of the scapula concurrent with diagonal abduction. (Muscles most involved appear in uppercase letters.) From Logan, *Adapted Physical Education.*

The main guiding force is derived from bilateral and equal tension between upper and lower fibers of the trapezius. This is due primarily to the fact that the lower fibers of the trapezius exert their force downward on the vertebral base of the scapular spine. The upper fibers exert a counterforce upward from the acromion area. The contralateral muscles for upward rotation are the pectoralis minor and rhomboid.

From a superficial muscle standpoint, the differences between upward rotation while the shoulder joints are being abducted and when they are flexed are apparent. The trapezius muscle is very prominent performing its upward rotation function during abduction. Conversely, the middle and lower fibers of the trapezius are in a position of disadvantage when flexion occurs at the shoulder joint. This means that the lower fibers of the serratus anterior become the muscle most involved when the shoulder joints are flexed against resistance through an anteroposterior plane of motion. These motions should be performed, and the trapezius and serratus anterior muscles should be palpated and observed to notice these differences.

Elevation

Lifting of the scapulae vertically without any rotation while in the anatomic position is elevation (fig. 8.9). The common shoulder "shrug" is an example of this motion. Elevation of both scapulae is observed during the butterfly stroke in swimming.

The muscles most involved for elevation are the levator scapulae, upper trapezius, and rhomboid. These muscles all have spatial relationships to the scapula which allow them to lift or elevate the scapula. The levator scapulae and upper trapezius are the guiding muscles. They work together to rule out their rotary components. The contralateral muscles for elevation are the lower trapezius and pectoralis minor.

Figure 8.9 shows an elevation exercise against resistance. The performer's right scapula is elevated.

The shoulder girdle motions can be observed in sequence in conjunction with shoulder joint motions. A key bone landmark to observe and to help determine shoulder girdle motion is the acromion process. Also, the extent of the range of motion of the shoulder joint will tell the observer which shoulder girdle motions are occurring, without seeing the actual clavicular-scapular motions. As an example, due to the extent of the shoulder joint motions by the basketball player executing the jump shot in figure 8.10, it is known that upward rotation and elevation of the shoulder girdles took place in that sequence. If those shoulder girdle motions did not occur concurrent with the shoulder joint motions, she would not have gotten the ball in that position for the shot.

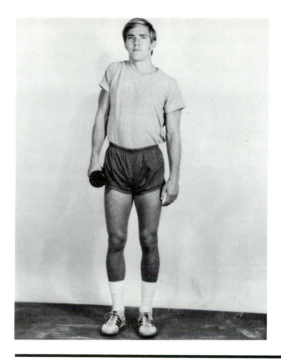

Figure 8.9. Elevation of the right scapula against resistance. From Logan, *Adapted Physical Education.*

Depression

The return of the scapulae to the anatomic position from elevation is known as depression. This is a motion most commonly performed by gravity when the individual is in the bipedal, upright stance.

When depression of the shoulder girdle is performed against resistance, such as during the so-called "dip" exercise on parallel bars, the muscles most involved are the lower trapezius and pectoralis minor. These posterior and anterior muscles literally pull downward on the scapular spine and coracoid process respectively during the concentric contractions. In so doing, the muscles most involved for depression serve as guiders inasmuch as their ability to upwardly and downwardly rotate the scapula has been ruled out.

Since shoulder girdle depression occurs most commonly with gravity, eccentric control of this motion is relatively frequent if the depression occurs slowly through its normal range of motion while the individual is standing. In that situation, the muscles most involved for controlling depression eccentrically would be the levator scapulae, upper trapezius, and rhomboid.

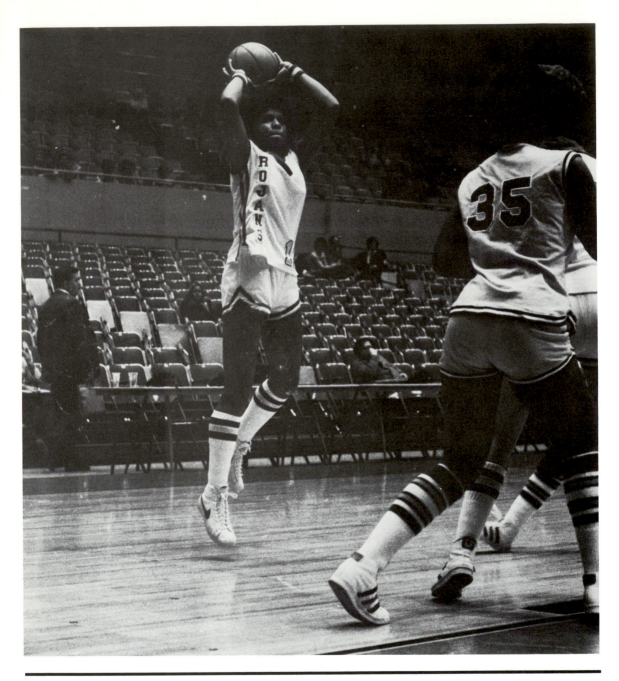

Figure 8.10. Kathy Haines (12), USC basketball player, executing a jump shot. Upward rotation and elevation have occurred in both shoulder girdles concurrent with left shoulder flexion and diagonal abduction of the right shoulder. Courtesy *USC Athletic News Service.*

Figure 8.11 shows a gymnast in a typical static maneuver on the still rings. The shoulder girdles are depressed concentrically when he exerts force downward on the rings lifting the body mass slightly. The shoulder girdles are also slightly abducted (protracted). No rotary motion of the shoulder girdles has occurred. This is deduced on the basis of the extended positions of both shoulder joints.

Figure 8.12 shows the attachments of the shoulder girdle musculature utilizing the traditional proximal to distal terminology. This provides the lines of pull for these muscles. Remember, if it is easier for the reader to conceptualize these, superior/inferior attachments and lateral/medial attachments may be substituted as follows:

Superior/Inferior Attachments   *Lateral/Medial Attachments*
    Pectoralis Minor   Serratus Anterior
    Levator Scapulae   Rhomboids
    Trapezius

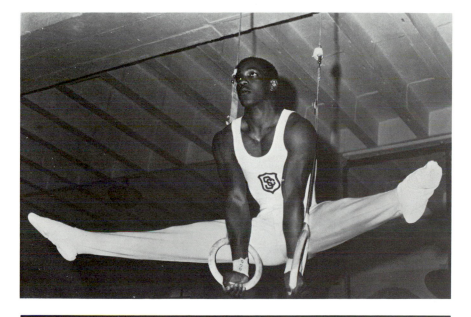

Figure 8.11. Jim Betters, USC gymnast, concentrically contracts the shoulder girdle depressors during this still ring maneuver. Courtesy *USC Athletic News Service.*

MUSCLES	PROXIMAL ATTACHMENT	DISTAL ATTACHMENT
I. Shoulder Girdle Musculature		
A. Abductors		
1. PECTORALIS MINOR	Upper, anterior aspects of ribs 3–5	Coracoid process of the scapula
2. SERRATUS ANTERIOR	Outer and lateral aspects of ribs 1–8	Anterior, vertebral scapula border
B. Adductors		
1. TRAPEZIUS a. (MIDDLE FIBERS)	Occipital protuberance; ligamentum nuchae and spinous process of the seventh cervical and all thoracic vertebrae	Scapular spine, superior border
2. RHOMBOID	Seventh cervical to the fifth thoracic spinous processes	Posterior, vertebral scapula border
C. Downward Rotators		
1. RHOMBOID	Seventh cervical to the fifth thoracic spinous processes	Posterior, vertebral scapula border
2. PECTORALIS MINOR	Upper, anterior aspects of ribs 3–5	Coracoid process of the scapula
D. Upward Rotators 1. TRAPEZIUS (ALL PARTS)		
a. UPPER FIBERS	Occipital protuberance; ligamentum nuchae and spinous process of the seventh cervical and all thoracic vertebrae	Posterior border of the lateral third of the clavicle and acromion process
b. LOWER FIBERS	Occipital protuberance; ligamentum nuchae and spinous process of the seventh cervical and all thoracic vertebrae	Medial aspect of the scapula spine
2. SERRATUS ANTERIOR (LOWER FIBERS)	Outer and lateral aspects of ribs 1–8	Anterior, vertebral scapula border

Figure 8.12. Shoulder girdle musculature. Muscles most involved or the motions against resistance are shown in uppercase letters.

Figure 8.12. Continued.

MUSCLES	PROXIMAL ATTACHMENT	DISTAL ATTACHMENT
E. Elevators		
1. LEVATOR SCAPULAE	Transverse processes of the first four cervical vertebrae	Superior angle of the scapula
2. TRAPEZIUS (UPPER FIBERS)	Occipital protuberance; ligamentum nuchae and spinous process of the seventh cervical and all thoracic vertebrae	Posterior border of the lateral third of the clavicle and acromion process
3. RHOMBOID	Seventh cervical to the fifth thoracic spinous processes	Posterior, vertebral scapula border
F. Depressors		
1. TRAPEZIUS (LOWER FIBERS)	Occipital protuberance; ligamentum nuchae and spinous process of the seventh cervical and all thoracic vertebrae	Medial aspect of the scapular spine
2. PECTORALIS MINOR	Upper, anterior aspects of ribs 3–5	Coracoid process of the scapula

Shoulder joint motions

With the evolution of the human from the quadrupedal to the bipedal stance, a number of changes have taken place within the shoulder joint. When man used the quadrupedal position, the bony structure and alignment of the scapulae and shoulder joint were highly stable for the performance of the weight-bearing function. However, in the bipedal or non-weight-bearing position, for the shoulder, the bony arrangement of the shoulder has changed. The shoulder joint is now free to perform a wide range and variety of motion. The motion demands placed on the muscles surrounding the shoulder joint call largely for a skilled or manipulative response; consequently, the muscles in the shoulder area tend to be developed below their potential strength in most men and women.

The shoulder joint is classified as an enarthrodial (ball-and-socket) joint (fig. 8.13). This bony arrangement makes it a multiaxial joint with movement potential through all planes. The term *ball-and-socket* is misleading, especially if the bony structure of the shoulder joint is compared to the hip joint. The bones involved at the shoulder joint are the humerus and scapula. From a bony standpoint, the shoulder joint is not a ball-and-socket type of arrangement, because the glenoid fossa does not receive the oval head of the humerus into it. The bony configuration of the glenoid fossa is not deep enough to be considered a natural socket. It becomes a socket by the addition of a ring of fibrocartilage material which, in effect, surrounds the glenoid fossa. This cartilaginous structure is triangular in cross section and is called the glenoid labrum. The glenoid labrum articulates with the head of the humerus. This arrangement of the shoulder joint provides little stability; therefore, the muscle stability at the shoulder joint is more important than at any other major joint of the body.

The articular capsule of the shoulder joint is very loosely oriented. As a result, it adds very little to the overall stability of the joint. Yet it does add to the motility function of the shoulder joint. In the anatomic position, the inferior aspect of the articular capsule actually hangs in folds.

The ligaments in and around the shoulder joint provide some stability. The major ligamentous support is derived from the coracohumeral ligament. This ligament supplies anterior and superior support from the coracoid process to the head of the humerus. The shoulder joint is also supported ligamentously on its anterior aspect by the transverse ligament.

The integrity of the shoulder joint is maintained primarily by the subscapularis, supraspinatus, infraspinatus, and teres minor muscles. These are called the *rotary cuff muscles,* and they attach to the head of the humerus via their distal attachments. Proximally, the rotary cuff muscles arise from the vertebral border of the scapula. The rotary cuff consists of the four tendons of these muscles as they surround and attach to the tubercles of the humerus. The

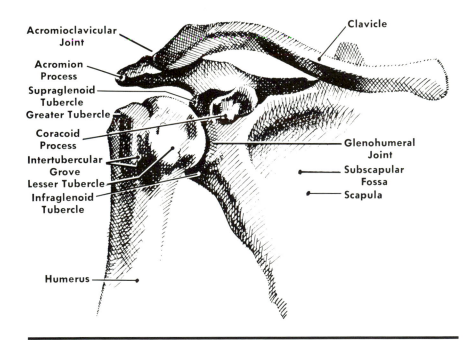

Figure 8.13. The right glenohumeral articulation—anterior view.

subscapularis attaches to the lesser tubercle anteriorly; the supraspinatus attaches to the greater tubercle from above, and the infraspinatus and teres minor muscles attach to the greater tubercle posteriorly. Thus, when all four muscles pull together they maintain the head of the humerus within the glenoid labrum. The anterior muscle provides a medial rotation function. The superior muscle works to abduct the arm, and the two posterior muscles serve the function of lateral rotation. The rotary cuff muscles are seen in figure 8.14.

Additional muscle support is provided by the remaining muscles which cross the shoulder joint. The tendon of the long head of the biceps brachii is of particular importance for anterior stability. In fact, anterior stability of the shoulder joint is probably its most important function.

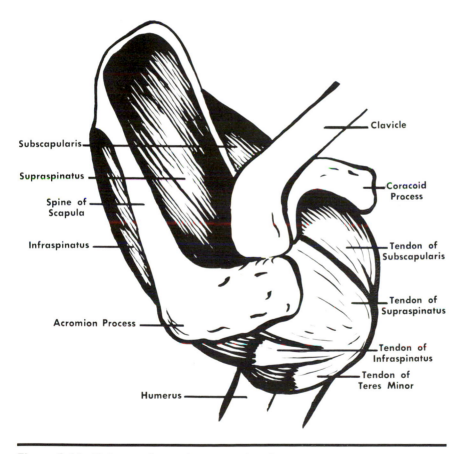

Figure 8.14. Rotary cuff muscles—superior view of the right shoulder. From Logan, *Adapted Physical Education.*

As stated previously, motions at the shoulder joint are accompanied by motions of the shoulder girdle. The shoulder girdle must be stabilized in order for the shoulder joint to move. This is a form of *dynamic stabilization;* that is, the fixing or stabilizing action of the scapula is continuous throughout the movement involved at the shoulder joint. The scapulae are relatively fixed during the first thirty degrees of shoulder abduction and during the first sixty degrees of shoulder flexion. *Beyond that point within these ranges of motion, movement occurs between the shoulder joint and the scapula at a ratio of two degrees to one degree.* For example, in arm abduction from thirty degrees to sixty degrees the humerus is moved thirty degrees, and the scapula is moved fifteen degrees. During the fifteen degrees of movement, the muscles moving the scapula continue to perform a dynamic stabilization function for shoulder joint movement.

Several myological and mechanical processes must occur to allow the humeral head to move freely without jamming it into the inferior aspect of the acromion process. An action of two forces pulling in opposite directions to perform one function has been defined as *force couple action.* This is an extremely important action at the shoulder joint.

Figure 8.15 provides an example of force couple action at the shoulder joint which allows the head of the humerus to rotate without contacting the inferior aspect of the acromion process. The deltoid muscle's line of pull is from the

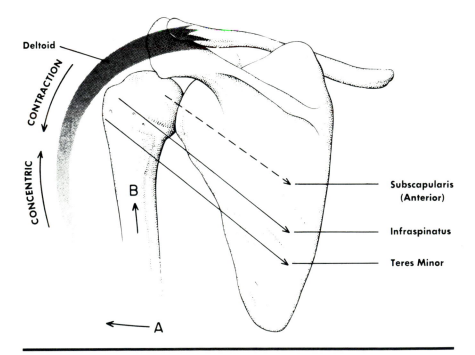

Figure 8.15. Force couple action in the left shoulder—posterior view—allowing the deltoid to abduct at the shoulder joint.

anterior clavicle, acromion and posterior scapular spine to the deltoid tuberosity on the humerus. It has a lateral spatial relationship to the shoulder joint; therefore, when it contracts concentrically with the proximal attachment stable it has a tendency to produce a desirable rotary force vector (A) and an undesirable verticle force component (B) as seen in figure 8.15. If this vertical force were not counteracted, it would jam the humeral head into the subacromial bursa lying immediately below the acromion process. Also, this vertical force (B) would limit the desired rotary force (A) which would produce abduction. In order to prevent the vertical displacement of the humerus due to the contraction of the deltoid, a counterforce is provided by the subscapularis (anterior) and the infraspinatus and teres minor muscles (posterior). These muscles contract together to position the scapula and depress the head of the humerus. This counterforce negates the vertical force vector (B) and allows the humeral head to rotate through the desired degrees of abduction (A). This action of two forces pulling in opposite directions—the deltoid pulling in one direction while the three humeral head and scapula depressors pull in another direction—to perform one function, is an example of force couple action (Inman, Saunders, and Abbott 1944).

Flexion

As an example, shoulder flexion is an essential motion for the basketball player in shooting a one-handed set shot from the free throw line or in executing a jump shot. The right-handed shooter will flex the right shoulder through approximately 120 degrees prior to release. This flexion at the shoulder is necessary for ball control when a defender is applying pressure, and it helps determine the accuracy of the shot by establishing the release angle and trajectory of the ball (fig. 8.10).

The flexion-extension movement pattern of the shoulder joints is very important in running. These rotary motions contribute to the force for linear motion. A more important function, however, is to help the runner maintain equilibrium. An example of this is shown in figure 8.16. The right shoulder of the sprinter is flexed at approximately sixty degrees while the left shoulder is hyperextended. The opposite motions are seen in the hip joint, i.e., the left hip is flexed while the right hip joint is extended. All of these alternating limb actions contribute to equilibrium and linear motion.

Figure 8.17 shows range-of-motion determination for flexion and extension at the shoulder.

The muscles most involved for shoulder flexion against resistance have anterior spatial relationships to the joint. These are the anterior fibers of the deltoid (fig. 8.18) and the upper fibers of the pectoralis major muscle (fig. 8.19). These are both large, superficial muscles with good leverage for flexion. The smaller corachobrachialis and biceps brachii (short head) muscles also contribute some force for shoulder flexion. They both have the same line of pull from the coracoid process to the humerus anterior to the shoulder joint. But, the biceps brachii continues to its distal attachment on the radial tuberosity while the corachobrachialis attaches distally to the humerus medial to the deltoid tuberosity.

The contralateral muscles for flexion are the lower fibers of the pectoralis major, latissimus dorsi, and teres major with help from the posterior deltoid and long head of the triceps brachii. (*In the shoulder joint, the position of the joint during movement and the effect this has on the lines of pull of muscles must be studied carefully.*) The guiding muscles for flexion are the medial and lateral rotators of the humerus.

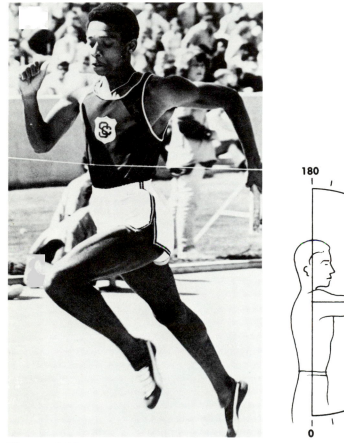

Figure 8.16.

Figure 8.17.

Figure 8.16. Shoulder flexion—hyperextension pattern during sprinting by Willie Deckard, USC sprinter. From Northrip, Logan and McKinney, *Introduction to Biomechanic Analysis of Sport.*

Figure 8.17. Shoulder joint flexion—extension range of motion determination.

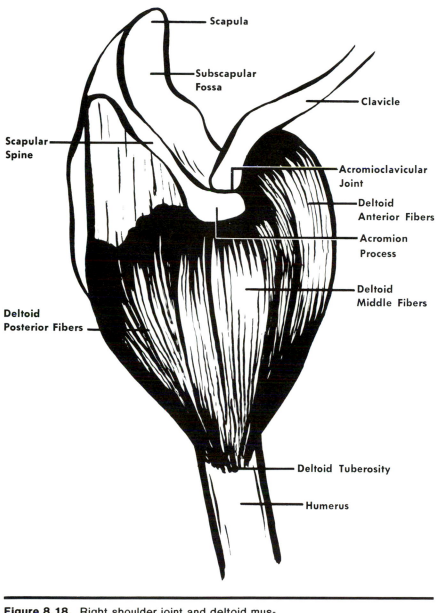

Scapula

Subscapular Fossa

Clavicle

Scapular Spine

Acromioclavicular Joint

Deltoid Anterior Fibers

Acromion Process

Deltoid Middle Fibers

Deltoid Posterior Fibers

Deltoid Tuberosity

Humerus

Figure 8.18. Right shoulder joint and deltoid muscle—lateral view. From Logan, *Adapted Physical Education.*

Extension

Shoulder extension is a motion which can be performed by gravitational force much of the time. As a result, the shoulder extensors need to be given special consideration for strength and muscle endurance, especially by performers who place considerable demand on the shoulder joint during their sport skills. An exercise such as the one shown in figure 8.20 works the extensors against resistance.

The muscles most involved for extension against resistance are the lower fibers of the pectoralis major (fig. 8.19), latissimus dorsi (fig. 8.20), and teres major (fig. 8.20). The posterior fibers of the deltoid (fig. 8.18) and long head of the triceps brachii (fig. 8.20) also contract concentrically to cause shoulder extension against a resistance. When the shoulder joint is in flexion, these muscles have spatial relationships posterior to the shoulder joint. The contralateral muscles are the anterior deltoid and upper fibers of the pectoralis major. The guiding muscles lie parallel to the anteroposterior plane of motion for extension at the shoulder joint. These are the medial and lateral rotators, which cancel out their rotary motions through the transverse plane as extension occurs.

If the shoulder joint is extended slowly with gravity, the muscles most involved in controlling this motion are the eccentrically contracting anterior deltoid and upper fibers of the pectoralis major.

Abduction

This lateral plane motion occurs through a 180-degree range of movement as indicated in figure 8.21 *if* lateral rotation occurs first. Lateral rotation is necessary to allow the humeral head to clear the inferior aspect of the acromion process as the humerus is being abducted.

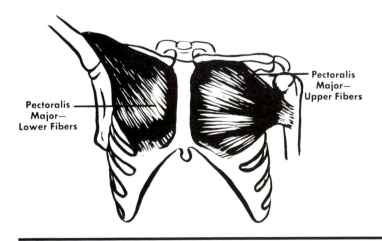

Pectoralis Major— Lower Fibers

Pectoralis Major— Upper Fibers

Figure 8.19. Pectoralis major—anterior view. From Logan, *Adapted Physical Education.*

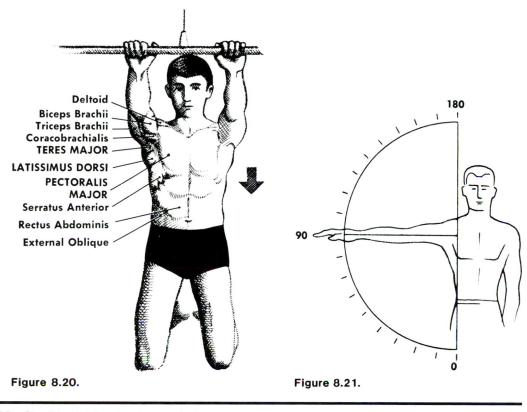

Deltoid
Biceps Brachii
Triceps Brachii
Coracobrachialis
TERES MAJOR
LATISSIMUS DORSI
PECTORALIS
MAJOR
Serratus Anterior
Rectus Abdominis
External Oblique

Figure 8.20.

180
90
0

Figure 8.21.

Figure 8.20. Shoulder joint extension against resistance. (Muscles most involved appear in uppercase letters.)

Figure 8.21. Shoulder joint abduction—adduction range of motion determination.

The deltoid (figs. 8.18 and 8.22) and supraspinatus (fig. 8.14) are the muscles most involved for shoulder abduction against resistance. These muscles have lateral spatial relationships to the shoulder joint. Figure 8.19 shows the pectoralis major. The upper fibers of the pectoralis major can also be considered as being actively involved in abduction when the arm is moved above the horizontal (ninety degrees of abduction). The middle fibers of the deltoid lie directly in the lateral plane of motion; therefore, this part of the muscle has the best leverage advantage. Under considerable resistance, however, all parts of the deltoid contribute to abduction as they apply force on the deltoid tuberosity.

The contralateral muscles for abduction have a medial spatial relationship to the shoulder joint when the humerus has been abducted. These are the latissimus dorsi, teres major, and lower fibers of the pectoralis major. The guiding force-counterforce is provided by the anterior and posterior fibers of the deltoid muscle. Figure 8.22 shows abduction against resistance. The deltoid can be palpated. The supraspinatus is a deep muscle lying in the supraspinous fossa of the scapula and attaching to the greater tubercle of the humerus laterally. It is a rotary cuff muscle.

The defensive basketball player in figure 8.23 has abducted her right shoulder joint approximately ninety degrees as part of her total body motion to divert the move to the basket by the offensive performer. Since this motion was against gravity, the muscles most involved contracting concentrically were the deltoid and supraspinatus. Using the ratio of motion discussed previously to define the interrelationship of motions between the shoulder joint and shoulder girdle, it can be assumed that the right shoulder girdle of the defensive player in figure 8.23 has upwardly rotated approximately thirty degrees for the glenoid fossa to functionally accommodate the humeral head during shoulder joint abduction of ninety degrees. (After the first thirty degrees of shoulder joint abduction, one degree of upward rotation of the shoulder girdle occurs for every two degrees of shoulder joint abduction. The sprinter's right shoulder girdle in figure 8.16 is beginning to upwardly rotate, because the shoulder flexion is just reaching the sixty degree position.)

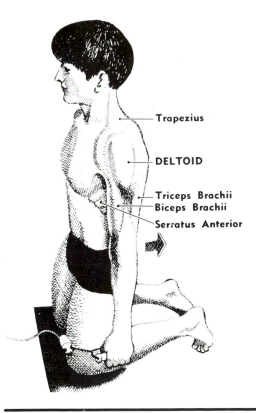

Figure 8.22. Abduction of the left shoulder joint against resistance. (Muscles most involved appear in uppercase letters.)

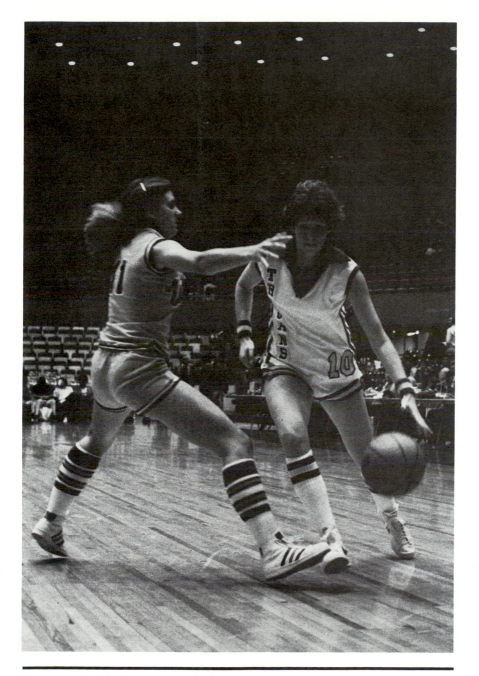

Figure 8.23. Kathy Hammond (10), USC basketball player, drives toward the basket against a determined defensive player who utilized right shoulder and hip joint abductions. The latter motion contributed to a foul. Courtesy *USC Athletic News Service.*

Adduction

The elementary backstroke in swimming, as one example, utilizes strong, concurrent adduction of the shoulder joints to produce linear motion through the water during the glide process. The water provides the resistive force. The muscles most involved for adduction against resistance have a medial spatial relationship to the joint, and they are the latissimus dorsi, teres major, and lower fibers of the pectoralis major. The long head of the triceps brachii also contributes to this motion. The guiding force is provided by the muscles most involved as they pull downward on the humerus at the intertubercular groove. The counter-force is provided by the long head of the triceps brachii posteriorly at the infraglenoid tubercle of the scapula.

Figure 8.24 shows a shoulder adductor weight-training exercise. These muscles need special attention, because they are not utilized too often in normal activities to work against gravity. If shoulder adduction is performed slowly with gravity, the eccentrically contracting deltoid and supraspinatus muscles are most involved for controlling the motion. Therefore, the muscles medial to the joint should be worked against resistance as shown in figure 8.24, especially by performers who place the shoulder area under considerable stress.

Medial rotation

A perfectly-timed medial rotation of the throwing limb's shoulder joint is essential in many skills if the performer desires to apply maximal or optimal forces to the thrown sport object. An example of this appears in figure 8.25. The shot putter

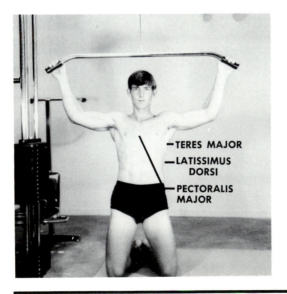

Figure 8.24. Adduction of both shoulders against resistance.

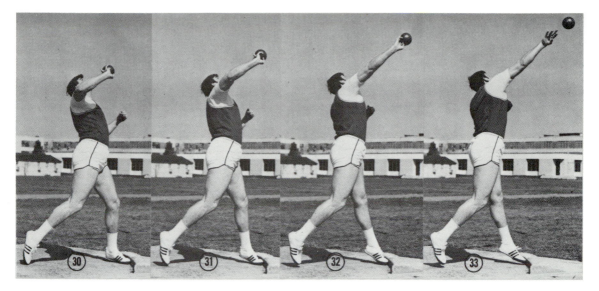

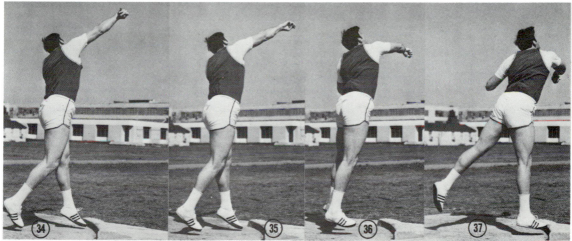

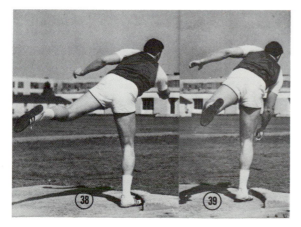

Figure 8.25. Right shoulder joint medial rotation by Randy Matson timed to culminate with the release of the shot. Courtesy Visual Track and Field Techniques, 292 South La Cienaga Boulevard, Beverly Hills, CA 90211. From Northrip, Logan and McKinney, *Introduction to Biomechanic Analysis of Sport.*

times his right medial rotation so it culminates at the time of release. His summated forces have been effectively applied to the shot. This sequential timing of joint motions was one reason for this performer being a "world class athlete."

If the medial rotation is poorly timed by the performer and appears exclusively in the follow-through phase of a throwing or striking skill, the contractions of the medial rotators cannot contribute functionally to the skill. Strong medial rotation is also seen as an integral aspect of many sport skills. The sport of arm wrestling, as one example, is based almost exclusively upon the strength within the medial rotators.

The muscles most involved for medial rotation against resistance are the latissimus dorsi (fig. 8.26), teres major (fig. 8.28), subscapularis (fig. 8.27), and pectoralis major (fig. 8.19). Generally, these muscles attach in the area of the intertubercular groove on the humerus. The subscapularis attaches to the lesser tubercle of the humerus. Their leverage advantage for medial rotation is excellent, especially when the limb is being diagonally adducted through the high diagonal plane of motion. That places them on maximum stretch when the diagonal motion is started.

Lateral rotation

A comparison of the mass of muscle for medial rotation with the muscles which serve a lateral rotation function indicates a considerable potential force difference in favor of the medial rotators. Fortunately, not much force is needed for many

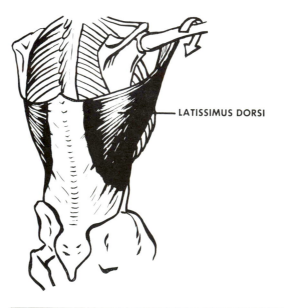

— LATISSIMUS DORSI

Figure 8.26. Latissimus dorsi. From Logan, *Adapted Physical Education.*

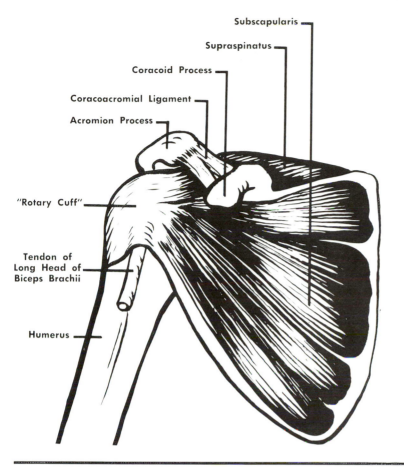

Subscapularis

Supraspinatus

Coracoid Process

Coracoacromial Ligament

Acromion Process

"Rotary Cuff"

Tendon of
Long Head of
Biceps Brachii

Humerus

Figure 8.27. Right shoulder musculature—anterior view. From Logan, *Adapted Physical Education.*

lateral rotations. As one example, lateral rotation during diagonal abduction of the racket limb of a tennis player serving requires very little, if any, muscle activity. This is due to the structure of the shoulder joint, momentum of the upper limb, and the literal weight of the moving limb and racket. The lateral rotation is very important in this type of skill, because that motion helps move the limb through a greater range of motion. This places the contralateral muscles (subsequent diagonal adductors and medial rotators) on stretch for increased force application over a greater distance. Thus, force can be applied to the upper limb for a longer period of time. This adds to limb velocity, which is very important in such ballistic skills as serving a tennis ball and throwing.

Figure 8.28 shows posterior musculature of the right shoulder joint. The muscles most involved for lateral rotation, the infraspinatus and teres minor, have posterior spatial relationships to the joint. They attach on the posterior aspect of the greater tubercle of the humerus, and are the two posterior muscles in the rotary cuff.

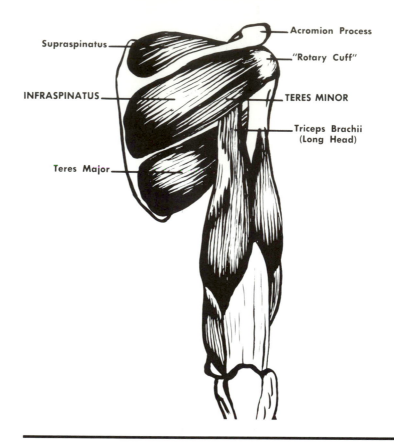

Supraspinatus

Acromion Process

"Rotary Cuff"

INFRASPINATUS

TERES MINOR

Triceps Brachii
(Long Head)

Teres Major

Figure 8.28. Posterior musculature of the right shoulder. (Muscles most involved for lateral rotation appear in uppercase letters.) From Logan, *Adapted Physical Education.*

Horizontal abduction

Movement of the shoulder joints through the transverse plane of motion are not too frequent in ballistic skills. Movements in this plane are common, however, in weight-training or calisthenic exercises as shown in figure 8.29. Moving a limb through this plane during a ballistic skill places considerable stress on the rotary cuff musculature. The centrifugal force is great, and the shoulder musculature can be traumatized easily by throwing "side arm." Most performers move their upper limbs through ranges of motion either above or below the transverse plane at the shoulder, depending upon the skill objective.

The spatial relationships of the horizontal abductors are posterior to the shoulder joint. The muscles most involved for this motion against resistance are the posterior and middle fibers of the deltoid, infraspinatus, and teres minor (fig. 8.29). These muscles can be palpated during the motion. The guiding muscles are the abductors and adductors.

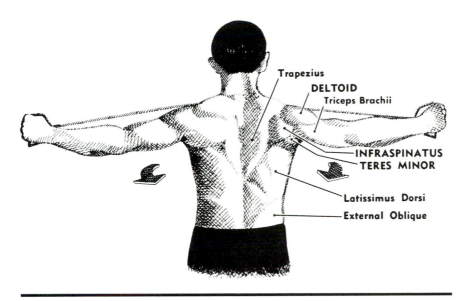

Figure 8.29. Shoulder joint horizontal abduction. (Muscles most involved appear in uppercase letters.)

Horizontal adduction

Figure 8.30 shows the final upper limb action of Jay Silvester, an Olympic athlete, throwing the discus. Observation of frame 33 only could lead to the erroneous conclusion that the discus had been moved through and released in a transverse plane, i.e., the right shoulder in that frame appears to be horizontally adducting. However, analysis of the preceding frames and frame 34 clearly shows that a diagonal plane of motion has been traversed by the throwing limb, which is rather common in skills of this nature.

The muscles most involved for horizontal adduction against resistance are the anterior deltoid, pectoralis major, and coracobrachialis. The short head of the biceps brachii is also involved in this motion. The guiding muscles are the adductors and abductors. An exercise for the horizontal adductors is shown in figure 8.31.

Diagonal abduction

Frame 27 of figure 8.30 shows the right shoulder joint of the discus thrower completely diagonally abducted through a low diagonal plane of motion. There are very few myologic differences between low and high diagonal abduction. Due to the resistance factor, high diagonal abduction elicits greater contractile forces in the MMI which, for these motions against resistance are the posterior fibers of the deltoid, infraspinatus, teres minor, and long head of the triceps brachii. If lateral rotation is an integral aspect of diagonal adbuction, the infraspinatus and teres minor can contribute the necessary force to rotate the humerus

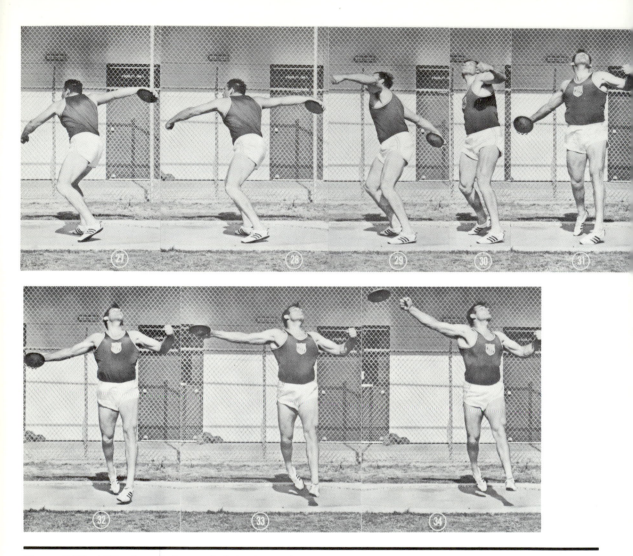

Figure 8.30. Utilization of diagonal abduction and diagonal adduction in the right shoulder by Jay Silvester. Courtesy Visual Track and Field Techniques, 292 LaCienaga Blvd., Beverly Hills, California 90211. From Northrip, Logan, and McKinney, *Introduction to Biomechanic Analysis of Sport.*

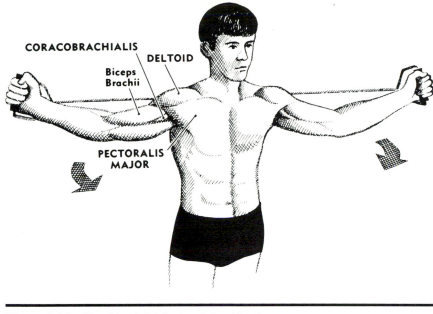

CORACOBRACHIALIS

DELTOID

Biceps
Brachii

PECTORALIS
MAJOR

Figure 8.31. Shoulder joint horizontal adduction.
(Muscles most involved appear in uppercase letters.)

in addition to abducting it through the diagonal plane. The spatial relationships
of these muscles to the shoulder joint are posterior (figs. 8.14 and 8.28).

Lateral rotation is often seen as a part of the diagonal abduction motion.
If the latter is a ballistic motion, internal force by the contracting infraspinatus
and teres minor most likely would not be necessary due to the structure of the
joint. It would probably rotate laterally due to the limb velocity during diagonal
abduction.

Figure 8.32 shows a posed diagonal abduction with lateral rotation in a
high diagonal plane. This is the starting point for a resistance exercise for the
diagonal adductors through a high diagonal plane of motion. The limb is moved
in diagonal adduction against the resistance of an Exer-Genie Exerciser. The
position of the shoulder joint must be taken into consideration in this type of
exercise in order to determine an appropriate weight load. The joint and rotary
cuff are highly vulnerable to injury in this position; consequently, a light weight
load (*two to three pounds*) is recommended for relatively strong performers.
This weight load will help the muscular endurance of the diagonal adductors if
multiple repetitions are used. Flexibility will be increased if the resistance is moved
through the complete range of motion. *Unilateral exercises against resistance
involving shoulder joints must be performed cautiously with very light weight
loads.*

Diagonal adduction

The discus thrower in figure 8.30, frames 28–34, is moving his right shoulder joint through a low diagonal plane of motion (diagonal adduction) against resistance. Myologically, this motion differs from diagonal adduction through a high diagonal plane of motion. The muscles most involved for a *low* diagonal adduction are the anterior deltoid, *upper fibers* of the pectoralis major, coracobrachialis, and short head of the biceps brachii. The guiding force-counterforce is provided by the adductors and abductors.

Figure 8.32 shows the start of *high* diagonal adduction against resistance. The arm would be moved diagonally across the midline of the body at the extreme end of the range of motion. There is only one muscular difference between low and high diagonal adduction, and that difference is seen within the pectoralis major (fig. 8.19). In low diagonal adduction, the *upper* or *clavicular fibers* lift and pull the humerus through the diagonal plane of motion. In high diagonal adduction, the lower fibers of the pectoralis major from the sternum exert the greatest force as the humerus is pulled through its range of motion. All other muscle involvement for these motions is the same.

Diagonal adduction may or may not include medial rotation at some point within the range of motion. The objective of the performance or skill would dictate

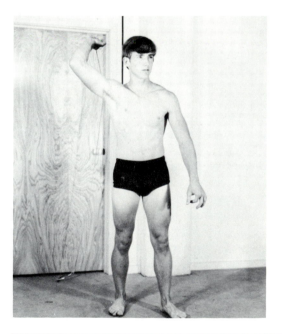

Figure 8.32. A high diagonal plane of motion exercise. The right shoulder has been diagonally abducted. Ultralight resistance is applied through the complete diagonal adduction range of motion.

whether or not medial rotation would be included. As discussed previously, a perfectly-timed medial rotation during diagonal adduction is important to throwing a sport object with high velocity. Since gravitational force contributes considerably to diagonal adduction when the performer is standing, medial rotation is observed during the follow-through portion of a diagonal limb movement. This could be due to the joint structure, limb velocity, and gravity instead of volitional contraction of the medial rotators. During the follow-through portion of diagonal adduction, muscles with posterior spatial relationships to the shoulder joint are contracting eccentrically to negatively accelerate the limb. This helps protect the joints involved and place muscles on stretch for subsequent motions if needed.

Figure 8.33 shows the lines of pull for the shoulder joint musculature.

MUSCLES	PROXIMAL ATTACHMENT	DISTAL ATTACHMENT
I. Shoulder Joint Musculature		
A. Flexors		
1. DELTOID (ANTERIOR FIBERS)	Anterior aspect of the lateral one-third of the clavicle, acromion and scapular spine	Deltoid tuberosity of the humerus
2. PECTORALIS MAJOR (UPPER FIBERS)	Anterior and medial half of the clavicle	Lateral to the intertubercular groove
3. Coracobrachi-alis	Coracoid process	Medial to the deltoid tuberosity
4. Biceps brachii (Short head)	Coracoid process	Radial tuberosity
B. Extensors		
1. PECTORALIS MAJOR (LOWER FIBERS)	Anterior sternum and cartilages of ribs four, five and six	Lateral to the intertubercular groove
2. LATISSIMUS DORSI	Spinous processes of thoracic vertebrae 7–12; all lumbar and sacral vertebrae; posterior lateral and iliac crest; four lower ribs posteriorly	Parallel to the pectoralis major tendon

Figure 8.33. Lines of pull for the shoulder joint musculature. Muscles most involved for each motion against resistance appear in uppercase letters.

Figure 8.33. Continued.

MUSCLES	PROXIMAL ATTACHMENT	DISTAL ATTACHMENT
3. TERES MAJOR	Inferior angle of the scapula posterior	Inferior to lesser tubercle of the humerus; medial to the latissimus dorsi
4. Deltoid (Posterior fibers)	Lower margin of scapular spine	Deltoid tuberosity of the humerus
5. Triceps brachii (Long head)	Infraglenoid tubercle of the scapula	Olecranon process—ulna
C. Abductors		
1. DELTOID (Mid)	Lateral clavicle and acromion process	Deltoid tuberosity of the humerus
2. SUPRASPINAT US	Supraspinatus fossa of the scapula	Greater tubercle of the humerus
3. PECTORALIS MAJOR (UPPER FIBERS)	Anterior and medial half of the clavicle	Lateral to the intertubercular groove
D. Adductors		
1. LATISSIMUS DORSI	Spinous processes of thoracic vertebrae 7–12; all lumbar and sacral vertebrae; posterior lateral and iliac crest; four lower ribs posteriorly	Parallel to the pectoralis major tendon
2. TERES MAJOR	Inferior angle of the scapula posterior	Inferior to lesser tubercle of the humerus; medial to the latissimus dorsi
3. PECTORALIS MAJOR (LOWER FIBERS)	Anterior sternum and cartilages of ribs four, five and six	Lateral to the intertubercular groove
4. Triceps brachii (Long head)	Infraglenoid tubercle of the scapula	Olecranon process—ulna
E. Medial Rotators		
1. LATISSIMUS DORSI	Spinous processes of thoracic vertebrae 7–12; all lumbar and sacral vertebrae; posterior lateral and iliac crest; four lower ribs posteriorly	Parallel to the pectoralis major tendon
2. TERES MAJOR	Inferior angle of the scapula posterior	Inferior to lesser tubercle of the humerus; medial to the latissimus dorsi

Figure 8.33. Continued.

MUSCLES	PROXIMAL ATTACHMENT	DISTAL ATTACHMENT
3. PECTORALIS MAJOR	Anterior clavicle and sternum	Lateral to the intertubercular groove
4. SUBSCAPU-LARIS	Medial two-thirds of the subscapular fossa	Lesser tubercle of the humerus
F. Lateral Rotators		
1. INFRASPINA-TUS	Upper two-thirds of the infraspinatus fossa—posterior	Posterior aspect of the greater tubercle of the humerus
2. TERES MINOR	Auxiliary border of the upper two-thirds of the scapula	Posterior aspect of the greater tubercle of the humerus
G. Horizontal Abductors		
1. DELTOID (POSTERIOR AND MIDDLE FIBERS)	Scapular spine, lateral clavicle and acromion process	Deltoid tuberosity of the humerus
2. INFRASPINA-TUS	Upper two-thirds of the infraspinatus fossa—posterior	Posterior aspect of the greater tubercle of the humerus
3. TERES MINOR	Auxiliary border of the upper two-thirds of the scapula	Posterior aspect of the greater tubercle of the humerus
H. Horizontal Adductors		
1. DELTOID (ANTERIOR FIBERS)	Anterior aspect of the lateral one-third of the clavicle, acromion and scapular spine	Deltoid tuberosity of the humerus
2. PECTORALIS MAJOR	Anterior clavicle and sternum	Lateral to the intertubercular groove
3. CORACO-BRACHIALIS	Coracoid process	Medial to the deltoid tuberosity
4. Biceps brachii (Short head)	Coracoid process	Radial tuberosity
I. Diagonal Abductors		
1. DELTOID (POSTERIOR FIBERS)	Lower margin of scapular spine	Deltoid tuberosity of the humerus
2. INFRASPINA-TUS	Upper two-thirds of the infraspinatus fossa—posterior	Posterior aspect of the greater tubercle of the humerus
3. TERES MINOR	Auxiliary border of the upper two-thirds of the scapula	Posterior aspect of the greater tubercle of the humerus

Figure 8.33. Continued.

MUSCLES	PROXIMAL ATTACHMENT	DISTAL ATTACHMENT
4. TRICEPS BRACHII (LONG HEAD)	Infraglenoid tubercle of the scapula	Olecranon process—ulna
J. Low Diagonal Adductors		
1. DELTOID (ANTERIOR FIBERS)	Anterior aspect of the lateral one-third of the clavicle, acromion and scapular spine	Deltoid tuberosity of the humerus
2. CORACO-BRACHIALIS	Coracoid process	Medial to the deltoid tuberosity
3. BICEPS BRACHII (SHORT HEAD)	*Short Head:* Coracoid process	Radial tuberosity
4. PECTORALIS MAJOR (UPPER FIBERS)	Anterior and medial half of the clavicle	Lateral to the intertubercular groove
K. High Diagonal Adductors		
1. DELTOID (ANTERIOR FIBERS)	Anterior aspect of the lateral one-third of the clavicle, acromion and scapular spine	Deltoid tuberosity of the humerus
2. CORACO-BRACHIALIS	Coracoid process	Medial to the deltoid tuberosity
3. BICEPS BRACHII (SHORT HEAD)	Coracoid process	Radial tuberosity
4. PECTORALIS MAJOR (LOWER FIBERS)	Anterior sternum and cartilages of ribs four, five and six	Lateral to the intertubercular groove

The elbow articulation is composed of three bones: the humerus, ulna, and radius. On the medial aspect, the humerus articulates with the ulna, and on the lateral side the humerus articulates with the radius. The bony articulation between the humerus and ulna tends to be stable. On the other hand, the articulation between the humerus and the radius lacks bony stability. The hinge arrangement of the elbow joint occurs at the articulation between the humerus and ulna. This deep articulation provides considerable bony stability. It also is a limiting factor as far as motion is concerned, because it only allows flexion and extension to occur within the elbow joint (fig. 8.34).

The ligamentous support of the elbow joint is provided by three ligaments. The lateral support is provided by the radial collateral ligament. Medial support is by the ulnar collateral ligament. The annular ligament maintains the position of the radius at its proximal head.

Hyperextension of the elbow is prevented in the normal upper limb primarily by the proximal end of the ulna contacting the olecranon fossa on the distal aspect of the humerus. Flexion, on the other hand, is limited by the size of the muscle mass on the anterior aspect of the proximal portion of the upper limb.

The elbow is well supplied with muscle to add stability to the joint. Anterior stability is provided by the biceps brachii, brachialis, and brachioradialis muscles. The major posterior stability is from the triceps brachii muscle. This muscular support is further enhanced by the proximal attachments of extrinsic muscles of the hand on the medial and lateral epicondyles of the humerus. The muscles arising from the medial epicondyle are the flexor carpi radialis, palmaris longus, flexor carpi ulnaris, pronator teres, and flexor digitorum superficialis (fig. 8.35). The lateral stability is provided by the extensor radialis longus, extensor carpi radialis brevis, extensor carpi ulnaris, humeral head of the supinator, extensor digitorum, and extensor digiti minimi. With the exception of the pronator teres and supinator muscles, these multiarticular muscles also act in the wrist and as extrinsic muscles for causing motions within the hand articulations.

Flexion

Figures 8.35 and 8.36 show the muscles with anterior spatial relationships to the elbow joint. The muscles most involved for elbow flexion against resistance are the biceps brachii, brachialis, and brachioradialis. The biceps brachii and brachialis both lie directly in the anteroposterior plane of motion for flexion at the elbow; consequently, the leverage advantage for this motion by the contraction of these muscles is excellent. Since the elbow is a uniaxial joint, allowing flexion and extension only, no guiding muscles are needed for flexion or extension.

The "biceps curl" is a common weight-training exercise for the elbow flexors (fig. 8.37). The muscles most involved for this flexion of the elbow can be palpated during concentric contraction. When the resistance is *lowered slowly,* these same muscles, by contracting eccentrically, serve as the muscles most involved for *elbow extension,* by controlling the speed and extent of motion. This is an example of reversal of the traditional function of muscle groups. The contralateral muscle for eccentric extension is the triceps brachii.

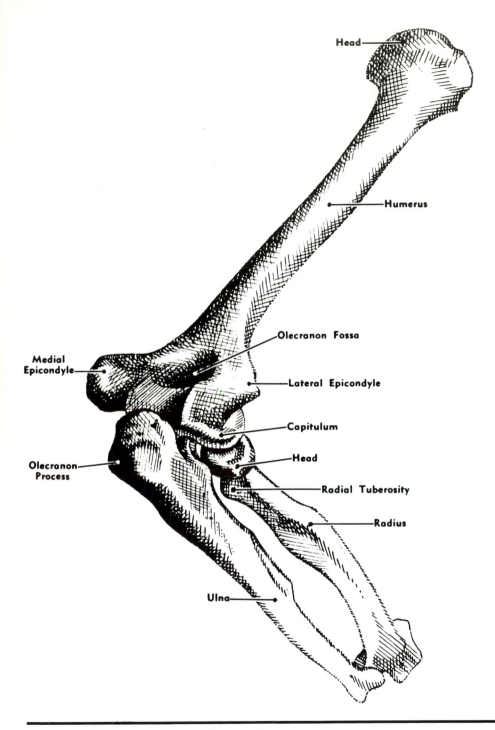

Head

Humerus

Olecranon Fossa

Medial
Epicondyle

Lateral Epicondyle

Capitulum

Head

Olecranon
Process

Radial Tuberosity

Radius

Ulna

Figure 8.34. Right elbow joint—diagonal view.

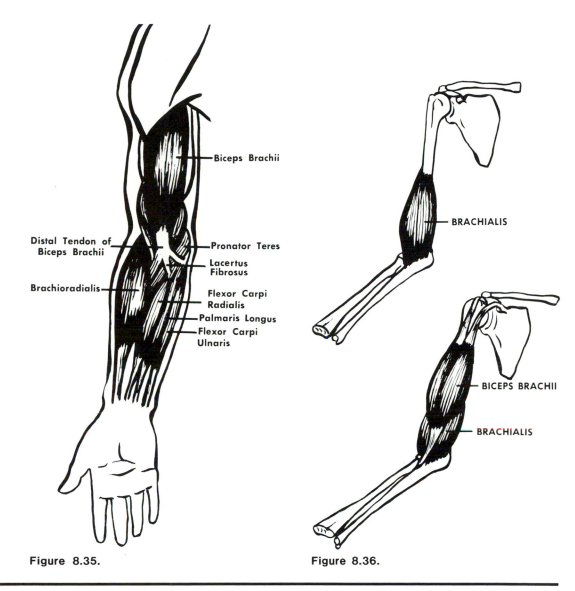

Figure 8.35.

Figure 8.36.

Figure 8.35. Right elbow musculature—anterior view. From Logan, *Adapted Physical Education*.

Figure 8.36. Elbow flexors—anterior view. From Logan, *Adapted Physical Education*.

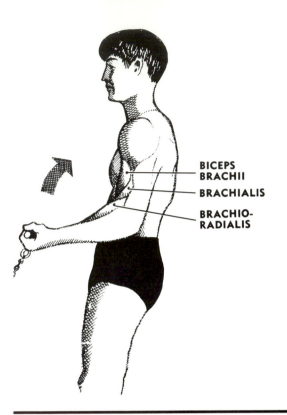

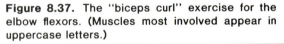

Figure 8.37. The "biceps curl" exercise for the elbow flexors. (Muscles most involved appear in uppercase letters.)

Extension

Elbow extension against resistance is observed in many exercises and skills. The common push-up exercise uses body weight as the resistance, and the push upward of the body is caused by elbow extension. The basketball player uses elbow extension during the jump shot. At the point of impact or release in many sport skills, it is common for the elbows to be extended.

The muscle most involved for elbow extension against resistance is the triceps brachii. It has a posterior spatial relationship to the elbow joint (fig. 8.38). This muscle has considerable strength potential, and is designed to develop limb speed when contracted.

The common push-up referred to above is a good exercise for the triceps brachii, especially when performed on a parallel bar. This increases the range of motion the body resistance must be moved through as compared to the floor push-up. If elbow flexion with gravity is performed to ease the body back to the starting position either on the floor or between the parallel bars, the triceps brachii controls this elbow flexion by contracting eccentrically. Therefore, the posterior elbow musculature can be worked during both extension and flexion motions of the elbow. An elbow extension exercise in a seated position with the subject working against an Exer-Genie Exerciser is shown in figure 8.39. Figure 8.40 provides the lines of pull of the elbow musculature.

There are two bony articulations within the radio-ulnar joint (fig. 8.41). These are described as the articulations between the radius and ulna proximally and distally. The radius and ulna articulate with each other proximally when the head of the radius contacts the radial notch of the ulna. Distally, the head of

Radio-ulnar joint motions

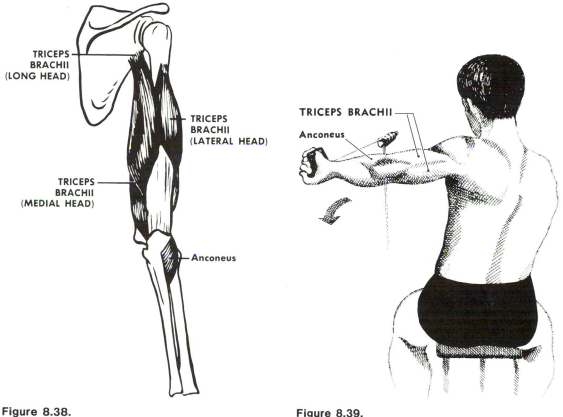

Figure 8.38.

Figure 8.39.

Figure 8.38. Posterior elbow musculature. (Muscles most involved for extension against resistance appears in uppercase letters.) From Logan, *Adapted Physical Education.*

Figure 8.39. Elbow extension. (Muscles most involved appear in uppercase letters.)

MUSCLES	PROXIMAL ATTACHMENT	DISTAL ATTACHMENT
I. Elbow Joint Musculature		
A. Flexors		
1. BICEPS BRACHII	*Short head:* Coracoid process *Long head:* Supraglenoid tubercle	Radial tuberosity
2. BRACHIALIS	Anterior and lower half of the humerus	Tuberosity of the ulna and the coronoid process
3. BRACHIORA-DIALIS	Upper two-thirds of the lateral supracondyloid ridge of the humerus	Lateral aspect of the styloid process of the radius
B. Extensor		
1. TRICEPS BRACHII (THREE HEADS)	*Long head:* Infraglenoid tubercle *Lateral head:* Superior half of the humerus to the greater tubercle *Medial head:* Medial-posterior two-thirds of the humerus	Olecranon process

Figure 8.40. Lines of pull of the elbow joint musculature. (Muscles most involved appear in uppercase letters.)

the ulna articulates with the ulnar notch of the radius. This is an unstable bony arrangement. Between these two proximal and distal articulations, the two bones do not come into direct contact with each other. Their relative relationship is maintained by means of an interosseous membrane. This interosseous membrane lies between the ulna and radius attaching these two bones together throughout their total length.

Ligamentous support of the radio-ulnar joints is provided by the annular ligament. The interosseous membrane also provides some support of the joint medially. There are anterior and posterior ligaments distally, which are called the volar radio-ulnar ligament and dorsal radio-ulnar ligament respectively. The ligamentous support within these joints must be relatively free to allow the bones to articulate with each other throughout the movements of pronation and supination.

The motion of pronation should not be confused with medial rotation at the shoulder joint, and supination is a distinct radio-ulnar joint motion independent of lateral rotation at the shoulder joint. If the relative position of the hands are

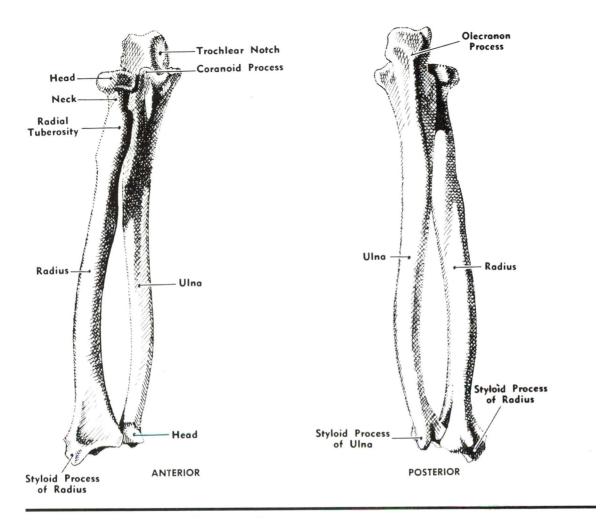

Figure 8.41. Right radio-ulnar joint—anterior and posterior views.

observed only, it is difficult to distinguish between shoulder and radio-ulnar joint motions. The joints must be observed to determine where the motions originate. The rotations of the shoulder joint as well as the motions of the radio-ulnar joint are important in many throwing and striking skills to impart spin to the sport object. Trajectory modifying spin of a sport object is important to achieve high levels of skill in many sports. While the objective is important, the motions of the shoulder, elbow, and radio-ulnar joints which cause the spin desired can traumatize the bones and other tissue within the limb.

Pronation

After the initiation of elbow flexion against resistance, the brachioradialis must be considered as a muscle most involved for both pronation and supination. From either the position of supination or pronation, the brachioradialis will tend to pronate or supinate the radio-ulnar joint to the mid-position when the elbow is flexed.

Trajectory modifying spin of a sport object is important to achieve high levels of skill in many sports. While that objective is important, the motions of the shoulder, elbow, and radio-ulnar joints which cause the spin can traumatize the bones and other tissue within the limb. This is especially true in performers who have not attained anatomic maturation. *As a result, the professional physical educator should not teach trajectory modifying spin skills until his or her students are anatomically mature enough to handle the stress.*

The muscles most involved to produce pronation against resistance are the pronator teres (fig. 8.35) and pronator quadratus. These muscles have anterior spatial relationships to the radio-ulnar joint. The pronator teres is located proximally on the radio-ulnar joint, and the pronator quadratus is positioned at the distal aspect of the radius and ulna. Since the radius and ulna literally wrap around each other during pronation, the contralateral muscles are the supinator and biceps brachii.

Guiding muscles are not required for radio-ulnar joint motions. Extraneous motions are not possible within the joint due to its structure.

Figure 8.42 shows a resistance exercise for pronation. The radio-ulnar joint is being moved from a position of supination to pronation. At the midposition, the brachioradialis muscle contracts with the pronator teres and pronator quadratus to overcome the resistance of the weight. The last few degrees of pronation in this example are due to gravitational force. The supinators can be exercised in the same manner by reversing the exercise. The elbow in this exercise should be flexed at ninety degrees.

Supination

The muscles most involved in supination against resistance are the biceps brachii and supinator. The line of pull of the supinator is from the lateral aspect of the humerus to the posterior portion of the radius. The line of pull of the biceps brachii for supination is posterior to anterior, since its distal attachment is on the radial tuberosity. The tendon of the biceps brachii wraps around the head of the radius during pronation; consequently, when the biceps brachii contracts concentrically to perform supination against resistance, the tendon of the biceps brachii literally "unwinds" and rotates the radius laterally around its longitudinal axis. The contralateral muscles for supination are the pronator teres and pronator quadratus.

The volleyball player (6), in figure 8.43 has moved her radio-ulnar joints into supination. One objective of this radio-ulnar position is to absorb the force of the ball upon impact. By supinating, she provides greater soft tissue surface area of the forearms over which the force of the ball can be more effectively dissipated. She also wants to control the angle of rebound of the ball so it can be passed to a teammate. These skill objectives are met by the stabilized and supinated radio-ulnar joints plus shoulder joint motions.

Figure 8.44 indicates the lines of pull for the radio-ulnar joint musculature.

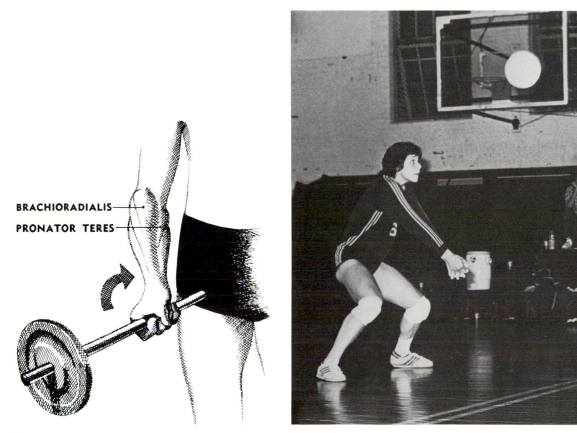

BRACHIORADIALIS
PRONATOR TERES

Figure 8.42.   **Figure 8.43.**

Figure 8.42. Pronation (superficial muscles involved appear in uppercase letters).

Figure 8.43. Anna Maria Lopez (6), USC volleyball player, using radio-ulnar joint supination to control the incoming force of the ball and the subsequent rebound angle. Courtesy *USC Athletic News Service.*

MUSCLES	PROXIMAL ATTACHMENT	DISTAL ATTACHMENT
I. Radio-Ulnar Joint Musculature		
A. Pronators		
1. PRONATOR TERES	*Humeral Head:* Medial epicondyle of the humerus *Ulnar Head:* Medial coronoid process of the ulna	Middle and lateral aspect of the radius
2. PRONATOR QUADRATUS	Lower one-fourth of the anterior ulna	Lower one-fourth of the anterior radius
3. BRACHIORA-DIALIS	Upper two-thirds of the lateral supracondyloid ridge of the humerus	Lateral aspect of the styloid process of the radius
B. Supinators		
1. SUPINATOR	Lateral epicondyle of the humerus	Lateral and upper third of the radius
2. BICEPS BRACHII	*Short Head:* Coracoid process *Long Head:* Supraglenoid tubercle	Radial tuberosity
3. BRACHIORA-DIALIS	Upper two-thirds of the lateral supracondyloid ridge of the humerus	Lateral aspect of the styloid process of the radius

Figure 8.44. Radio-ulnar joint musculature. Muscles most involved for the motions against resistance appear in uppercase letters.

Wrist joint motions

The wrist joint consists of the articulations between the distal end of the radius, navicular, lunate, and triangular carpal bones (figures 8.45 and 8.46).

From a bony standpoint, the wrist is a stable structure. The three carpal bones are received into the radius in a deep ovoid structure. This articulation allows flexion, extension, radial flexion, and ulnar flexion. The latter two movements can be considered as abduction and adduction movements; consequently, circumduction is also possible at the wrist joint.

The wrist is stable due to the arrangement of the ligaments surrounding the joint. There is anterior, posterior, lateral, and medial ligamentous support. Anterior ligamentous support is maintained by the volar radiocarpal ligament. Posterior support is offered by the dorsal radiocarpal ligament. The ulnar collateral ligament provides support medially, and the radiocarpal ligament maintains support laterally.

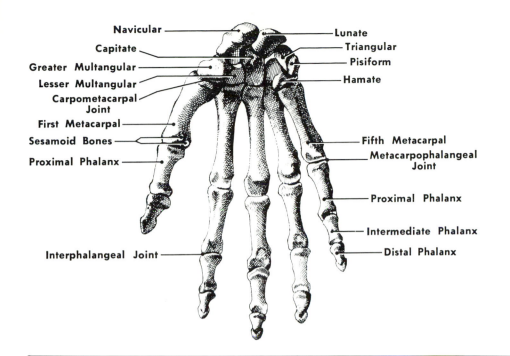

Figure 8.45. Palmar surface—right hand.

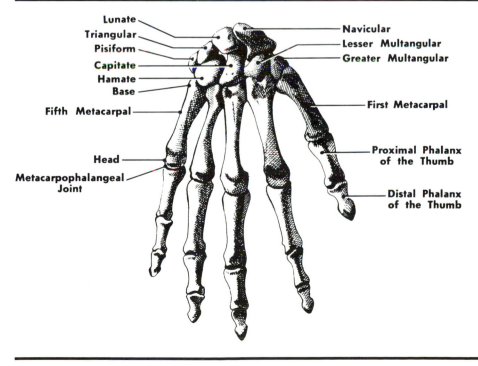

Figure 8.46. Dorsal surface—right hand.

The wrist joint is amply provided with muscular support. There are fifteen *extrinsic muscles* of the hand located on the anterior, posterior, medial, and lateral aspects of the wrist joint. The spatial relationships of these extrinsic muscles to the wrist joint are shown in figure 8.47. This figure shows a cross section of the left wrist with the palm facing upward. The tendons of the muscles are included where they cross the joint enroute to their distal attachments. Figure 8.47 can be utilized to conceptualize the spatial relationships of the muscles which cross the reader's right wrist by observing the anterior aspect of the joint. The discussion of wrist and hand motions is delimited to these muscles only. The intrinsic muscles of the hand are not included.

Muscles in figure 8.47 with anterior spatial relationships to the axis of the wrist joint are flexors when they contract concentrically. Conversely, the posterior muscles extended the wrist joint when they contract against resistance. The medial muscles on the ulna are the ulnar flexors, and the five flexors with the greatest lateral spatial relationships are the radial flexors against resistance.

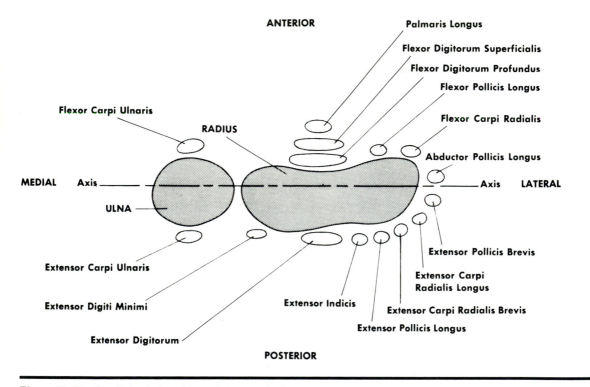

Figure 8.47. Spatial relationships of the extrinsic muscles of the hand to the wrist joint—left wrist seen in cross section with the palmar surface rotated upward due to radio-ulnar supination.

Flexion

The proximal attachments of the wrist flexors are located on or near the *medial epicondyle* of the humerus. These muscles form the contour of the anterior, medial aspect of the forearm. As can be seen in figure 8.47, the wrist flexors against resistance (medial to lateral) are the flexor carpi ulnaris, palmaris longus, flexor digitorum superficialis, flexor digitorum profundus, flexor pollicis longus, and flexor carpi radialis. The contralateral muscles are posterior.

The guiding muscles for flexion and extension at the wrist are located medially and laterally. They rule out ulnar and radial flexions during wrist flexion if desired. The medial guiders are the flexor carpi ulnaris and extensor carpi ulnaris. Laterally, the guiders are the flexor carpi radialis, abductor pollicis longus, extensor pollicis brevis, extensor carpi radialis longus, and extensor carpi radialis brevis.

Extension

The proximal attachments of many of the wrist extensors are located on or near the *lateral epicondyle* of the humerus. These muscles form the contour of the posterior, lateral aspect of the forearm. The posterior spatial relationships to the wrist joint of the extensor carpi ulnaris, extensor digiti minimi, extensor digitorum, extensor indicis, extensor pollicis longus, extensor carpi radialis brevis, and extensor carpi radialis longus make them the muscles most involved for wrist extension against resistance. (The extensor pollicis brevis extends the thumb.)

Exercises for the wrist flexors and extensors are shown in figure 8.48.

Radial flexion

This is movement of the thumb side of the hand toward the forearm. The range of motion for radial flexion is extremely limited. The wrist motion is used, as one example, by a baseball pitcher to apply "screwball spin" to the ball at the time of release; that is, the righthander will apply a counterclockwise rotation on the ball which causes its trajectory to move inward on a right-handed hitter. This is accomplished by using medial rotation and diagonal adduction of the shoulder joint and radial flexion. Due to the structures of the radio-ulnar and wrist joints, the rotation of the ball is around an axis at an angle to the earth instead of parallel to it.

Applying trajectory-modifying spin to sport objects by utilizing radial or ulnar flexion should only be done by adults. These motions, along with the sequential motions in the shoulder, elbow, and radio-ulnar joints, produce great stress on the upper limb. The elbow joint is particularly vulnerable, especially in children and young adults who have not reached anatomic maturation. A radial flexion with shoulder medial rotation and pronation puts the elbow under stress as it extends. The same phenomenon occurs with ulnar flexion, lateral rotation at the shoulder, and supination (curve ball). The ossification of bones in the upper limb is not complete until the individual is twenty to twenty-one years of age; consequently, epiphyseal growth centers are still open in parts of the humerus, ulna, and radius until that age. To avoid permanent damage to the elbow joint and bones in the upper limb, young performers under the age of twenty in sport areas such as baseball and tennis should not be taught to apply trajectory modifying spins to baseballs or tennis balls. The teaching-coaching emphasis during the performer's athletic and anatomic formative years in these and other sports should be on *accuracy and consistency* while using motions which minimize upper limb stress.

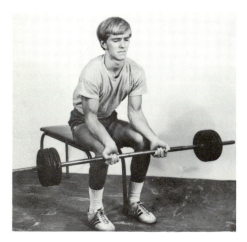

Wrist flexion—Start

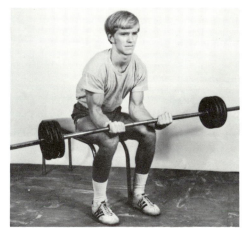

Wrist flexion—Finish

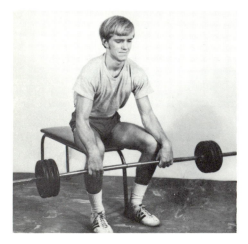

Wrist extension—Start

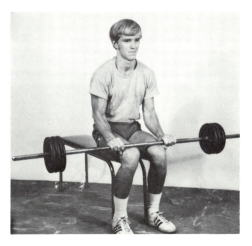

Wrist extension—Finish

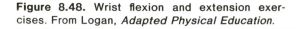

Figure 8.48. Wrist flexion and extension exercises. From Logan, *Adapted Physical Education.*

The muscles most involved for radial flexion against resistance have lateral spatial relationships to the wrist joint as shown in figure 8.47. These are the flexor carpi radialis, extensor carpi radialis longus, extensor carpi radialis brevis, extensor pollicis brevis, and abductor pollicis longus.

The guiding function for radial flexion is provided by the flexor carpi radialis anteriorly. The extensor carpi radialis longus, extensor carpis radialis brevis, and extensor pollicis brevis apply the counterforce posteriorly.

An exercise to develop strength and/or muscular endurance in the radial flexors is shown in figure 8.49. As the weight is moved as shown through the range of motion for radial flexion against resistance, the muscles most involved contract concentrically. If the return to the neutral position and into ulnar flexion is performed slowly, these same muscles on the lateral aspect of the wrist will be the muscles most involved for controlling the motion by contracting eccentrically.

Ulnar flexion

Study of figure 8.47 shows that the two muscles most involved for ulnar flexion, the flexor carpi ulnaris and extensor carpi ulnaris, have medial spatial relationships to the wrist joint. They also guide the wrist through ulnar flexion by ruling out their flexion and extension capabilities. The flexor carpi ulnaris is anterior to the lateral plane of motion, and the extensor carpi ulnaris is posterior. The contralateral muscles are the muscles with medial spatial relationships to the wrist joint.

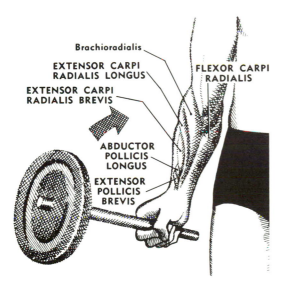

Figure 8.49. Radial flexion. (Muscles most involved appear in uppercase letters.)

Figure 8.50 shows a basic weight-training exercise designed to develop strength and/or muscular endurance in the ulnar flexors. As the resistance is moved through the range of motion for ulnar flexion, the flexor carpi ulnaris and extensor carpi ulnaris muscles contract concentrically. If the weight is lowered slowly to the midposition and into radial flexion, the flexor carpi ulnaris and extensor carpi ulnaris would be the muscles most involved controlling the motion by contracting eccentrically.

Figure 8.51 delineates the lines of pull for the wrist joint musculature.

Metacarpophalangeal and interphalangeal motions

Discussion of the extrinsic muscles of the hand is limited to flexion and extension at the metacarpophalangeal and interphalangeal joints. It is recognized, of course, that some of these extrinsic muscles are also involved with the intrinsic muscles of the hand to perform abduction and adduction of the digits as well as extension of the interphalangeal joints.

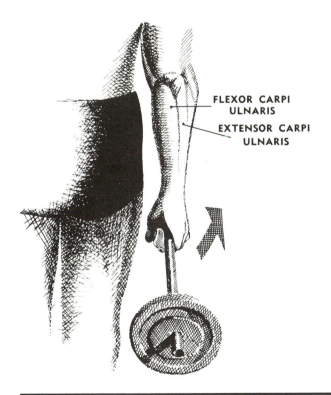

FLEXOR CARPI ULNARIS

EXTENSOR CARPI ULNARIS

Figure 8.50. Ulnar flexion against resistance— posterior view.

MUSCLES	PROXIMAL ATTACHMENT	DISTAL ATTACHMENT
I. Wrist Joint Musculature		
A. Flexors		
1. FLEXOR CARPI ULNARIS	*Humeral head:* Medial epicondyle of the humerus *Ulnar head:* Medial olecranon and upper two-thirds of the ulna	Pisiform, hamate and fifth metacarpal—palmar surface
2. PALMARIS LONGUS	Medial epicondyle of the humerus	Anular ligament and palmar aponeurosis
3. FLEXOR DIGITORUM SUPERFICIALIS	Medial epicondyle of the humerus and the radial tuberosity	Via four tendons into each side of the medial phalanx of the four fingers
4. FLEXOR DIGITORUM PROFUNDUS	Upper anterior and medial ulna	Via four tendons to the distal phalanx of the four fingers
5. FLEXOR POLLICIS LONGUS	Volar surface of the radius below the radial tuberosity and medial epicondyle of the humerus	Base of the distal phalanx of the thumb
6. FLEXOR CARPI RADIALIS	Medial epicondyle of the humerus	Bases of the first and second metacarpals
B. Extensors		
1. EXTENSOR CARPI ULNARIS	Lateral epicondyle of the humerus	Ulnar side of the base of the fifth metacarpal
2. EXTENSOR DIGITI MINIMI	Common extensor tendon of the extensor digitorum	Dorsal aspect of the proximal phalanx of the little finger
3. EXTENSOR DIGITORUM	Lateral epicondyle of the humerus	Via four tendons to the dorsal surface of the distal phalanx of each finger
4. EXTENSOR INDICIS	Dorsal aspect of the ulna	Via the extensor digitorum tendon to the index finger
5. EXTENSOR POLLICIS LONGUS	Middle third of the dorsal aspect of the ulna	Base of the distal phalanx of the thumb

Figure 8.51. Wrist joint musculature. The muscles most involved for the motions against resistance are shown in uppercase letters.

Figure 8.51. Continued.

MUSCLES	PROXIMAL ATTACHMENT	DISTAL ATTACHMENT
6. EXTENSOR CARPI RADIALIS BREVIS	Lateral epicondyle of the humerus	Radial and dorsal aspects of the base of the third metacarpal
7. EXTENSOR CARPI RADIALIS LONGUS	Lower third of the lateral supracondylar ridge of the humerus	Radial and dorsal aspects of the base of the second metacarpal
C. Radial Flexors		
1. FLEXOR CARPI RADIALIS	Medial epicondyle of the humerus	Bases of the first and second metacarpals
2. EXTENSOR CARPI RADIALIS LONGUS	Lower third of the lateral supracondylar ridge of the humerus	Radial and dorsal aspects of the base of the second metacarpal
3. EXTENSOR CARPI RADIALIS BREVIS	Lateral epicondyle of the humerus	Radial and dorsal aspects of the base of the third metacarpal
4. EXTENSOR POLLICIS BREVIS	Dorsal aspect of the radius	Base of the proximal phalanx of the thumb
5. ABDUCTOR POLLICIS LONGUS	Lateral and dorsal aspect of the ulna, middle third of the dorsal aspect of the radius	Radial aspect of the base of the first metacarpal
D. Ulnar Flexors		
1. FLEXOR CARPI ULNARIS	*Humeral Head:* Medial epicondyle of the humerus *Ulnar Head:* Medial olecranon and upper two-thirds of the ulna	Pisiform, hamate and fifth metacarpal—palmar surface
2. EXTENSOR CARPI ULNARIS	Lateral epicondyle of the humerus	Ulnar side of the base of the fifth metacarpal

The muscles most involved in metacarpophalangeal and interphalangeal flexion against resistance are the flexor digitorum profundus, flexor digitorum superficialis, and flexor pollicis longus. These muscles have a spatial relationship anterior to the joint, i.e., they are located on the volar surface of the hand. The contralateral muscles for metacarpophalangeal and interphalangeal flexion are the extensor digitorum, extensor indicis, extensor digiti minimi, extensor pollicis longus, and extensor pollicis brevis. Guiding action within this area must be considered in terms of the metacarpophalangeal joints only. The guiding force for flexion at the metacarpophalangeal joints of the fingers is provided by the abductors and adductors of the metacarpophalangeal joints. The metacarpophalangeal joint of the thumb does not require guiding action because it only allows flexion and extension.

The muscles most involved in metacarpophalangeal and interphalangeal joint extension are the extensor digitorum, extensor indicis, extensor digiti minimi, extensor pollicis longus, and extensor pollicis brevis. It is essential for extension within the interphalangeal joints that these extrinsic muscles work with the intrinsic muscles of the hand. The extrinsic muscles have a posterior spatial relationship to the wrist joint and to the metacarpophalangeal and interphalangeal joints. The contralateral muscles for metacarpophalangeal and interphalangeal joint extension are the flexor digitorum profundus, flexor digitorum superficialis, and the flexor pollicis longus. Guiding action is performed by the abductors and adductors of the metacarpophalangeal joints of the four fingers as described above.

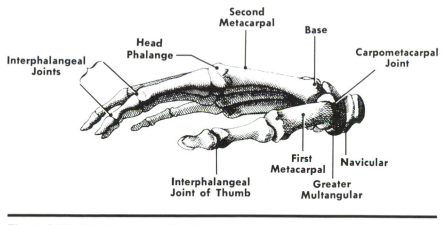

Figure 8.52. Right hand—radial view.

The metacarpophalangeal and interphalangeal motions are critical for the grips utilized to control sport objects and sport implements. An example of this is seen in figure 8.53. This excellent quarterback, a Rhodes Scholar as well as an All-American football player, utilizes metacarpophalangeal abductions and interphalangeal joint flexions to grip and control the football for passing.

The lines of pull for the extrinsic muscles of the hand which cause and control metacarpophalangeal and interphalangeal motions are listed in figure 8.54.

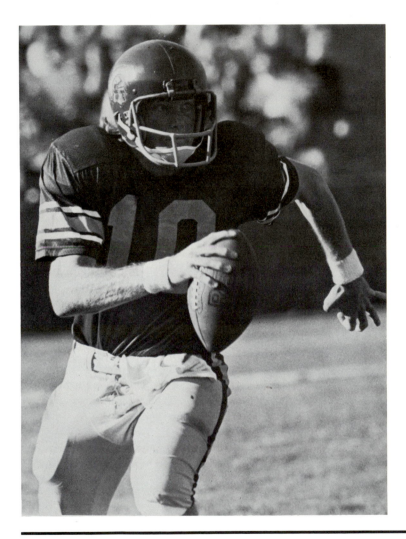

Figure 8.53. Pat Haden, USC quarterback, utilizes metacarpophalangeal abductions and interphalangeal flexions to grip the football for passing. Courtesy *USC Athletic News Service.*

MUSCLES	PROXIMAL ATTACHMENT	DISTAL ATTACHMENT

I. Metacarpophalangeal and Interphalangeal Musculature (extrinsic)

A. Flexors

1. FLEXOR DIGITORUM PROFUNDUS	Upper anterior and medial ulna	Via four tendons to the distal phalanx of the four fingers
2. FLEXOR DIGITORUM SUPERFICIALIS	Medial epicondyle of the humerus and the radial tuberosity	Via four tendons into each side of the medial phalanx of the four fingers
3. FLEXOR POLLICIS LONGUS	Volar surface of the radius below the radial tuberosity and medial epicondyle of the humerus	Base of the distal phalanx of the thumb

B. Extensors

1. EXTENSOR DIGITORUM	Lateral epicondyle of the humerus	Via four tendons to the dorsal surface of the distal phalanx of each finger
2. EXTENSOR INDICIS	Dorsal aspect of the ulna	Via the extensor digitorum tendon to the index finger
3. EXTENSOR DIGITI MINIMI	Common extensor tendon of the extensor digitorum	Dorsal aspect of the proximal phalanx of the little finger
4. EXTENSOR POLLICIS LONGUS	Middle third of the dorsal aspect of the ulna	Base of the distal phalanx of the thumb
5. EXTENSOR POLLICIS BREVIS	Dorsal surface of the radius and interosseous membrane	Base of the first phalanx of the thumb

Figure 8.54. Lines of pull for the metacarpophalangeal and interphalangeal musculature.

Selected references

Bankoff, Dalla, et. al. "Simultaneous EMG of Latissimus Dorsi and Sternocostal Part of Pectoralis Major Muscles During the Crawl Stroke." *Electromyography and Clinical Neurophysiology*, 18 (June-August, 1978):289-295.

Barnes, W. J., et. al. "Isometric Torque of the Finger Extensors at the Metacarpophalangeal Joints." *Physical Therapy*, 58 (January, 1979):42-45.

Basmajian, John V., and Travill, Anthony. "Electromyography of the Pronator Muscles in the Forearm." *Anatomical Record* 139 (1961) :45–49.

Basmajian, John V., and Griffin, W. F. "Function of the Anconeus Muscle." *Journal of Bone and Joint Surgery* 54-A (1972) :1712–14.

Bearn, J. G. "An Electromyographic Study of the Trapezius, Deltoid, Pectoralis Major, Biceps and Triceps Muscles During Static Loading of the Upper Limb." *Anatomical Record* 140 (June 1961) :103–7.

————. "Function of Certain Shoulder Muscles in Posture and in Holding Weights." *Annals of Physical Medicine* 6 (August 1961) :100–104.

Buller, N. P., et. al. "Recording of Isometric Contractions of Human Biceps Brachii Muscle." *Journal of Physiology,* 277 (April, 1978):11–12.

Clarke, H. Harrison, et al. "Conditions for Optimum Work Output in Elbow Flexion, Shoulder Flexion and Grip Ergography." *Archives of Physical Medicine and Rehabilitation* 39 (August) 1958) :475–81.

Coppock, D. E. "Relationship of Tightness of Pectoral Muscles to Round Shoulders in College Women." *Research Quarterly* 29 (May 1958) :139–45.

Dempster, Wilfrid T. "Mechanisms of Shoulder Movement." *Archives of Physical Medicine and Rehabilitation* 46 (January 1965) :49–70.

DeSousa, O. Machado, et al. "Electromyographic Study of the Brachioradialis Muscle." *Anatomical Record* 139 (1961) :125–31.

Diviley, Rex L., and Meyer, Paul W. "Baseball Shoulder." *Journal of the American Medical Association* 171 (November 1959) :12 :1959–61.

Duvall, E. N. "Critical Analysis of Divergent Views of Movement at the Shoulder Joint." *Archives of Physical Medicine* 36 (1955) :149–54.

Ekholm, J., et. al. "Shoulder Muscle EMG and Resisting Moment During Diagonal Exercise Movements Resisted by Weight-and-Pulley-Circuit." *Scandinavian Journal of Rehabilitation Medicine* 10 (1978):179–185.

Hayes, K. C., et al. "Passive Visco-elastic Properties of the Structures Spanning the Human Elbow Joint." *European Journal of Applied Physiology and Occupational Physiology* 37 (December, 1977):265–274.

Inman, Verne T.; Saunders, J. B. DeC.M.; and Abbott, Leroy C. "Observations on the Function of the Shoulder Joint." *Journal of Bone and Joint Surgery* 26 (1944) :1–30.

Ismail, H. M., et. al. "Isometric Tension Development in a Human Skeletal Muscle in Relation to its Working Range of Movement: The Length-Tension Relation of Biceps Brachii Muscle." *Experimental Neurology* 62 (December, 1978):595-604.

Ketchem, L. D., et. al. "The Determination of Moments of Extension of the Wrist Generated by Muscles of the Forearm." *Journal of Hand Surgery* 3 (May, 1978):205-210.

Landa, Jean. "Shoulder Muscle Activity During Selected Skills on the Uneven Parallel Bars." *Physical Therapy* 46 (1974) :120-27.

Little, Ann D., and Lehmkuhl, Don. "Elbow Extension Force." *Physical Therapy* 46 (January 1966) :7-17.

Long, Charles, and Brown, Mary Eleanor. "Electromyographic Kinesiology of the Hand: Muscles Moving the Long Finger." *Journal of Bone and Joint Surgery* 46-A (December 1964) :1683-1705.

Marmor, L., et al. "Pectoralis Major Muscle." *Journal of Bone and Joint Surgery.* 43-A (1961) :81-87.

McCloy, C. H. "The Apparent Importance of Arm Strength in Athletics." *Research Quarterly* 5 (March 1934) :3.

McCraw, Lynn W. "Effects of Variations of Forearm Positions in Elbow Flexion." *Research Quarterly* 35 (December 1964) :504-10.

McFarland, G. B.; Krusen, U. L.; and Weathersby, H. T. "Kinesiology of Selected Muscles Acting on the Wrist: Electromyographic Study." *Archives of Physical Medicine and Rehabilitation* 43 (April 1962) :165-71.

Nelson, Richard C., and Fahrney, Richard A. "Relationship Between Strength and Speed of Elbow Flexion." *Research Quarterly* 36 (December 1965) :455-63.

Ordway, George A., Kearney, Jay T. and Stull, G. Alan. "Rhythmic Isometric Fatigue Patterns of the Elbow Flexor and Knee Extensor." *Research Quarterly* 48 (December, 1977):734-770.

Poppen, N. K., et. al. "Forces at the Glenohumeral Joint in Abduction." *Clinical Orthopaedics and Related Research* 135 (September, 1978):165-170.

Provins, K. A., and Salter, N. "Maximum Torque Exerted About the Elbow Joint." *Journal of Applied Physiology* 7 (1955) :393-98.

Ramsey, Robert W., et al. "An Analysis of Alternating Movements of the Human Arm." *Federation Proceedings* 19 (March 1960) :254.

Rasch, Philip J. "Effect of the Position of Forearm on Strength of Elbow Flexion." *Research Quarterly* 27 (1956) :333-37.

Ray, Robert D.; Johnson, Robert J.; and Jameson, Robert M. "Rotation of the Forearm." *Journal of Bone and Joint Surgery* 33-A (1951) :993-96.

Reeder, Thelma. "Electromyographic Study of the Latissimus Dorsi Muscle." *Journal of the American Physical Therapy Association* 43 (March 1963) :165-72.

Schenker, A. W. "Finger Joint Motion: A New, Rapid, Accurate Method of Measurement." *Military Medicine* 131 (January 1966) :22-29.

Shaver, Larry G. "Relation of Maximum Isometric Strength and Relative Isotonic Endurance of the Elbow Flexors of Athletes." *Research Quarterly* 43 (1972) :82-88.

Sigerseth, P. O., and McCloy, C. H. "Electromyographic Study of Selected Muscles Involved in Movements of Upper Arm at the Scapulohumeral Joint." *Research Quarterly* 27 (December 1956) :409.

Sills, Frank D., and Olson, A. L. "Action Potentials in the Unexercised Arm When Opposite Arm Is Exercised." *Research Quarterly* 29 (May 1958) :213-21.

Slaughter, Duane R. "Electromyographic Studies of Arm Movements." *Research Quarterly* 30 (October 1959) :326-37.

Sullivan, P. E., et. al. "Electromyographic Activity of Shoulder Muscles During Unilateral Upper Extremity Proprioceptive Neuromuscular Facilitation Patterns." *Physical Therapy* 60 (March, 1980) :283-288.

Sullivan, W. E., et al. "Electromyographic Studies of M. Biceps Brachii During Normal Voluntary Movement at the Elbow." *Anatomical Record* 107 (1950) :243-51.

Taylor, Craig L., and Schwartz, Robert J. "The Anatomy and Mechanics of the Human Hand." *Artificial Limbs* 2 (1955) :22-35.

Travill, A. A. "Study of the Extensor Apparatus of the Forearm." *Anatomical Review* 144 (1962) :373-76.

Travill, Anthony, and Basmajian, John V. "Electromyography of the Supinators of the Forearm." *Anatomical Record* 139 (1960) :557-60.

Van Linge, B., and Mulder, J. O. "Function of the Supraspinatus Muscle and Its Relation to the Supraspinatus Syndrome." *Journal of Bone and Joint Surgery* 45-B (1963) :750-54.

Weathersby, Hal T., et al. "The Kinesiology of Muscles of the Thumb: An Electromyographic Study." *Archives of Physical Medicine and Rehabilitation* 44 (June 1963) :321-26.

Whitley Jim D., and Smith, Leon E. "Measurement of Strength of Adduction of the Arm in Various Positions." *Archives of Physical Medicine and Rehabilitation* 45 (July 1964) :326-28.

Wiedenbauer, M. M., and Mortensen, O. A. "An Electromyographic Study of the Trapezius Muscle." *American Journal of Physical Medicine* 31 (1952) :363-73.

Yamshon, L. J., and Bierman, W. "Kinesiologic Electromyography, I. The Trapezius." *Archives of Physical Medicine* 24 (1948) :647-51.

————. "Kinesiologic Electromyography, III. The Deltoid." *Archives of Physical Medicine* 30 (1949) :286-89.

9

Antigravity Musculature

Aggregate muscle action refers to the general concept that muscles work in groups rather than independently to achieve a given joint action. Muscles have two major functions: (1) to pull on bony levers to cause motion at articulations, and (2) to maintain the body in a variety of positions both moving and relatively stationary against the pull of gravity. The first function of muscles was discussed in chapters 5 through 8. The second function is discussed in this chapter.

The term *aggregate muscle action* is used to denote the muscular teamwork necessary at joints in order to perform a specific movement. There is also seen within the human organism another type of teamwork between or among muscles within muscle groups. One of these functions involves the maintenance of the upright, or bipedal, position. This requires a considerable amount of integrated activity among several large and important muscle groups of the body. These muscle groups are primarily the extensors of the major joints of the body. The individual in a normal upright stance will exhibit a very slight amount of flexion at the ankle, knee, and hip joints. Furthermore, there is also a slight forward lean of the trunk in the normal upright stance. There are at least two major reasons for these tendencies toward flexion. Flexion occurs due to the: (1) anatomic or bony structure of the joints at the ankle, knee, hip, and spinal column, and (2) effect of the downward pull of gravity on these joints. Furthermore, the slight amount of flexion observed is necessary for subsequent movements on the part of the individual. What appears to be static stabilization occurring at the major joints of the body is a form of dynamic stabilization, because the body is in constant motion as it reacts to the force of gravity. Each person has a posture to handle this constant force.

It is believed by some physical educators that there is a standard by which posture can be measured for all individuals. This so-called standard is based largely on aesthetics. Historically, it can be traced to studies done in Germany during the nineteenth century by Braune and Fischer. Braune and Fischer calculated the center of gravity of the total body and its limbs by making calculations on two frozen, dissected cadavers. These researchers were not studying posture per se. They compared their findings with a photograph of a living soldier, and they observed that there was considerable similarity between their cadaver findings and the picture of the soldier. Consequently, they stated that the original position of their cadavers could be considered normal. Unfortunately, some physical educators erroneously interpreted the findings of Braune and Fischer to mean that all people considered to be normal from a postural standpoint should conform to the "Braune and Fischer Measurements." Thus, the measurements of Braune and Fischer on cadavers have become "posture standards" in some physical education programs (Rasch and Burke 1978).

Metheny's comments exemplify current trends and practices—there should be no rigid posture standards for all people. She emphasized that each person has one body, and must make the most of it. Posture is a highly individual matter (Metheny 1952).

Although it is obvious that "good posture" is desirable from an aesthetic standpoint, it does not follow that the individual with good posture will be a better athlete because of posture. The mature athlete tends to have a posture related to his or her particular sport if that individual has trained for years to become expert in a specific position or event.

The reason for this phenomenon is the fact that the body tends to adjust or adapt to the various stresses or demands imposed upon it as a result of prolonged muscular activity. Wallis and Logan have called this the *SAID Principle:* SAID is an acronym for Specific Adaptations to Imposed Demands (Wallis and Logan 1964). The great variety of postures observed among athletes is due to the specific bodily adaptations made by each to imposed demands and skill requirements of their various individual sport positions or events—which result in changes in strength, local muscular endurance, cardiovascular endurance, and flexibility. These "postural deviations" from so-called ideal posture standards seen in the athlete as a result of adaptations to imposed demands are not abnormal or pathologic in nature. As a matter of fact, these specific changes at times tend to enhance the skill level of the performer at his position. On the other hand, there are times when such deviations within the "normal individual" or nonathlete may be contraindicated.

Anteroposterior antigravity muscles

The antigravity muscles are the most important muscle groups which make possible the maintenance of body postures in sport, exercise, and dance situations. The antigravity musculature must be considered both from anteroposterior as well as lateral standpoints. Because of the body's tendency toward flexion, as noted above, the anteroposterior antigravity muscles must be considered most important. *Anteroposterior antigravity muscles serve as a "foundation" for the superimposition of skilled movements. Therefore, all of the anteroposterior antigravity muscles must be given prime consideration in conditioning and/or weight-training programs for performers of both sexes.*

There are four major groups of muscles which work together to keep the body in the bipedal position against gravity. These are the triceps surae, quadriceps femoris muscle group, the gluteus maximus and erector spinae muscle group (fig. 9.1). The rectus abdominis muscle is also considered to be an antigravity muscle from a reflex standpoint. The triceps surae muscles, the gastrocnemius and soleus, perform an antigravity function at the ankle joint through plantar flexion. However, it must be noted that the soleus provides most force

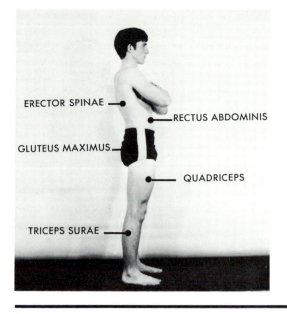

ERECTOR SPINAE

RECTUS ABDOMINIS

GLUTEUS MAXIMUS

QUADRICEPS

TRICEPS SURAE

Figure 9.1. Anteroposterior antigravity musculature.

for this because the gastrocnemius has a function at the knee as well as the ankle. At the knee, the quadriceps femoris muscle group acts as a functional unit to extend the knee against gravity. Within this muscle group, the three vasti muscles are primarily involved in the antigravity function because the rectus femoris is a biarticular muscle acting at the hip as well as the knee. At the hip joint, the antigravity function is performed primarily by the gluteus maximus muscle. Extension of the spine is maintained primarily by the erector spinae group contracting equally and bilaterally. This muscle group is assisted in the antigravity function by the deep posterior spinal muscles.

During the concentric contraction of the erector spinae muscles and the deep posterior spinal group while maintaining the spinal column in the antigravity position, the rectus abdominis contracts reflexly to maintain a relatively constant position between the rib cage and pelvic girdle. Thus, the rectus abdominis also serves an anteroposterior antigravity function. The concentric contraction function of the rectus abdominis muscles is to flex the lumbar-thoracic spine. The antigravity role by these muscles involves eccentric contraction. If equilibrium is lost posteriorward, as an example, these abdominal muscles will eccentrically contract to control extension-hyperextension of the lumbar-thoracic spine with gravity. Within limits, this will help the individual maintain the upright position. If the individual wishes to return to the anatomic position from lumbar-thoracic hyperextension while standing, this involves equal, bilateral concentric contraction of the rectus abdominis muscles. These are the ways in which these muscles perform their anteroposterior antigravity function.

The work of the anteroposterior antigravity muscles is minimized when body equilibrium is maintained as efficiently as possible during motion. This is one reason why a runner, as an example, should be taught to keep his or her center of mass over the base of support as much as possible. The runner should be coached to keep the lumbar-thoracic and cervical spine segments extended. These body segments must be dynamically stable over the pelvic girdle throughout as much of the race as possible. This principle applies just as much to sprinting (figure 9.2) as it does to distance running (figure 9.3). The spinal column must not be hyperextended during a race, and flexion of the lumbar-thoracic segment is contraindicated.

There is a myth that world class sprinters run with a "forward lean" involving lumbar-thoracic flexion in particular throughout the event. The sprinter in figure 9.2 was an Olympic athlete, and his stride and body position is typical of athletes who can attain exceptional linear velocity. The better sprinters simply do not overwork the antigravity musculature by using a "forward lean" once they are in full stride. A forward lean would shorten the stride and reduce speed. Sprinters are slightly flexed at the lumbar-thoracic spine at the start when moving out of the blocks, and there are times when lumbar-flexion will be used at the finish line. However, the "lean at the tape" is a questionable technique and may have a negative effect on time.

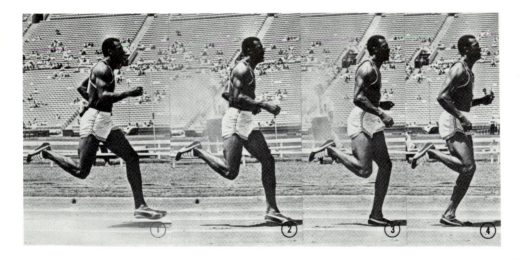

Figure 9.2. The sprinting technique of John Carlos, USA Olympic team, typifies the stereotype of perfect mechanics for running. The extended lumbar-thoracic spine is effective. A "forward lean" would be ineffective, because the anteroposterior antigravity muscles would have to contract eccentrically to help maintain motion equilibrium. Courtesy Visual Track and Field Techniques, 292 South LaCienaga Boulevard, Beverly Hills, California 90211.

If runners move the spinal column posterior or anterior during any event from forty meters to the marathon, the demands on the antigravity muscles are increased dramatically. A "forward lean" involving lumbar-thoracic flexion would mean that the anteroposterior antigravity muscles would have to undergo extensive eccentric contraction to help the runner maintain equilibrium. The erector spinae, as one example, would be conducting excessive eccentric work.

Professionally competent track coaches try to modify running techniques of their sprinters and distance runners to keep their bodies in a state of moving equilibrium as much as possible. That minimizes the need for excessive eccentric control by the antigravity muscles. The athlete is more efficient when the anteroposterior antigravity muscles are utilized primarily to extend the ankle, knee, hip, and spinal column against gravity during a performance.

Figure 9.2. Continued.

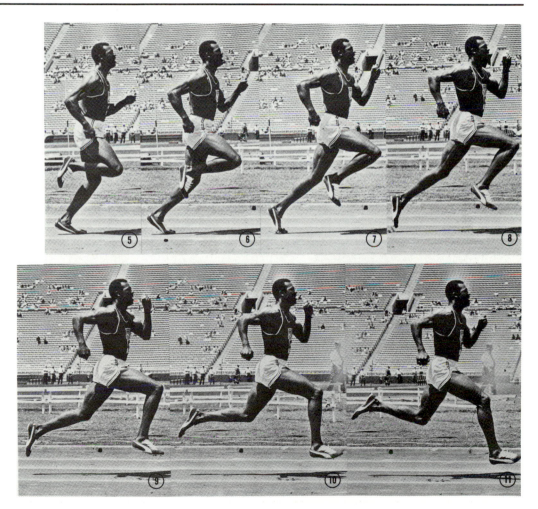

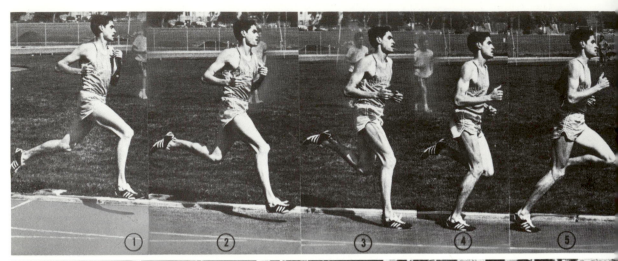

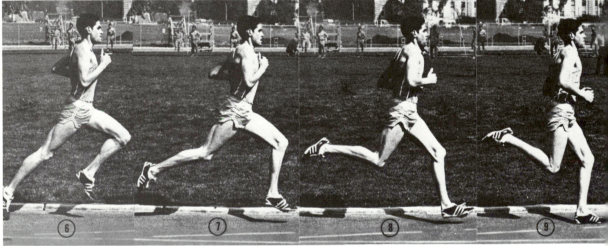

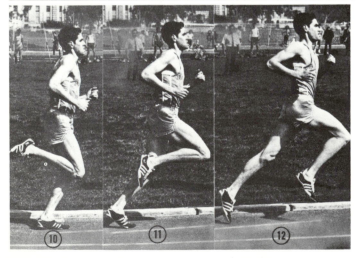

Figure 9.3. The distance running technique of
Ryun, one of America's premier milers of this c
tury. Courtesy Visual Track and Field Techniq
292 LaCienaga Boulevard, Beverly Hills, Califo
90211.

The reader should compare and contrast the running techniques shown in figures 9.2 and 9.3. Both were Olympic athletes. The athlete in figure 9.3 was the premier miler in America for several years. Although the events of the two athletes differed considerably, there are more similarities than differences in their running styles. That is one reason for their athletic success!

The previous discussion regarding running and the anteroposterior anti-gravity musculature relates to linear body motion on flat land. Adjustments in technique must be made for running up and down hills and mountains. As one example, stride length is usually shortened during the ascent on mountain runs, and the stride is lengthened on the descent to accommodate the greater speed as one moves under control with help from gravity.

Uphill running places maximum demands on the anteroposterior antigravity musculature. Figure 9.4 shows runners on the Barr Trail on the Mount Manitou Incline, the first part of the Pike's Peak Marathon. They started at an elevation of 6,336 feet above sea level, and there is a 2400 foot elevation during the first four miles! The 14.3 mile ascent portion of this very difficult ultramarathon takes the runners to the top of Pike's Peak at 14,110 feet above sea level. The Pike's Peak Marathon runner must move his or her body 7,774 feet vertically during the ascent!

Stride length is shortened to move more effectively over the steep trail with its roots, rocks and shale. Due to the body lean, there is a tendency to adjust the center of mass forward over the base of support. As can be seen in figure 9.4, there is slight lumbar-thoracic flexion with gravity requiring extra eccentric work by the erector spinae and other antigravity muscle groups. The stride length adjustment plus the forward lean shifts the foot strike primarily to the metatar-sophalangeal joint level of the foot. This increases the demands on the triceps surae for plantar flexion. The work load increases for the concentrically contracting quadriceps and gluteus maximus at the extending knee and hip joints respectively. These same muscle groups also exert eccentric control over the moderate and sequential flexions at the ankle, knee, and hip joints during this locomotor activity. The abdominal and erector spinae muscles are dynamically stabilizing the pelvic girdle to enhance a functional force-counterforce relationship for body motion between the earth and the marathoner. The runner must have good strength and muscular endurance in the anteroposterior antigravity muscles, excellent cardiovascular endurance, and a spirit of adventure to complete the round trip of the Pike's Peak Marathon!

The easiest part of hill and mountain running is the uphill or ascent portion of the event. The descent is less demanding on the cardiovascular system, but, running downhill is very demanding on the bone, contractile, and noncontractile tissues. The anteroposterior antigravity muscles are placed under great stress during a downhill run. The stride is usually lengthened; there is a slight poste-riorward adjustment of the spinal column by some runners (which may be a mistake if hyperextension occurs); and there is greater body speed moving down the incline with gravity.

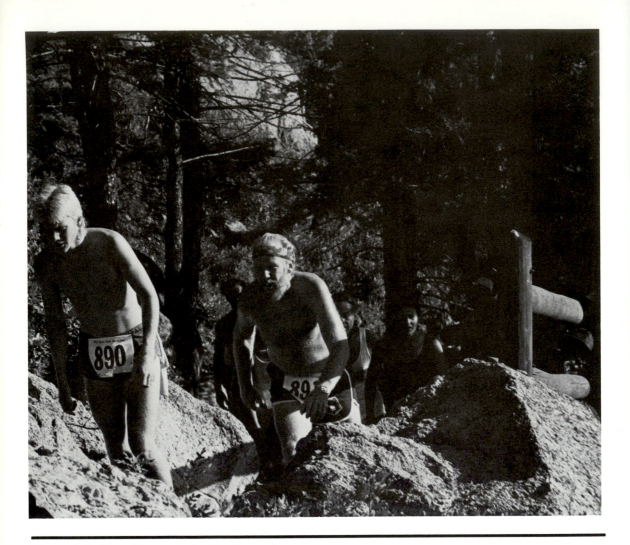

Figure 9.4. The Pike's Peak Marathon places great concentric and eccentric contraction demands on the anteroposterior antigravity musculature. Jon McKinney (890) utilizes the characteristic forward lean and shortened stride during the ascent portion of this race on the Mount Manitou Incline. This ultramarathon starts at an elevation of 6,336 feet above sea level. The ascent on Barr Trail is 14.3 miles to the summit at 14,100 feet. The 14 mile descent is more difficult than the ascent in terms of the stress on bone, contractile and noncontractile tissues. Photo by David Earl Cameron.

To protect the major joints in the lower limbs and to help maintain equilibrium, the anteroposterior antigravity muscle groups must undergo extensive eccentric contraction to meet these objectives during a downhill run. If the downhill run is lengthy (14 miles in the Pike's Peak Marathon), the runner most likely will have some localized muscle soreness in the gluteus maximus, quadriceps femoris, and triceps surae muscles for the next few days.

There is a myth believed by some people that muscle soreness after a downhill run is due to the fact that they "used different muscles." The fact of the matter is that the same anteroposterior antigravity muscles were used on both the ascent and descent. The causes of muscle soreness after long downhill runs are: (1) prolonged, sequential eccentric contraction of large antigravity muscles; (2) unusual joint angle utilization due to increased stride length causing unaccustomed stress within contractile and noncontractile tissues; (3) increased linear velocity of the body with gravity which must be eccentrically controlled primarily; and (4) lack of downhill training. If trained, *specific adaptations* could be made by the muscle-tendon tissue to accommodate prolonged eccentric contraction. Noncontractile tissue of the joints would adapt to the internal and external forces brought on by the *imposed demands* of downhill running (SAID Principle). There is great specificity in training for any performance. One does not learn how to play a trumpet by beating a bass drum!

The reader should compare and contrast the running techinques of the sprinter in figure 9.2 and the flat land distance runner in Figure 9.3 with the form of the mountain marathon runners in figure 9.4. Training for mountain marathons should be done in the mountains for specific ascent and descent work by the antigravity musculature. A track sprinter should run on a flat track to meet the specific demands on those same muscle groups in that environment. All athletes, however, can benefit by first developing these muscles from strength and endurance standpoints through weight training. That will be discussed later in this chapter.

Lateral antigravity musculature

Playing an important antigravity function, but perhaps less important than anteroposterior antigravity musculature, is the lateral antigravity musculature (fig. 9.5). These antigravity muscles perform their movements at the ankle, hip, lumbar, and cervical spinal segments. These muscles help maintain equilibrium and stability of the body laterally when the individual is in an upright or vertical position.

The lateral antigravity muscles at the subtalar and transverse tarsal joints are the inverters and everters. There is a force-counterforce relationship between the medial tibialis anterior and tibialis posterior muscles and the lateral peroneal muscles. This helps provide an antigravity function when the center of mass of the body is displaced laterally.

The knee, owing to its structure, has most of its lateral support provided by the anteroposterior antigravity musculature. There is considerable lateral stability provided by the iliotibial tract and biceps femoris. Medially, the semimembranosus and semitendinosus provide the greatest muscular support to the knee.

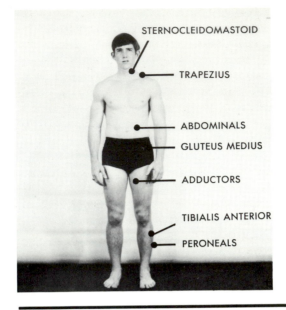

STERNOCLEIDOMASTOID

TRAPEZIUS

ABDOMINALS

GLUTEUS MEDIUS

ADDUCTORS

TIBIALIS ANTERIOR

PERONEALS

Figure 9.5. Lateral antigravity musculature.

The medial and lateral muscular support at the hip joint is provided by the adductors and abductors respectively. Medially, the muscle mass of the adductor brevis, adductur longus, and adductor magnus is considerable. The gluteus medius is the main lateral antigravity muscle at the hip, but it does receive assistance for this function from the lateral fibers of the other two gluteal muscles.

The lateral antigravity support of the lumbar-thoracic spine is provided by the anterior anteroposterior antigravity muscles of the spinal column, i.e., these muscles serve a dual role in the trunk area. The posterior erector spinae plus the three pairs of abdominal muscles provide the lateral antigravity function. Of these, the internal and external obliques have lateral to medial, diagonal lines of pull and provide support in the lateral plane of motion.

The cervical spine's lateral antigravity support comes primarily from the sternocleidomastoid muscles and the erector spinae. The sternocleidomastoid muscles cross through the lateral plane by virtue of their diagonal line of pull. They work with the erector spinae unilaterally to laterally flex the cervical spine.

When considering total body movements in relation to the earth, the terms *vertical* and *horizontal* are used because of the downward pull of gravity. Body position must be described as being either vertical, horizontal, or in a position between these two extremes in relation to the surface of the earth.

When the body is in a vertical position, the anteroposterior and lateral antigravity groups are working together to maintain the position of extension at the joints involved. In any vertical position relative to the earth's surface, the antigravity musculature is mainly involved to maintain extension within the various joints. During a sport skill or exercise, any movement from the vertical to the horizontal position requires an interaction of the antigravity muscles with other muscle groups to maintain the desired position against the pull of gravity in order to complete the sport skill or exercise volitionally initiated. An example of this change of position from the vertical to the horizontal is exemplified when the gymnast, working on the parallel bars, moves from a vertical handstand to a full horizontal body position. It is obvious that during kinesiologic analyses a consideration of gravitational pull must be taken into account when the body is moving through space. Movement problems in outer space are considerably different from movements through space on or near earth. Also, movements within inner space, aquatic movements, are considerably different from movements on land, or in outer space. In all three of these situations there is a distinctly different problem as far as gravity is concerned. The physical educator must be primarily concerned about movement on or near the surface of the earth or within water. And, body position and base of support are also major considerations.

Antigravity muscle strength development

The importance of the anteroposterior antigravity muscles is often overlooked by physical educators during the physical conditioning or training process of students. *These antigravity muscle groups and their contralateral muscles must always receive primary consideration when designing physical fitness programs for physical education students and athletic conditioning programs for student-athletes.* Conditioning is the most important sport fundamental!

Strength of the antigravity muscles is basic, because they serve vital movements and stabilization functions. The strong antigravity musculature serves as a *foundation* for skilled performance. If this foundation is weak in any performer, the potential for excellence will be reduced significantly.

Strength development exercises for the anteroposterior antigravity musculature are performed against gravity through the anteroposterior plane of motion. Movement through the anteroposterior plane against gravity imposes a demand on the muscles bilaterally. Strength development for the lateral antigravity musculature involves movement against gravity through the lateral plane of motion. This type of exercise develops strength within the muscle groups most involved in unilateral or one-side movement. This means that exercises to develop lateral antigravity musculature must be done bilaterally.

To develop maximum strength within the shortest period of time, a bout of exercise consisting of *eight to twelve repetitions* with maximum weight should be done daily. Maximum weight is determined by the individual's ability to complete a minimum of eight repetitions through the desired range of motion. If eight repetitions cannot be completed, too much weight is being used. On the other hand, if the individual can perform more than twelve repetitions, weight should be added to enable the performer to work within the eight-to-twelve repetition range. This procedure should be followed for each exercise in a general strength development regimen designed to improve performance. After the initial muscle soreness, which accompanies any new exercise program, is overcome, the performer will have no adverse physiologic effects from daily strength development exercise. Some people advocate that strength development exercises should be done on alternate days. The basic rationale for alternating days is that it reduces boredom. However, the motivated performer will benefit more from a daily program during the off-season. The type and intensity of daily activity may be alternated, if desired, to prevent boredom. Three sets of each exercise should be completed during each workout period.

Proper execution of resistance exercise should be taught to insure that the most beneficial results will accrue. This should be done according to the best kinesiologic principles to avoid injury. *One repetition weight lifting with maximum weight should be avoided.* It is true that this is the way weights are handled in the sport of weight lifting, but this is done only after the weight lifter has spent years developing overall strength.

Breathing while doing resistive exercises for strength development purposes should be done as normally as possible. The breath should not be held during the more difficult part of the exercise, and there should not be a rapid series of inhalations and breath-holding prior to the lifting of the weight. Holding the breath increases the interabdominal and interthoracic pressures, which may lead to injury.

Figures 9.6 through 9.10 provide examples of weight training exercises for the anteroposterior antigravity muscles. These or comparable exercises for the muscle groups should be included in physical fitness and athletic conditioning programs. In addition, weight or resistance exercises must also be included in these programs concurrently for the contralateral muscles of the antigravity

Muscles most involved
- *GASTROCNEMIUS*
- *SOLEUS*

Contralateral muscles
- *Tibialis anterior*
- *Extensor hallucis longus*
- *Extensor digitorum longus*
- *Perones tertius*

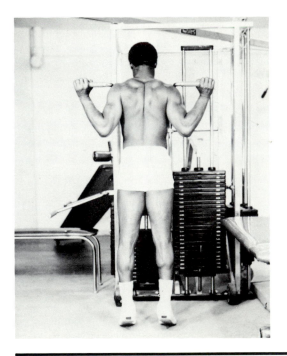

Figure 9.6. The heel raise—plantar flexion against resistance.

muscle groups. It is very important to maintain a functional strength ratio between these muscle groups at all times. As an example, figure 9.7 shows an exercise for the quadriceps femoris muscle group which works these muscles eccentrically and concentrically. The "hamstring muscles" also need to be exercised concentrically and eccentrically during the same workout period. This practice helps maintain the optimal strength ratio between the two muscle groups and contributes to flexibility. (See figure 6.27 for an appropriate knee flexion exercise.)

Figure 9.6 shows an exercise designed to develop strength in the triceps surae muscle group. The tricep surae muscles can be worked during both aspects of this exercise—they contract concentrically during plantar flexion against resistance on the "up phase," and they will control the motion by contracting eccentrically on the "down phase" if the motion is performed slowly to minimize the gravitational effect.

A board approximately two inches thick can be used during this exercise to increase the number of degrees traversed during plantar flexion. The feet should be placed approximately at shoulder width with the toes pointed straight ahead—there should be no medial or lateral rotation at the hip joint.

An exercise to strengthen the dorsiflexors should be included. As an example, there is a "barbell boot" made of metal which holds weight plates. The appropriate strength load can be placed on the boot, and the ankle can be dorsiflexed against that resistance.

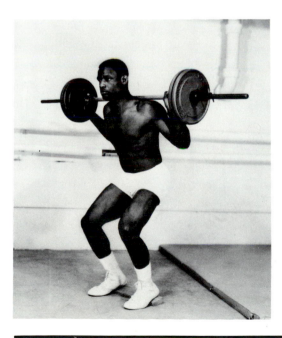

Muscles most involved
- *RECTUS FEMORIS*
- *VASTIUS MEDIALIS*
- *VASTUS INTERMEDIUS*
- *VASTUS LATERALIS*

Contralateral muscles
- *Biceps femoris*
- *Semitendinosus*
- *Semimembranosus*

Figure 9.7. The half squat—knee extension against resistance (Ardie McCoy).

An exercise for the quadriceps femoris muscle group is shown in figure 9.7. The key motion is knee extension against resistance, but this particular exercise also involves some hip extension. Consequently, the gluteus maximus receives some reciprocal benefits. If this exercise is performed properly, the return to knee flexion slowly with gravity will also be controlled by the eccentrically contracting quadriceps femoris muscle group.

There are safer ways to work the quadriceps femoris muscle group. If this method is used, the board should be placed beneath the heels for stability as shown. Also, a chair should be placed behind the performer to insure that the knee flexion does not go beyond ninety degrees. In a class or athletic training situation, there should be a spotter on each side of the barbell to remove it when the performer becomes fatigued or completes the repetitions.

Another knee extension exercise is shown in figure 6.25. If the quadriceps are strengthened, it is essential to include concurrent strength work for the "hamstrings." An exercise to meet that objective is shown in figure 6.27.

A hip extension exercise is shown in figure 9.8. For most individuals, the weight of the legs would not be enough resistance for a strength development weight load. Consequently, added resistance would have to be applied. This could be done, as examples, either with a "barbell boot" or pulley device. The hip joints are extended simultaneously to the position shown and then they are lowered slowly. The latter motion also involves the gluteus maximus and hamstring mucles. This slow hip flexion with gravity is controlled by the muscles with posterior spatial relationships to the hip joint contracting eccentrically.

Muscles most involved
- *GLUTEUS MAXIMUS*
- *BICEPS FEMORIS (LONG HEAD)*
- *SEMIMEMBRANOSUS*
- *SEMITENDINOSUS*

Contralateral muscles
- *Iliopsoas*
- *Pectineus*
- *Rectus femoris*

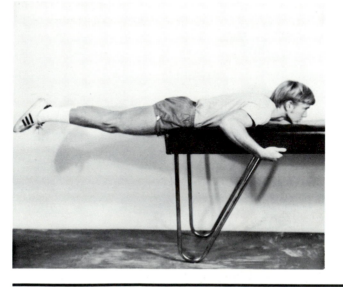

Figure 9.8. Double-leg hip extension against resistance. From Logan, *Adapted Physical Education.*

Since the hip extensors are strengthened, a hip flexor strengthening exercise should also be included in the program. These muscles have an anterior spatial relationship to the hip joint, and may be strengthened as shown in figure 6.34. An Exer-Genie Exerciser is being utilized to strengthen the hip flexors in figure 6.34.

Figure 9.9 shows an exercise to develop abdominal strength. This exercise may be performed on a flat surface. When it is performed on an incline board with the feet held under an object as shown, the holding of the feet involves the iliopsoas as a muscle which contributes some force to the motion. Resistance can be added by: (1) raising the angle of the incline board, (2) moving the buttocks closer to the heels, (3) adding weight behind the head as shown, and (4) adding weight on a barbell.

The abdominal muscles contract concentrically during the lumbar flexion phase of the sit-up. The lumbar extension should be performed slowly. If this is done, the abdominals are controlling the motion by contracting eccentrically. This is the way they perform their antigravity function. When the center of mass starts to fall backward outside of the base of support while an individual is in the bipedal position, the abdominals contract eccentrically to pull the thoracic area back over the pelvis.

Figure 9.10 shows an exercise to develop strength within the erector spinae muscle group. A padded table must be used, and the feet are anchored as shown. For strength development, weight must be added behind the neck as shown in order to decrease the repetitions to eight. During the initial workouts when strength in the erector spinae may be relatively low, the individual should move into a position of lumbar extension only. However, when strength has improved appreciably, the individual may move through the complete range of motion as shown in figure 9.10.

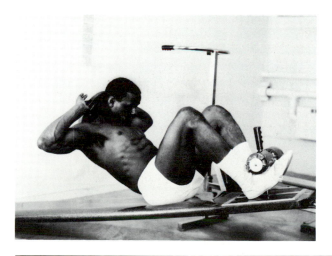

Muscles most involved
- *RECTUS ABDOMINIS*
- *EXTERNAL OBLIQUES*
- *INTERNAL OBLIQUES*

Contralateral muscles
- *Erector spinae*

Figure 9.9. Hook-lying sit-up—lumbar flexion against resistance (Ardie McCoy).

Muscles most involved
• *ERECTOR SPINAE*

Contralateral muscles
• *Rectus abdominis*
• *External oblique*
• *Internal oblique*

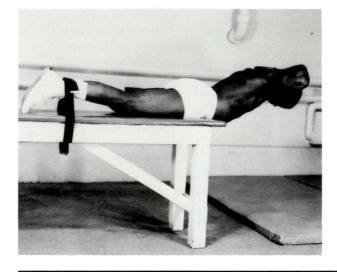

Figure 9.10. Back raise—lumbar extension against resistance.

The erector spinae muscles contract concentrically in an equal and bilateral manner during lumbar extension. This rules out spinal column rotations or lateral flexions. Lumbar flexion with gravity is also a part of this exercise, and this motion needs to be performed slowly to prevent (1) hitting the face on the table, and (2) dizziness and nausea. The muscles most involved for lumbar flexion performed slowly with gravity are the erector spinae contracting eccentrically.

The erector spinae muscle group does not have to work significantly to maintain spinal extension if the center of mass lies within the base of support. They are called upon to perform their antigravity function as the body mass moves forward from the base of support. They must contract eccentrically in this case to help the individual maintain the upright position.

As noted, the erector spinae are the reciprocally innervated contralateral muscles working with the abdominals during the exercise shown in figure 9.9. The situation is reversed during spinal extension shown in figure 9.10. *In summary, physical fitness and athletic conditioning programs should have a core of eight basic antigravity exercises to strengthen:*

1. Plantar flexors
2. Dorsi-flexors
3. Knee extensors
4. Knee flexors
5. Hip extensors
6. Hip flexors
7. Lumbar-thoracic flexors
8. Lumbar-thoracic extensors

Once strength has been developed in the antigravity muscles of performers, the foundation for other conditioning or training parameters is established. This makes it easier to help the performers improve skills and reach their potentials.

Physiologic conditioning is the number one fundamental in all performance areas. The starting point to develop this fundamental is to strengthen the afore-mentioned anteroposterior antigravity muscle groups plus those muscle groups positioned contralateral to them. This conditioning process must also include appropriate flexibility, cardiovascular endurance, muscular endurance, and skill development activities concurrently. Each performer has different and very specific conditioning requirements based on several factors such as the sport played, position requirements, bilateral strength differences in the same muscle groups, and range of motion limitations in joints critical to his or her performance. There-fore, the athletic conditioning program for an individual athlete should be in the form of an *exercise prescription* after the fitness parameters and skill problems have been diagnosed (measured and analyzed) by the professional physical educator. *For example, it is an insult to condition all members of an American football squad exactly the same during an off-season conditioning program.* This approach overlooks the individual needs of the athletes; it is based on the illogical assumptions that all athletes are the same and the position demands are the same for all the players. Beyond the core of eight antigravity exercises, the exercise prescription must become very specific for the student-athlete, if im-proved performance is the main objective. This concept will be discussed further in Chapter 13.

Selected references

Agan, T., et al. "A Method of Measuring Postural Attitudes."
    Ergonomics 8 (April 1965) :207-22.
Basmajian, J. V. "Weight Bearing by Ligaments and Muscles."
    Canadian Journal of Surgery 4 (1961) :166-70.
————. "Man's Posture." *Archives of Physical Medicine* 46 (1965)
    :26-36.
Costill, D. L., et. al. "Adaptations in Skeletal Muscle Following Strength
    Training." *Journal of Applied Physiology* 46 (January, 1979)
    :96-99.
Fenn, W. O. "Work Against Gravity and Work Due to Velocity Changes
    in Running." *American Journal of Physiology* 95 (1930) :433-62.
Flint, M. Marilyn, and Diehl, Bobbie. "Influence of Abdominal Strength,
    Back Extensor Strength and Trunk Strength Balance Upon Antero-
    Postero Alignment of Elementary School Girls." *Research
    Quarterly* 32 (December 1961) :490-98.
Ganslen, Richard V. "Do Athletes Defy the Law of Gravity?" *Sports
    College News,* (October 1955).
Gersten, J. W. "Mechanics of Body Elevation by Gastrocnemius-Soleus
    Contraction." *American Journal of Physical Medicine* 35 (1956)
    :12-16.
Greene, P. R., et. al. "Reflex Stiffness of Man's Anti-gravity Muscles
    During Kneebends While Carrying Extra Weights." *Journal of
    Biomechanics* 12 (1979) :921-928.
Gromback, J. V. "The Gravity Factor in World Athletics." *Amateur
    Athlete* 31 (1960) :24-25.

Hallen, L. G., and Lindahl, O. "The Lateral Stability of the Knee Joint." *Acta Orthopaedica Scandinavica* 36 (1965) :179-91.

Hellebrandt, F. A., and Fransun, E. B. "Physiological Study of the Vertical Stance of Man." *Physiological Review* 23 (1943) :220.

Houtz, S. J.; Lebow, M. J.; and Beyer, F. R. "Effect of Posture on Strength of the Knee Flexor and Extensor Muscles." *Journal of Applied Physiology* 11 (November 1957) :475-80.

Margaria, R., and Cavagna, G. A. "Human Locomotion in Subgravity." *Aerospace Medicine* 35 (December 1964) :1140-46.

Metheny, Eleanor. *Body Dynamics.* New York: McGraw-Hill, Inc., 1952.

Portnoy, H., and Morin, F. "Electromyographic Study of Postural Muscles in Various Positions and Movements." *American Journal of Physiology* 186 (1956) :122-26.

Rasch, Philip J., and Burke, Roger K. *Kinesiology and Applied Anatomy.* Philadelphia: Lea & Febiger, 1978.

Slater-Hammel, A. T. "Action Current Study of the Rectus Abdominalis As a Postural Muscle in Arm Movements." *Research Quarterly* 14 (March 1943) :96.

Wallis, Earl L., and Logan, Gene A. *Figure Improvement and Body Conditioning Through Exercise.* Englewood Cliffs, N.J.: Prentice-Hall, 1964.

Wortz, E. C., and Prescott, E. J. "Effects of Subgravity Traction Simulation on the Energy Costs of Walking." *Aerospace Medicine* 37 (December 1966) :1217-22.

10

The Serape Effect

The serape is a brightly colored woolen blanket worn as an outer garment by people who live in Mexico and other Latin-American countries. A serape is designed to hang around the shoulders and cross diagonally on the anterior aspect of the trunk of the wearer. This is analogous to the direction of pull of a series of four pairs of muscles in the same general region covered by a serape. The four pairs of muscles are: (1) rhomboids, (2) serratus anterior, (3) external obliques, and (4) internal obliques (figs. 10.1 and 10.2).

Synchronized contractions by these four pairs of muscles cause interrelated motions within the pelvic girdle, lumbar-thoracic spine, shoulder girdle and shoulder joint during throwing, striking, and kicking ballistic skills. These motions if great enough can produce the Serape Effect. (It is recognized that external forces and other muscles also contribute some force for the critical segment motions which result in the Serape Effect.) The Serape Effect is a synthesis of several principles from anatomic kinesiology and biomechanics (Logan and Wallis, 1960).

The importance of the Serape Effect lies in the fact that performers who use it during a ballistic skill are almost always more skilled than athletes who either do not use the motions in proper timed sequence or minimize the ranges of motion within and between the segments. (The Serape Effect is a maximum force concept; therefore, it applies only to throwing, striking and kicking ballistic skills.)

The critical moving segments which produce the Serape Effect are the transverse plane rotations of the pelvic girdle and lumbar-thoracic spine. The transverse rotation of the lumbar-thoracic spine during throwing and striking skills utilizing the upper limbs is helped by shoulder girdle and shoulder joint motions within the limb being used in the skills. The timing of the pelvic girdle and lumbar-thoracic spine transverse rotations is critical. They must be observed during the *preparatory phase* of the ballistic skill immediately prior to the start of the motion phase. Furthermore, these two major segments must rotate in *opposite directions* (torque-countertorque) during the preparatory phase of the skill. In throwing skills where the upper limb is moved through a high diagonal plane, as one example, a left-handed performer must have right transverse pelvic girdle rotation concurrent with left transverse rotation of the lumbar-thoracic spine during the preparation phase of the throw (figure 10.4). If that sequence of motions within those segments has occured, this produces the Serape Effect.

The *effect* of the perfectly timed torque-countertorque of the pelvis and lumbar-thoracic spine during the early stage of ballistic skills is to place the muscles to be used during the critical motion phase on maximum stretch. *That is the Serape Effect.* The *effect* of the two body segments rotating in opposite directions concurrently through the transverse plane places abdominal and shoulder girdle-joint muscles on stretch. The force exerted by a muscle is in direct proportion to its length-tension at the time of contraction (muscle length-force ratio). The "stretched muscles" during the preparatory phase become the "force muscles" during the motion phase. (Three examples of the Serape Effect are provided for the reader later in this chapter.)

In throwing, striking, and kicking skills where maximal to near maximal forces and velocities of limbs, sport objects, and sport implements are desired, the Serape Effect adds significantly to the summation of force. As an example, there is an efficient transfer of force from the large, stretched muscles of the trunk, once they contract to initiate the motion phase, into the smaller muscle mass at the shoulder which moves the throwing limb. From a biomechanic standpoint, this is an effective manner in which to summate and transfer force.

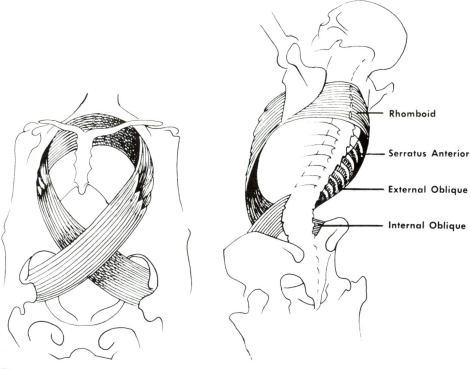

Rhomboid

Serratus Anterior

External Oblique

Internal Oblique

Figure 10.1.   **Figure 10.2.**

Figure 10.1. Serape muscles—anterior view.

Figure 10.2. Serape muscles—posterior view.

In order to describe fully the Serape Effect, the functional relationship of the "serape muscles" on either side of the body must be considered. Starting with the rhomboids, which have a downward and lateral direction and attach proximally to the spinal column and distally to the vertebral border of the scapula, there is a functional completion of these muscles in the serratus anterior. The serratus anterior also attaches at the vertebral border of the scapula. The serratus anterior continues diagonally and downward as it attaches to the rib cage laterally and anteriorly. These two pairs of muscles work together on the vertebral border to move the scapula. Therefore, these "serape muscles" provide dynamic stability as well as movement of the scapula (figs. 10.1 and 10.2).

Continuing in a circular downward and diagonal direction on the rib cage is the external oblique on one side which *functionally* (not literally) continues into the internal oblique on the opposite side. The internal obliques terminate on the pelvis. When the bilateral pairs of these four muscles are considered, there are two diagonals crossing in front of the body working in conjunction with each other. This is a "muscular serape" wrapping diagonally around the trunk (fig. 10.3).

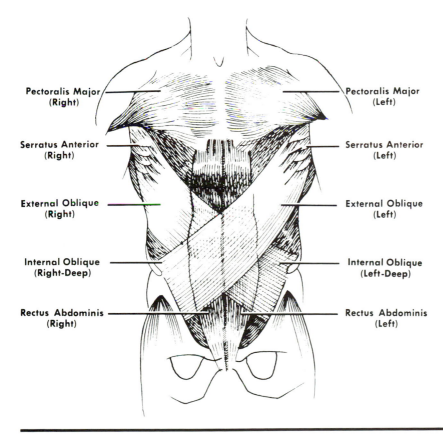

Figure 10.3. Interaction of "serape muscles" with other anterior muscles of the trunk.

Figure 10.4 provides an excellent example of a performer who utilizes the Serape Effect. As noted, the motions which produce the Serape Effect must be observed in the preparatory phase of a ballistic skill. The left handed pitcher in figure 10.4 has just completed that phase, and he is starting to take advantage of the effect of stretched muscles during the motion phase of the pitch.

The pelvic girdle is rotated right through the transverse plane concurrent with left lumbar-thoracic rotation in figure 10.4. Those motions occured during the unilateral weight shift from the left to the right leg during the preparatory phase of the skill. The lumbar-thoracic rotation was assisted by the diagonal abduction momentum of the left upper limb at the shoulder girdle-joint segment. The effect of these motions was to place the right transverse plane rotators of the lumbar-thoracic spine on maximum stretch. The Serape Muscles involved for the latter motion are the left external oblique and right internal oblique muscles. These were reciprocally innervated contralateral muscles during the torque-countertorque of the pelvic and spinal segments in the preparatory phase of the pitch.

As the pitcher in figure 10.4 starts his motion phase, the pelvic girdle is dynamically stabilized throughout the completion of the pitch (DeMille 1962). The lumbar-thoracic spine is rotated right by the stretched muscles noted above plus the right erector spinae. The left shoulder girdle-joint musculature contracts to diagonally adduct and bring the left upper limb through a high diagonal plane of motion. The reader should observe figure 10.4 closely and try to conceptualize the stretch placed on the left pectoralis major, anterior deltoid, coracobrachialis, and biceps brachii (short head) by the action of the left shoulder girdle-joint diagonal abduction plus the pelvic and spine rotations during the preparatory phase for the pitch. Those muscles with the anterior spatial relationship to the shoulder joint are the important diagonal adductors used in the motion phase. They must be placed on maximum stretch to functionally summate force within the total kinetic chain of this skill.

The sequence of motions by the pitcher in figure 10.4 shows good utilization of the timing and ranges of motion at the segments and joints involved to produce the Serape Effect. His only technique problem in figure 10.4 is related to the placement of the right foot during the unilateral weight shift during the preparatory phase. His line of thrust should be toward the hitter. There appears to be lateral rotation of the knee causing a lateral displacement of the foot. This could dissipate some of his summated forces in a tangent away from the home plate area. It could be a control factor in this skill. For those reasons, a coach should adjust the skill by eliminating lateral rotation of the right knee *if* that is a consistant motion problem which reduces some of his overall effectiveness.

A second example will further illustrate how the Serape Effect is utilized by a skilled athlete. This is done through a *basic cinematographic analysis* of a javelin throw (figure 10.5). *Segmental analysis* techniques are utilized in these observations which combine concepts from anatomic kinesiology and biomechanics (Northrip, Logan and McKinney, 1979). The sequence of motions in figure 10.5 should be examined frame by frame by the reader while studying the text of this example of a basic cinematographic analysis.

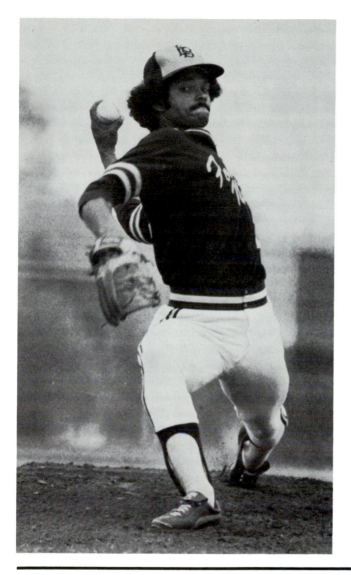

Figure 10.4. Rich Rivera, California State University-Long Beach pitcher, demonstrates a classic example of the serape effect. The right transverse lumbar-thoracic spine rotators and left shoulder joint diagonal adductors have been placed on maximum stretch due to the concurrent torque-countertorque of the pelvic girdle and lumbar-thoracic spine segments plus left shoulder diagonal abduction during his preparatory motion for the pitch. He is just starting into the motion phase. Photo by Bruce Hazelton. Reprinted with permission of the Sports Information Bureau, California State University, Long Beach.

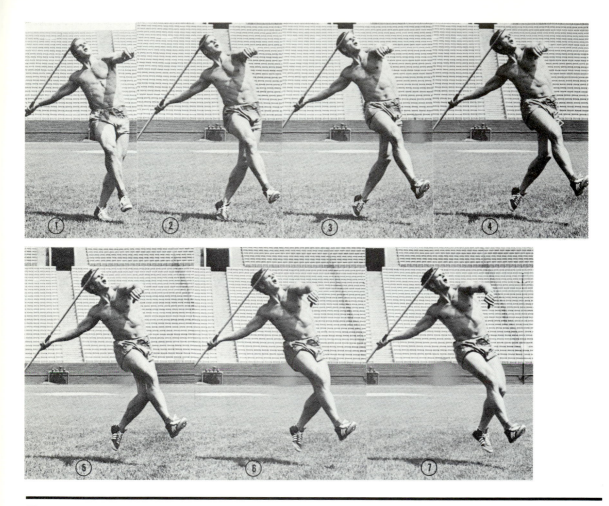

Figure 10.5. The javelin throw as executed by Janis Lusis, USSR. Preparatory phase: frames 1–20. Motion phase: frames 21–25. Follow-through: frames 26–30. From Northrip, Logan and McKinney, *Introduction to Biomechanic Analysis of Sport.* Courtesy Visual Track and Field Techniques, 191 La Cienaga Blvd., Beverly Hills, CA 90211.

Figure 10.5. Continued.

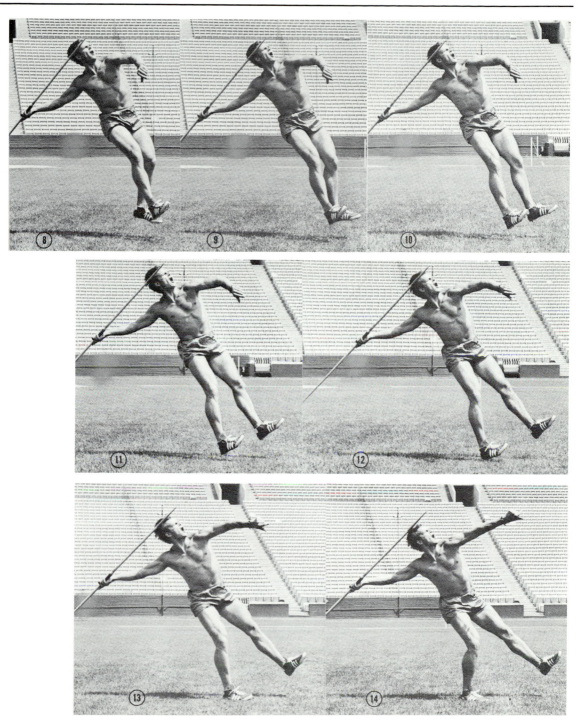

Figure 10.5. Continued.

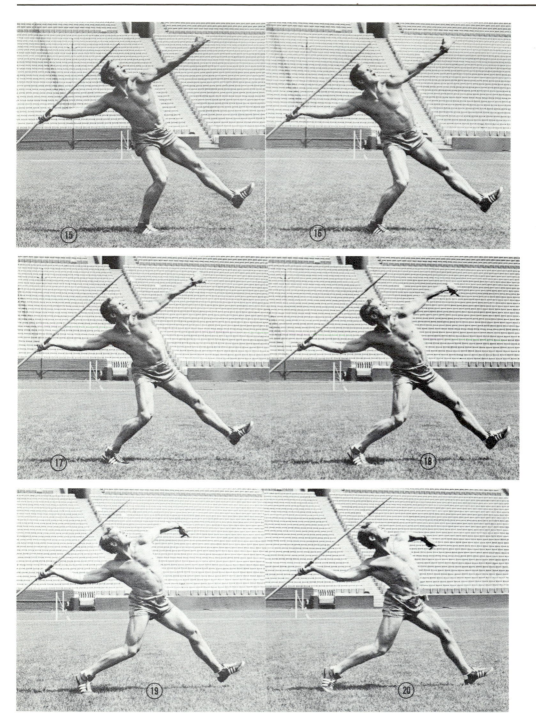

Figure 10.5. Continued.

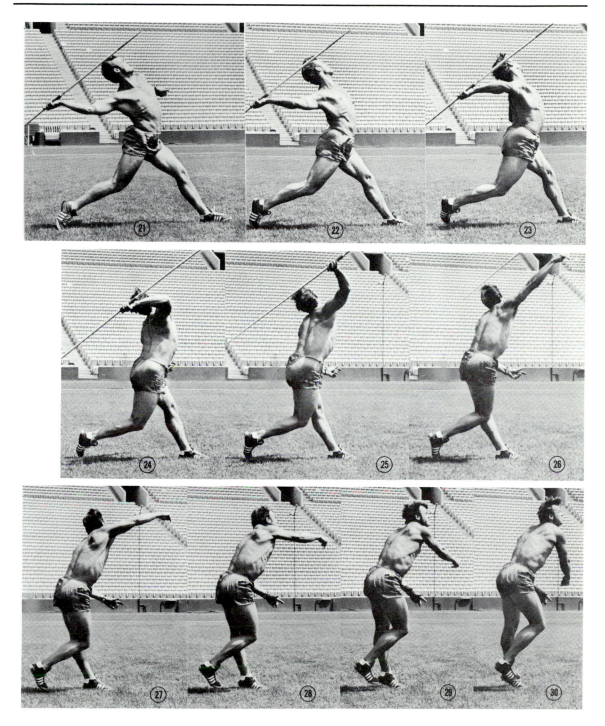

The *preparatory phase* is extended from frames 1–20. Actually, the preparatory phase would begin before frame 1 in the preliminary run which is not shown in these photographs. This extended preparatory phase is a necessary part of the javelin throw because of the complex relationship between the various segment motions which must be synchronized in order to achieve an optimum velocity and release angle of the javelin. Because of the length of the javelin, it is awkward to place the body in the correct position with the proper muscles on stretch in order to achieve a final optimum velocity. Also, this velocity needs to be directed at an angle between thirty and forty-five degrees above the horizontal, and the javelin needs to be tilted slightly above the line of motion in order to achieve proper flight interaction with the air. This means that a very complex combination of rotational movements between the pelvic girdle, spinal column, and right shoulder joint must be used.

Following the extended preparation phase, the *motion phase* is extremely short. The motion phase occurs in frames 21–25, a total time of about one-eighth of a second. After release following frame 25, frames 26–30 show the beginning of the *follow-through*. The follow-through is designed to prevent the javelin thrower from fouling by crossing the line. No formal recovery phase is required since the performance is completed with the follow-through.

The motions of the pelvic region and lumbar-thoracic spine are extremely important in the javelin throw during the final aspect of the preparatory phase and give an excellent example of the Serape Effect.

During the crossover-step portion of the preparatory phase, the coach should observe the magnitude of the vertical lift of the body. If this is excessive, it means that a portion of the kinetic energy gained during the initial run is being converted into vertical motion rather than being retained as horizontal motion. In the example, the maximum vertical position occurs near frame 6, but can be seen to be only four to six inches above the average vertical position throughout the sequence. Throughout the preparation phase, the *lumbar-thoracic spine* is held dynamically stable in lateral flexion combined with a slight rotation to the right. This stability exists through frame 16, at which time both lateral flexion and rotation are increased as the muscles are placed on stretch in preparation for the motion phase. This lateral flexion of the lumbar-thoracic spine is essential in order to correctly establish the subsequent angle of release of the javelin.

Frames 17–20 illustrate the Serape Effect as used by this performer. Left transverse pelvic rotation is occurring in this unilateral weight bearing or weight shifting position. The "serape muscles" involved for this motion are the left external oblique and right internal oblique. There is a concurrent right lumbar-thoracic rotation with right lateral flexion. These motions occur together, due to the nature of the curvatures within the spinal column. The "Serape Muscles" involved for right lumbar-thoracic rotation are the left external oblique and right internal oblique. These musclss are assisted with this rotation by the momentum of diagonal abduction occurring within the right shoulder. The right serratus anterior and rhomboids are functioning as muscles most involved and contra-lateral muscles respectively to upwardly rotate the right scapula at this point in the throw.

The Serape Effect on the *left* lumbar-thoracic spinal rotators can be appreciated by observing frame 20 and their subsequent activity in the frames which follow. Left lumbar-thoracic rotation is the critical force movement during the motion phase. The "serape muscles" involved for this motion are the right external oblique and left internal oblique. During the preceding left transverse pelvic and right lumbar-thoracic rotations (torque-countertorque), these muscles served as contralateral muscles during the motions. Consequently, these muscles were placed on maximum stretch during the preparatory phase of the throw. This is of utmost importance to the outcome of the performance. *Muscles must be placed on their greatest length in order to exert the greatest internal force.* If left transverse pelvic rotation and right lumbar-thoracic rotation were eliminated or minimized during the preparation phase of the throw, the left lumbar-thoracic spinal rotators would not be placed on their greatest length. Thus, potential force to be applied to the javelin at release would be decreased, resulting in a loss of velocity and a decrease in distance. Pragmatically, the Serape Effect in ballistic skills is very important.

The placement of the *base of support*, especially during the final step, is important in allowing the proper set of rotations to take place without loss of either linear or angular momenta. The final placement of the right foot in this sequence is observed in frame 13. It would appear that during this performance, placement was made with the foot somewhat far forward with respect to the center of gravity of the performer. As observed in frame 13, the backward lean of the performer would mean that any forces being transferred from the ground would have a horizontal component which would tend to cancel a part of the horizontal velocity gained during the run. It probably would be better if the landing could occur with the total body position being more as observed in frame 14.

Placement of the left foot during the final weight-shifting process, as observed in frame 20, is very important. The foot must be to the left of the midline of the body and pointed in the intended direction of the throw in order to provide stability and allow pelvic and spinal rotations to occur. Foot placements need to be made with a timing which allows a smooth shifting of weight from one to the other with minimum loss of horizontal velocity.

The *head and cervical spine* are maintained in a relatively stable position through most of the preparatory phase, as indicated in frames 1–20. In frames 21–25, an extreme cervical rotation is observed. This adds to the rotation of the lumbar-thoracic region and also aids in diagonal adduction of the right shoulder joint. This is another example of the use of the torque-countertorque principle in order to ultimately increase the total velocity of the throwing limb. At the point of release seen in frame 26 in this sequence, the performer is not looking in the direction the javelin will fly. If he attempts to look in the direction of motion too soon, the summation of motions critical to this event will be interrupted. The head does not return to the position which allows the performer to observe javelin flight until frame 28, or approximately one-tenth of a second *after* release.

The functions of the *left arm* throughout this performance are to help provide balance and add to the torque-countertorque sequence of motions within the final throwing phase. Throwing with force involves both arms.

In frames 1–10, the left shoulder is in a position of diagonal adduction as an aid to equilibrium of the body during this phase of the performance. In frames 11–21, the left shoulder is diagonally abducted, and the left elbow moves into extension. This places muscles on stretch and aids in the final production of torque within the spinal column for rotation of the lumbar-thoracic spine and the final medial rotation and diagonal adduction of the right shoulder. In frames 22–30, although the left arm is hidden by the body, the left shoulder is adducted through the lateral plane in order to provide a balance mechanism to offset ballistic motions of other body segments. Flexion occurs at the left elbow as a result of the ballistic motion of the right arm through the crossed-extensor relfex.

Throughout the initial phases of the performance, through frame 16, the *right arm* is diagonally abducted in a stable position. The wrist is also stabilized in slight hyperextension in order to maintain the desired angle for the javelin with respect to the horizontal. Any wobbling motion of the javelin during the preparatory phase results not only in inefficient uses of energy by the performer, but also may contribute to poor flight characteristics of the javelin after release. Since orientation of the javelin is so critical and a spin about the longitudinal axis must be given in the motion phase, it is highly important that the orientation of the javelin during the preparatory phase be a fixed part of the performance.

Frames 17–25 provide an example of development of angular momentum through adduction of the right shoulder joint through a high diagonal plane. There is a subsequent increase in limb velocity by a decrease of the moment of inertia through flexion at the right elbow. This flexion is observed in frames 23 and 24 of the sequence. Also occurring in frames 24 and 25 is medial rotation of the right shoulder joint. This provides a final velocity increase prior to release of the javelin. As discussed previously, it is necessary to observe that this medial rotation takes place *before* the *release* of the object. If it is delayed until the follow-through phase, it cannot contribute any forces and increase velocity of the sport object. At that point, medial rotation of the throwing limb would contribute to the aesthetic aspect of the performance and negative acceleration of the throwing limb.

During the crossover, diagonal action of the *legs,* the performer in this sequence is minimizing vertical lift while maintaining a horizontal velocity by an inversion of the left transverse tarsal and subtalar joints. A complete plantar flexion of the left ankle at this point would provide an undesired vertical component of velocity. This would result in a loss of horizontal velocity. During the landing on the right foot, as observed in frames 13–15, it is necessary that the right knee joint undergo flexion. This motion is eccentrically controlled by the right quadriceps muscle group. This places these muscles on stretch for subsequent powerful extension of the right knee joint observed in frames 18–21. This knee extension provides the push against the ground and precedes the pelvic rotation so vital to the Serape Effect. Frame 20 shows the leg position which provides the optimal horizontal force component for initiating this rotation.

At the same time, there is a minimizing effect on any vertical component of motion at this stage of the performance. If the performer simply pivots through this step, it will be extremely difficult to obtain the necessary pelvic rotation to provide an optimum Serape Effect and subsequent ballistic rotations.

In frames 18–20, the left hip is placed in slight flexion, with the knee stabilized in an extended position. This provides the fulcrum over which the final rotation takes place. As the body moves forward, the hip gradually returns to an extended postion.

The javelin throw is an excellent example of the concept of a sequence of motions timed to produce a skilled performance. An optimum performance requires a force generated from the right leg which provides a rotation for the pelvic region. In turn, this produces rotations of the lumbar-thoracic spine followed by diagonal-plane motions at the shoulder and a flexion at the elbow. All these motions must be performed in proper sequence in order to obtain a maximum performance.

The Serape Effect also plays a major role in forceful or ballistic movements of the lower limbs. When forceful movements of the lower limbs are seen, such as in punting or kicking, there is a reversal of the sequential movements of body segments. For example, during a ballistic kicking motion, transverse rotation of the lumbar-thoracic spine (torque) occurs before the opposite direction transverse rotation within the pelvic gridle (countertorque). The effect, however, remains the same. The critical muscles for the motion phase are placed on stretch. This adds to the potential force which gives the kicking limb greater velocity.

Some American football coaches teach their punters to move the kicking limb through an anteroposterior plane of motion. Although this concept is taught to some athletes, in reality the movement pattern of the kicking limb in the skilled punter is diagonal in nature. The reason for this lies in the fact that the spatial relationship of the muscles to the hip joint, particularly the adductors, will tend to pull the kicking lower limb through the diagonal plane of motion at the hip. Another factor contributing to this movement through a diagonal plane is the multiaxial arrangement of the hip joint.

Since the soccer style of kicking obviously generates more force and employs diagonal plane motion by the kicking limb (figure 10.6), it will be used as the third example of the Serape Effect.

Figure 10.6 is actually four frames of sixteen millimeter film taken from analysis film of a soccer-style place kicker during skill drills from short yardage for field goals in American football. The end of the preparatory phase is shown in (a). The start and end of the motion phase is depicted in (b) and (c) respectively, and the follow-through is seen in (d). The quality of the film is not too good, but it is included because it is typical of film or videotape taken for the purpose stated above. The reader should refer to figure 10.6 as needed while reading the text material explaining how the Serape Effect is derived by this kicking style.

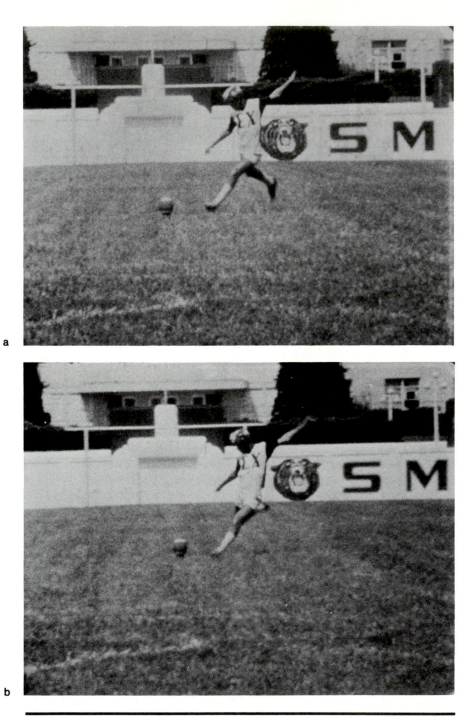

a

b

Figure 10.6. The soccer-style kick: (a) preparatory phase, (b) motion phase, (c) impact, and (d) follow-through.

Figure 10.6. Continued.

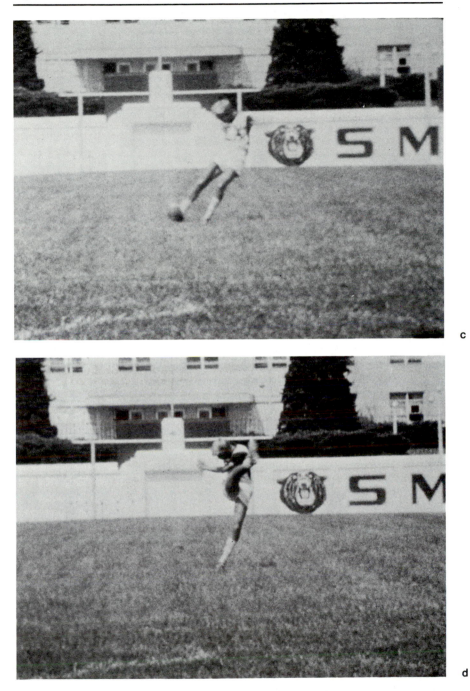

c

d

When the kicker transfers weight (unilateral weight shift) to the left lower limb or supportive limb during the preparatory phase, it should be noted that the left shoulder joint is being diagonally abducted rather forcefully. This is an important motion often overlooked by coaches. The combination of force from this shoulder motion plus concurrent concentric contraction of the right external oblique and left internal oblique Serape Muscles causes left lumbar-thoracic rotation through the transverse plane. The left external and right internal oblique muscles are being reciprocally innervated and placed on stretch. There is concurrent right pelvic girdle rotation caused primarily by muscular action and the force of right hip joint diagonal abduction during the preparatory phase.

The torque-countertorque of the left transverse rotation of the lumbar-thoracic spine and right transverse rotation of the pelvic girdle has the effect of placing the right internal oblique and left external oblique on stretch. While the range of motion in these moving segments are not as great as those seen in the two previous throwing skill examples, the effect of the muscular stretch as it relates to subsequent force summation and transfer to the kicking limb is equally important.

The Serape Effect result is seen in the motion phase as the stretched Serape Muscles of the pelvis and spine contract concentrically to cause left transverse rotation of the pelvis and right transverse rotation of the lumbar-thoracic spine. Most of these forces generated in this kinetic chain are ultimately transferred to the kicking limb to move it into a high velocity diagonal adduction. The ball is the recipient of these internally and externally generated forces.

It is interesting to note the total contribution of the *left upper limb* to the kicking performance seen in figure 10.6. The diagonal abduction-diagonal adduction sequence contributes to the summation of forces, spinal rotation, and dynamic equilibrium. The action-reaction of left upper limb and right lower limb in the follow-through is very important for equilibrium and skilled performance.

The Serape Effect is a synthesis of a few major principles of analytic kinesiology designed to assist in the conceptualization of several interrelated aspects of anatomy and biomechanics. The idea of the Serape Effect relates mainly to the function of abdominal muscles when maximum force is desired in the use of the limbs. The purpose of presenting the Serape Effect is to provide the learner with a visual illustration indicating the function and importance of the interrelationship of pelvic girdle and spinal column motions when the upper and lower limbs are used in ballistic skills. The intricate timing of these rotations is a prerequisite to skilled performance in ballistic activities.

Selected references   DeMille, Rosalind. Personal Communication, 1962.

Logan, Gene A. "Movement in Art." *Quest* 2 (April 1964) :42–45.

————. *Adaptations of Muscular Activity.* Belmont, Calif.: Wadsworth Publishing Company, 1964.

Logan, Gene A., and Wallis, Earl L. "Recent Findings in Learning and Performance." Southern Section Meeting, California Association for Health, Physical Education and Recreation, October, 1960, at Pasadena City College.

Logan, Gene A., end McKinney, Wayne C. "The Serape Effect." *Journal of Health, Physical Education, Recreation* 41 (February 1970) :79-80.

Northrip, John W.; Logan, Gene A.; and McKinney, Wayne C. *Introduction to Biomechanic Analysis of Sport.* Dubuque, Iowa: Wm. C. Brown Company Publishers, 1979.

part 3

Application of Kinesiology Theory

11

Analytic
Kinesiology
Techniques

Teaching neuromuscular skills is based on: (1) knowledge of the skill being taught from technical as well as scientific points of view; (2) insight regarding the performer's strengths, limitations, and potentials in the skill area being taught; (3) ability of the physical educator to utilize analytic kinesiology techniques; and (4) versatility of the physical educator in communicating pertinent facets of the skill analyses to the learners. *Analysis of the performance of the learner must precede teaching. Verbal and/or nonverbal communication of analytic information designed to have a positive effect on the learner is teaching.* Informing a performer that he or she has numerous faults without indicating how improvement can be made is known as incompetence! Negative information relayed to a performer is usually counterproductive to effective teaching.

Skills should be analyzed by merging knowledge of the technique of the performer's skill with the accepted stereotypes of perfect mechanics. (Stereotypes of perfect mechanics should constantly be undergoing critical evaluations.) This technical information is analyzed in turn by the physical educator in terms of scientific movement principles derived from anatomic kinesiology, biomechanics, and other sciences related to motion. It is this ultimate synthesis of technical and scientific knowledge which provides the foundation for professionally analyzing and improving the performances of students, whether they are involved in physical education classes or athletic programs. The technical knowledge (techniques) of a performance is essential to an understanding of *how* it is accomplished. The scientific knowledge derived from kinesiology provides the understanding of motion necessary to decide *why* a given movement is either functional or extraneous for the performance under analysis.

The *professional* physical educator has backgrounds in both the technical and scientific dimensions of exercise, sport, and dance. Neither of these dimensions should be considered subordinate to the other. The ability to analyze from a scientific standpoint is learned in such courses as kinesiology, biomechanics, exercise physiology, and motor learning, among others. Techniques are learned in sport techniques and theory courses. The best way to learn the technical dimension of physical education is to be a "thinking performer" in a wide variety of activities including at least one sport (intercollegiate athletics) or dance area where a good level of excellence is achieved. The success and frustration experienced while pursuing excellence can make a positive contribution to the teaching effectiveness of the future physical educator.

Hierarchy of analyses

Northrip, Logan, and McKinney introduced a hierarchy of analytic techniques for use in kinesiology and teaching in 1974. There are four levels in this hierarchy, based on frequency of usage of the analytic techniques in practice: (1) noncinematographic analysis, (2) basic cinematographic analysis, (3) intermediate cinematographic analysis, and (4) research. Out of absolute necessity, the practicing physical educator will utilize the first level in teaching and coaching situations most of the time. Basic cinematographic analyses can be used extensively in classes and coaching situations to analyze performances of students (on videotape) or athletes (on game film). Intermediate cinematographic analysis is utilized less frequently since this technique involves mathematically objectifying observations which tend to be subjective in nature during a basic cinematographic analysis. Research in biomechanics and anatomic kinesiology is the most sophisticated level, and is not utilized too frequently in the direct context of teaching neuromuscular skills.

Noncinematographic analysis

As the term implies, neither film nor videotape is utilized during this analysis technique. This means that the physical educator must have a disciplined approach for observing and analyzing motions at various body articulations. Without a structured analytic technique for observing live performers in classes and athletic situations, it is doubtful that the skill-improvement objective of physical education would be met. This analytic technique should be used during each physical education class and athletic practice session.

To analyze a skill, the performance should be observed critically several times before any teaching or coaching suggestions are made. This is an important principle. The individual who only watches one performance, then gives the performer extensive advice regarding what is being done correctly and incorrectly, does a disservice to the performer. There are at least two factors to consider in such a case. First, there is variability among performances by the same performer executing a skill. Lower skilled individuals in particular exhibit great variability between performances. It is entirely possible that a consistent or major problem may not be observed or identified during one performance.

The second factor to consider relates to determining which portion of the analysis should be communicated to the performer and how this should be accomplished. A detailed discussion of all the faults observed will only tend to confuse and discourage many performers psychologically. Negative communication such as this will impede motor learning. The emphasis during teaching should not be on the faults observed. *Teaching should be directed positively towards ways and means of eliminating the most significant motion problem.* This will lead to improved performance.

There is a definite analogy between teaching physical education activities and the work of a physician in diagnosing and curing an illness. A physician usually will not give heavy medication to a patient initially because it could mask symptoms and prevent or delay an accurate diagnosis. A physical educator must observe and analyze a performer many times to see if major faults (symptoms or a syndrome) are occurring consistently. When the major faults have been recognized or diagnosed, a "prescription" is then provided for specific improvement of the performance. Guesswork on the part of the physical educator at any time during this process could result in permanent skill problems on the part of the student performer. The combination of technical and scientific knowledge utilized during a disciplined noncinematographic analysis tends to eliminate ineffective teaching.

There are various ways in which a physical educator can observe human motion. The following systematic approach to observing sport skills is based on viewing body segments specifically during the performance. This segmental approach to observing sport skills is applicable to basic cinematographic analysis as well as noncinematographic analysis. Experience has indicated that a performer should be observed many times prior to making any teaching suggestions. The observations for each trial would be directed to the: (1) total performance, (2) pelvic area and rib cage, (3) base of support or feet, (4) head and shoulders, (5) arm and hand, (6) knees and hips, (7) follow-through, and (8) total performance once again (Rose 1959). The following are *examples* of the types of questions which should be asked and ultimately answered. It should be noted that questions would differ, depending upon the skill under observation; consequently, the physical educator should make a check list for each skill under study. Examples of this systematic, segmental analysis technique are found in chapters 10 and 12.

I. Total Performance **Observations**
  A. What is the general timing on the part of the athlete for the total skill?
  B. What was the outcome of the performance?
II. Pelvic Area and Rib Cage. The pelvic girdle is a relatively slow movement area and a good orientation point for analysis when compared to limb actions.
  A. How high is the pelvic girdle from its base?
  B. What is the critical motion of the pelvic girdle?
  C. Does the critical path change during any phase of the movement?
  D. What is the extent and direction of the total pelvic action?
III. Base of Support
  A. How does the body weight shift at the start, during, and at the finish of action?
  B. What is the line of projection for efficient action?
  C. Does the line of projection during the performance change?
  D. In what direction(s) do the feet point prior to, during, and at the completion of the performance?
  E. Are the feet too far apart or too close together during the performance?
  F. What is the position of the feet immediately prior to the action?

IV. Head and Shoulders
- A. Is the head in the proper position at the start, during, and at the end of the action?
- B. Are both eyes focused on the objective?
- C. Which is the performer's preferred eye?
- D. Were the eyes open or closed during the crucial phase of the performance?
- E. Is there any abnormal movement at the start of the performance which would have an adverse effect on subsequent movements?
- F. In cases where an implement is used, are the eyes focused on the object to be hit at the moment of impact?

V. Arm and Hand
- A. In what direction do the arms move during the action?
- B. Are the arms too close or too far from the body for effective movement?
- C. Are the arms moving diagonally or in flexion-extension patterns?
- D. In cases where an implement is used, is the proper grip taken initially and held throughout the performance?
- E. In cases of impact, was the implement released at the point of impact?
- F. Was the total range of motion of both arms adequate?
- G. Are both arms rotated properly?

VI. Knees and Hips
- A. In what direction do the legs move during the action?
- B. Are the knee flexion angles consistent with the skill to be performed?
- C. Are there any rotational movements at the hips which might inhibit performance?
- D. Is there any indication of inadequate flexibility at the hip joints?
- E. If impact is an integral part of the skill, what are the knee and hip actions immediately prior to, during, and following impact?
- F. Are the legs moving diagonally or in flexion-extension patterns?

VII. Follow-through and/or Recovery
- A. What is the extent, direction, and pattern of the follow-through?
- B. Is there any evidence that muscular tension impeded the follow-through? If so, in what body segments?
- C. If an implement was used, how did it react at the point of impact and during the follow-through?
- D. Was the follow-through continuous?
- E. Was the recovery related to subsequent movements?

VIII. Total Performance
- A. Was there an effective summation of internal forces?
- B. Was the objective of the skill met?

The evaluation of responses to questions of this nature must be based on the overall performance objective(s). These objectives should be stated in terms of the individual performer. *What needs to be done specifically in terms of joint motion adjustments to make the performer more efficient?* That is *the critical question* which must be asked and answered by the professional physical educator when working with students in classes and student-athletes on teams.

Following these observations, several faults will undoubtedly be observed in the average performance. These will need to be corrected in order to improve the individual's overall performance. One important human trait must be considered: *A human being concentrates on one thing at a time.* This means that the physical educator should not disclose all analytic findings to the athlete.

Teaching takes place following the analysis. The physical educator must use professional judgment in placing the performance faults on a priority list, that is, the most flagrant fault must head the list, and other faults would be listed in diminishing order of importance. The most serious fault should receive immediate attention. The physical educator should give help in the form of *specific* changes in technique, body mechanics, skill drills, development exercises, or whatever is indicated, to correct the most serious fault, and ultimately improve the performance.

When working with small classes in a physical education instructional program or with athletic teams, correction of major performance faults is enhanced if the physical educator *writes an exercise prescription* for each student or athlete following analyses of the performance. This requires considerable time and effort, so the procedure is not readily applicable in all class situations. But, it can be used extensively in athletics. The exercise prescription must be written to meet the specific needs of each student, i.e., one "exercise prescription" should not be written for an entire team to follow. That procedure would not allow for such factors as individual differences in the fitness parameters and fundamental skills plus the different demands of team positions. *The exercise prescription for the student must include the following:*

1. Specific types of activities for improving the fitness parameters and the fundamental skill where the major problem was noted;
2. Intensity of those exercises and skill drills;
3. Duration of the exercises and skill drills;
4. Frequency of the exercises and skill drills.

This technique is of great value, as one example, for offseason and preseason athletic conditioning.

The exercise prescription should be communicated in writing and verbally in language that the performer can understand. It could be counterproductive to write it in detailed scientific terms if the student lacks the sophistication to understand the concepts presented. Therefore, the exercise prescription should be based on the kinesiologic analyses of the performance and scientific principles to improve the performer, but it may be written in very basic language for communicative purposes. *It is important for the physical educator to know the specific outcome desired for each exercise and drill written on the exercise prescription.*

One of the greatest sources of irritation and frustration for the student in a physical education class or for a student-athlete in an athletic situation, is for a physical educator to generalize consistently and call it teaching. *Teaching-coaching suggestions based on the analytic findings must be specific for each individual.* A swimming instructor, for example, who starts a beginning swimming class prematurely with the front crawl stroke and instructs students to "relax" while they are almost drowning is not teaching. Many skill progressions must be learned by the swimmers prior to the teaching of the stroke. Students do not need a generalization as a teaching suggestion! They do need specific instructions regarding such things as arm action, cervical spine motions, leg movement, etc. If the physical educator is critically analyzing by using the noncinematographic technique, specific suggestions can be made to students which will help them improve their skills.

Basic cinematographic analysis

The only difference between this technique and noncinematographic analysis is that it involves utilization of film or videotape. The use of film tends to objectify, substantiate, or refute what has been seen noncinematographically. One major limitation of the latter technique is the difficulty in actually seeing detailed motions in limbs *during* ballistic skills. *Film allows the observer to see what has actually occurred rather than what the observer thinks took place.* There is quite a difference—a difference that is important in terms of teaching-coaching.

Basic cinematographic analysis does not involve utilization of mathematical computations to objectify observations made on film. Joint motions are analyzed, and judgments are made regarding the effectiveness or ineffectiveness of the total skill. The performance faults are placed in rank order for each performer, and decisions are then made as to how each fault can best be eliminated in subsequent classes or athletic practice sessions.

This type of analytic technique, involving a combination of technical and scientific knowledge, should be used extensively by coaches analyzing individual skills of athletes on game film. Obviously, game film will not meet the very rigid film criteria established for biomechanic research. Nevertheless, while recognizing the fact that such film does have limitations, one can make very significant and critical analyses, even on a basic level, to help improve performances.

Just one example of how this is done: the very effective use of this technique in eradicating baseball hitters' "slumps." Game film of a hitter should be taken when he is hitting for a good percentage. This film should be filed according to such factors as date, pitching situation, and the result of the swing or swings of the bat as shown on the film. It can subsequently be utilized for comparison and contrast with what appears on film taken during a game situation when the same hitter is performing poorly. Similar or identical game situations can be analyzed independently or concurrently. For example, two stop-action projectors can be utilized concurrently, and the hitter's mechanics can be analyzed frame by frame at synchronized times during both hitting processes. Motion variations can be noted in such factors as total body position in the batting stance, motion variations during the preparatory phase of the swing, angular velocity of the pelvic and spinal column rotations, bat velocity and variations in the follow-through actions. On the basis of this type of basic cinematographic analysis, positive decisions can be reached by the coach with regard to readapting the individual's hitting style to its previous mechanics when he was hitting for a good average. These coaching adjustments would be made during the next practice.

Having a permanent record of both performances on film tends to eliminate any guesswork on the part of the coach. By using noncinematographic techniques only, the coach would have to rely on his memory to tell him what the student-athlete had been doing as a hitter several weeks previously. The human brain is simply not capable of retaining precise images over a period of time. This is one reason the physical educator must rely on film periodically for analytic purposes, especially in athletic situations.

Can the basic cinematographic analysis technique be used in the average elementary and secondary school? The answer is an emphatic *yes!* Most school districts or systems have audiovisual equipment. Many secondary schools have their own audiovisual departments with all kinds of cameras, projectors, television videotape recorders, television monitors, and other photographic paraphernalia. Consequently, the tools are available for performing basic cinematographic analysis, particularly in light of the fact that this technique does not involve the use of expensive cameras and projectors. If a camera is available to record preformances on film or videotape, the analysis can be made, utilizing the segmental technique recomended previously for noncinematographic analysis.

In practice, the physical educator reviews the film numerous times, making notes regarding the various joint or body segment motions during the performance phases. Observations are also made regarding the effectiveness of the total motion, and whether or not motion principles were violated, causing the performer to be ineffective. If so, the joint motions causing the problem are noted. This is followed by planning for future drills, exercises, and technique adjustments to ameliorate the condition within the performer. Many coaches use basic cinematographic analysis techniques to grade their athletes' performances during an athletic contest. That serves two purposes: (1) motivation for the athlete to improve, or reward for an excellent performance, and (2) provides a positive base and direction for the coach to make suggestions for improvement.

For the kinesiology student, the basic cinematographic analysis technique involves reviewing the film numerous times while making general observations as previously discussed. Following these general observations, the film should be analyzed frame-by-frame, with a record made of each joint motion during each phase of the performance. Ranges of motion should be noted, as well as whether or not the motion was against resistance or with gravity. This helps to define muscle contraction; moreover, the muscles most involved for causing or controlling the motion can be determined readily if the spatial relationship concept is understood. Implications of the extraneous motion observed, if any, should be evaluated in terms of the performance objectives. Finally, the faults should be ranked, and teaching suggestions written to eliminate each fault.

For specific joint analysis, there are two general techniques that may be employed. These may be done in conjunction with each other or separately. The most commonly used technique is a tracing of the *contour* or body outline on paper (figs. 12.1–12.9). A workable image size should be projected and drawn. For individual contour drawings, 8½-by-11-inch paper is adequate. These drawings can be done on transparencies of approximately the same size for subsequent projection using an overhead projector. The advantage of the transparency is that the total number of drawings may be superimposed for multiple-image projection. Artistic ability is not essential for this process; however, the tracing should be accurate enough to determine joint angles. It should be reemphasized, however, that attainment of absolute joint angles is impossible with photographic techniques, due primarily to perspective error. However, enough joint angle accuracy can be determined to conduct a basic cinematographic analysis if the analyzer is cognizant of bone landmarks and joint motion.

The second analysis procedure is called *the point-and-line* technique. In this technique, a point is used to indicate the estimated center of a joint or *anatomic landmark*, and the lines that connect these points indicate body segments. It is essential that one of the points be utilized to indicate the center of the pelvic segment. This can be used to make an estimate of the line of movement. This technique provides a less cluttered multi-image picture and more accurate joint angle measurements (figs. 12.10 and 12.11). On the other hand, the image of the performer is lost.

It is obvious that doing a contour drawing or a point-and-line drawing of every frame is unnecessary. There are two suggested ways for selecting frames to be analyzed and drawn. First, a decision should be made based on the number of total frames analyzed for the skill under study. For example, if the total skill consists of thirty-two frames, and eight drawings are desired, this would mean that every fourth frame will be drawn. This procedure has the advantage of a consistent time interval between drawings. The second procedure consists of determining *crucial phases* of the performance after the film has been observed several times. This technique actually places the emphasis at the crucial points of the skill where the performer's faults may be more obvious. Using the first procedure, a crucial movement might be missed. To assist in the subsequent analysis, the frame number should be included on each drawing.

Intermediate cinematographic analysis

This technique is a functional progression into the research level; however, it can be utilized in the teaching-coaching situation. This level of analysis requires more precision in calculating such factors as joint ranges of motion per time unit, angular velocity of joint and body segments, linear velocity, and accelerations. As a result, more care must be taken during the filming process with reference to such factors as camera angle, critical planes of motion of the performance, background, and filming-speed rates. Some "game film" can be used for analytic purposes, but it must be interpreted with care.

The above factors tend to limit the use of this technique in practice. Therefore, the emphasis in this book is on the first two levels in the analysis hierarchy. The reader interested in examples of intermediate cinematographic analyses is referred to Northrip, Logan, and McKinney, 1979.

Research

This level on the hierarchy is presented simply to inform the reader that research is an ongoing process which is extremely important in advancing knowledge in the areas of anatomic kinesiology and biomechanics. Research involves sophisticated instrumentation. Most of this equipment can only be found in a very few specialized laboratories within universities. High-speed cameras for triaxial cinematographic analysis, with associated velocity measurement devices, stroboscopic devices, electromyographic units, electrogoniometers, force plates, force transducers, and computers are not commonly found in elementary- and secondary-school situations. These and other types of equipment are absolutely essential to the conducting of research.

Research techniques bring a great amount of precision to the task of solving a motion problem. Also, research facilitates discovery of new knowledge in the area of kinesiology. When research techniques are utilized, considerable attention is given to working with a delimited portion of the motion problem. This is conducive to a deeper understanding of the factors underlying the motion observed. This may or may not contribute to teaching-coaching.

Cameras

Whether or not to use eight- or sixteen-millimeter equipment depends primarily upon funds and equipment available. Sixteen-millimeter is preferred over eight-millimeter equipment for cinematographic analysis for at least two reasons: (1) the image is larger and provides greater detail, and (2) most educational institutions are equipped to work with sixteen-millimeter as opposed to eight-millimeter film. Some institutions do not provide cinematographic equipment for their personnel; consequently, the physical educator who employs cinematographic techniques will usually purchase eight-millimeter cinematographic equipment for his or her personal use. Analyses can be made professionally, and money can be saved while using eight-millimeter equipment.

A camera should have variable speeds up to sixty-four frames per second for analysis purposes. Basic cinematographic analysis can be done effectively by using thirty-two to sixty-four frames per second during the filming process. Film taken at less than thirty-two frames per second will be too blurred during maximum velocity performances of the limbs. There will be some blurring in film taken at thirty-two and sixty-four frames per second, but it is not enough to preclude its use. Film taken at thirty-two frames per second will permit the user to visualize the movement occurring frame-by-frame while observing the film with a stop-action projector. The perception of movement occurring within various body segments is less pronounced as the frames per second are increased. Also, it is economically more feasible to use thirty-two or sixty-four frames-per-second camera settings. Cameras are available with variable speeds to thousands of frames per second.

**Cinematographic
analysis equipment**

Figure 11.1 shows a functional and popular sixteen millimeter camera used to take performance film for analytic kinesiology purposes.

An interchangeable lens system is also recommended on a camera used for cinematographic analyses purposes. A telephoto lens with "zoom" capabilities is of particular importance. The use of a telephoto lens will reduce the amount of parallax. Parallax involves a perspective error when the camera is relatively close to the subject being filmed. The telephoto lens will reduce this error by enabling the photographer to be farther from the subject. Perspective errors are recorded by the camera lens because it does not have the ability to make size adjustments as the human eye does. The human makes automatic perspective adjustments with the eyes as he or she moves closer to or farther from the object. This is a learned phenomenon, and it has not been duplicated in camera lenses. An ideal camera with a multiple lens apparatus should have

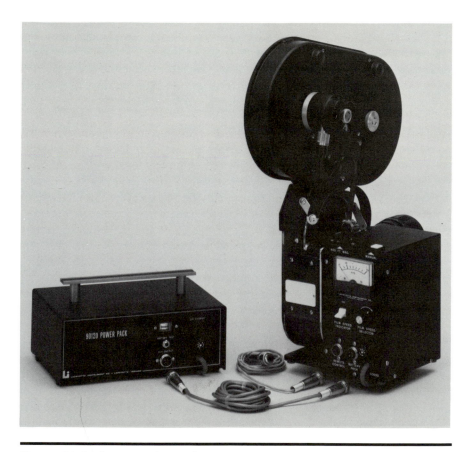

Figure 11.1. A commonly used 16mm game film camera system. Bolex Rex-5 with Lafayette power pack and camera drive. Compliments of Lafayette Instrument Company, Lafayette, IN.

the following f stops: (1) The standard lens should have a f stop range from 1.9 to 22; (2) The wide-angle lens should have f stop settings from 1.8 to 16; and (3) The telephote lens should have an f stop setting from 2.5 to 32. This combination of lenses will provide efficient filmmaking for types of film speeds recommended and varying light conditions.

Several factors must be considered prior to photographing the subject to be analyzed. These include the position of the camera relative to the performer, the height of the camera in relation to the center of mass of the individual to be filmed, the actual distance of the camera from the performance, the size of the performer in relation to the viewfinder, and the time taken to perform the skill. *If only one sequence is to be filmed, the camera should be placed at a ninety-degree angle in relation to the most important plane of motion.*

For analytic purposes, multiple views are preferred. Ideally, these should be taken from the side, front, back, and above the performer. Photographing two views of the same subject on one frame can be accomplished by using a dichroic mirror and photographing the individual from above, the side, or in front (Cooper and Sorani 1965). To further reduce distortions, the height of the camera should be centered on the object to be photographed. To maintain a constant level as well as stability for the camera, it is recommended that a stable tripod be used during the photographic process. It is difficult to control the distance of the camera from the performing subject, especially when the subject is filmed during an athletic contest. However, it is essential to have at least one known distance for future reference when analyzing the film. It is also important to have an actual measurement of some part of the performer. For example, the length of the forearm might be measured between two anatomic landmarks. This can be used for future reference to assist the observer in determining the velocity of linear motion as well as the actual size of the object in various positions and the range of motion of the joints involved. When the size of a body part is known, the projected image can be scaled to determine its actual size.

Timing within film is another very essential aspect. There is disparity between cameras, because some cameras are motor-driven while other cameras are spring-driven. The timing factor is relatively constant in motor-driven cameras, as opposed to spring-driven cameras. Motor-driven cameras are expensive; consequently, they are not used as frequently for cinematographic analysis purposes as the less expensive spring-driven cameras. To insure accuracy in timing when using spring-driven cameras, it is essential to include a timing device in the film. The timing device should be a clock readable to .01 of a second. This will serve as a check on the accuracy of the frames-per-second setting of the camera. If it is not possible to include a timing device in a film, the operator of the spring-driven camera should take care to have maximum tension on the spring mechanism by having it fully wound before each photographic session.

Ultra-high-speed cameras are available for cinematographic research purposes. These motor-driven cameras have special sprocket systems which allow filming of athletic performances within the range of 100 to 32,000 frames per second. Obviously, the use of this type of camera is unrealistic for the average person interested in using film analysis in school situations.

Cameras are also available with stroboscopic light attachments. This type of camera gives the individual a sequential multiple image on one photographic print. Some of these cameras will produce multiple pictures of the same performance on separate photographs. The multiple image and instant developing features on this camera are useful tools in the analysis-teaching process. However, it has the disadvantage of producing a relatively small image.

There are photographic equipment accessories which should be included to insure adequate results during the filming process. It is recommended that the camera be purchased with a good light meter system built into it. This will avoid many filming difficulties, especially for the novice photographer. To insure good pictures indoors, it is advisable to have at least five photo floods on stands strategically placed during photographic sessions. It is recommended that the floods be placed as follows: (1) two on both sides at forty-five degree angles, knee level to the performer; (2) two on both sides at forty-five degree angles, chest level to the performer, and (3) one high enough to spotlight the head. These would be of particular value to coaches in such sports as basketball, wrestling, and gymnastics. However, photo floods are of little practical value during the filming of an actual contest since they would be in the way.

It is essential to provide a known measurement in the background of films used for cinematographic analysis. One way of doing this is to photograph a subject in an athletic practice situation and include a portable grid screen in the background. A grid screen can be constructed from 4 feet by 8 feet Masonite or plyboard panels. Tempered Masonite is recommended because it is lighter in physical weight than plyboard. The grid squares should be at least four inches, marked off in contrasting colors with lines of no less than ⅛-inch width. The overall size of the total grid screen would depend upon the athletic skill to be photographed. It must be remembered that there will be a slight amount of perspective error when using a grid screen; consequently, it should be used only as a rough guide for a known measurement.

The problem of having a known background measure is more difficult when filming during an actual athletic contest. However, there is usually one part of the physical surroundings which can be measured prior to or following the filming, in order to provide a known measurement. This might be a part of the stands, a goalpost, or other constant aspects within the surroundings.

Projectors

Several essential criteria must be considered prior to selecting a motion analysis projector: (1) single frame stop-action with the facility for holding a picture indefinitely without film damage from heat; (2) single frame-by-frame advance feature without flicker; (3) forward and reverse capabilities at multiple speeds; (4) constant illumination; (5) constant focus; (6) a frame counter that will add, subtract, and reset; and (7) a remote control allowing the operator to control all speeds, stop-action, and forward and reverse motion. Although motion analysis can be done with regular and slow-motion projectors, the features listed above are needed to perform a complete analysis. Eight-millimeter and sixteen-millimeter projectors which include these features are available.

The projector shown in figure 11.2 meets and exceeds the above criteria. Projectors of that calibre are essential in order to conduct basic and/or intermediate cinematographic analyses.

Another piece of photographic equipment which can be used to analyze film at a low-budget level is the editor-viewer. There are several models available to accommodate eight- and sixteen-millimeter film. The major consideration in regard to film analysis, however, is the size of the projected image on the viewing screen. The screens on editor-viewers are built into the total apparatus; consequently, the size of the projected image cannot be changed. A good editor-viewer is a recommended piece of equipment, even though a high-quality motion analysis projector is available. The editor-viewer will permit editing, splicing, and preparing film for the library for future reference.

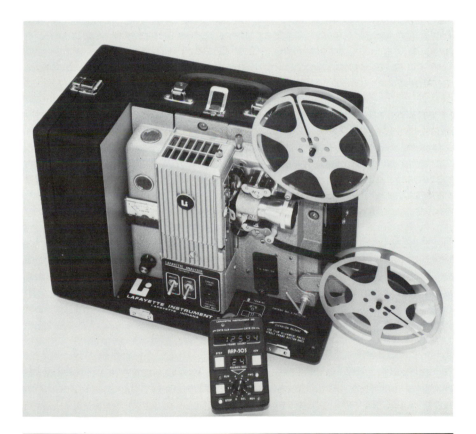

Figure 11.2. Basic cinematographic analysis 16mm projector, Lafayette Analyzer with digital frame counter. Compliments of Lafayette Instrument Company, Lafayette, IN.

Microfilm readers may also be used for motion analysis purposes. One limitation of the microfilm reader is that the projected image cannot be enlarged or reduced as needed.

For sophisticated motion analysis research, there are very expensive motion analyzers available. Essentially, these units consist of a projector and angle measurement read-out screen which works automatically to gather data and feed these data into a computerized system for analysis purposes. This computerized unit can be programmed to provide an automatic read-out of all visible joint movements performed by the subject being analyzed.

Film

The choice of film for analysis is dependent upon the nature of the desired outcome. Film makers are constantly improving their products. The choice of film, therefore, should be based upon the camera used, film speeds, lighting conditions, and the ultimate objective for use of the film. For analysis purposes, black-and-white film is preferred to colored film, since better contrasts are seen in black-and-white film. However, if the film is to be used within a class for instructional purposes in order to illustrate a kinesiologic principle, color film might well be used.

Television equipment

Use of television and videotape for basic *cinematographic analysis* purposes has potential. There are three pieces of television equipment necessary for kinesiologic analysis. These are: video camera, video recorder, and video monitor-receiver. The overall cost of these three items is comparable to an adequate camera and projector for motion analysis.

There are several advantages of videotape over eight- or sixteen-millimeter film. The major advantage is that videotape can be taken of a performer and replayed instantly for analysis purposes. In addition, and supplemental to the instant replay, is the fact that verbal comments can be recorded simultaneously with the videotape. Instant videotape and sound recording are very useful from analysis and teaching standpoints. For example, the athlete can be shown a major problem immediately. The coach can make specific teaching suggestions to help the athlete improve. The coach can record noncinematographic observations verbally while videotaping the athlete's performance initially. These spontaneous remarks by the coach can be retained and used later in a more detailed approach to the analysis. This means that the coach can make a more functional use of the observation check list referred to previously.

There are other advantages in using videotape. Light is a less crucial factor, videotape is less expensive than most film, and all television cameras are motor-driven. There are no spring-driven television cameras with the inconsistent speed factor. The television camera does not have a frame-by-frame timing element as does a sixteen- or eight-millimeter camera; however, videotape moves through the camera at a set rate of inches per second. The inches-per-second recording is made on the videotape recorder, and this information can be utilized to assist in the timing process of the kinesiologic analysis. For further timing accuracy a .01 second clock can be included in the televised picture. Since videotape has some advantages over eight- or sixteen-millimeter film, it should be used for kinesiologic analyses to enhance the instructional process.

The television camera should be portable and capable of filming athletic performances in a wide variety of situations. It should have a speed device to allow videotape to move at a preset speed in inches per second through the camera. The camera should be fully automatic in regard to its video- and audio-level controls.

The most important item of television equipment for analytic purposes is the videotape recorder. It is absolutely essential that this piece of equipment have full-stop motion features. It should have slow motion and instant playback capabilities both in forward and reverse. Furthermore, videotape and audio channels should be capable of operation by remote control.

The television monitor-receiver should be a lightweight, portable unit. It should have quality video input and output systems as well as audio input and output systems. It is recommended that the *minimum* diagonal screen size for analysis purposes be eighteen inches. Some very large screens are now available with some TV units.

This brief discussion of cinematographic analysis equipment and its use pertains primarily to the practical or day-to-day needs of the physical educator in class or athletic situations. Most of the equipment and techniques recommended would only meet the criteria for performing basic cinematographic analyses designed to facilitate the teaching-coaching process. This use of kinesiology theory in daily practice is the major theme of the book in hand. It is recognized that more sophisticated techniques and equipment are needed to conduct complete intermediate cinematographic analyses and research projects in anatomic kinesiology and biomechanics. These levels on the analysis hierarchy are also important in the teaching of neuromuscular skills, but in a less direct manner.

Selected references

Bergemann, Brian W. "Three Dimensional Cinematography: A Flexible Approach." *Research Quarterly* 45 (1974): 302–9.

Bevan, Randall J. "A Simple Camera Synchronizer for Combined Cinephotography and Electromyographic Kinesiology for Use with a Pen Recorder." *Research Quarterly* 43 (1972): 105–12.

Biscan, Dianne V. and Hoffman, Shirl J., "Movement Analysis as a Generic Ability of Physical Education Teachers and Students." *Research Quarterly* 47 (May, 1976): 161–163.

Cooper, John M., and Sorani, Robert P. "Use of the Dichroic Mirror as a Cinematographic Aid in the Study of Human Performance." *Research Quarterly* 36 (May 1965): 210–11.

Cureton, T. K. "Elementary Principles and Techniques of Cinematographic Analysis." *Research Quarterly* 10 (May 1939): 3.

Davis, Robert; Wehrkamp, Robert; and Smith, Karl U. "Dimensional Analysis of Motion: I. Effects of Laterality and Movement Direction." *Journal of Applied Psychology* 35 (October 1951): 363-66.

Deshon, Deans E., and Nelson, Richard C. "A Cinematographical Analysis of Sprint Running." *Research Quarterly* 35 (December 1964); 451-55.

DeVries, Herbert A. "A Cinematographical Analysis of the Dolphin Swimming Stroke." *Research Quarterly* 30 (December 1959): 413-22.

Fenn, W. O. "Mechanical Energy Expenditure in Sprint Running as Measured by Moving Pictures." *American Journal of Physiology* 90 (1929): 343-44.

Lockhart, Aileene. "The Value of the Motion Picture as an Instructional Device in Learning a Motor Skill." *Research Quarterly* 15 (May 1944): 181-87.

Northrip, John W.; Logan, Gene A.; and McKinney, Wayne C. *Introduction to Biomechanic Analysis of Sport.* Dubuque, Iowa: Wm. C. Brown Company Publishers, 1974.

————. *Introduction to Biomechanic Analysis of Sport* (Second Edition). Dubuque, Iowa: Wm. C. Brown Company Publishers, 1979.

Plagenhoef, S. C. "Methods for Obtaining Kinetic Data to Analyze Human Motions." *Research Quarterly* 34 (March 1966): 103.

Rock, I.; Tauber, E. S.; and Heller, D. P. "Perception of Stroboscopic Movement." *Science* 147 (February 1965): 1050-51.

Rose, Jack. "Analysis of Track and Field Performances." Unpublished paper. California State College at Long Beach, 1959.

Steben, Ralph E. "A Cinematographic Study of Selective Factors in the Pole Vault." *Research Quarterly* 41 (1970): 95-104.

Terauds, Juris (ed.). *Science in Biomechanics Cinematography.* Del Mar, CA: Academic Publishers, 1979.

VanGheluwe, Bart. "Errors Caused by Misalignment of the Cameras in Cinematographical Analyses." *Research Quarterly* 46 (1975): 153-61.

12

Skill Analysis

Four analysis levels for analytic kinesiology were described in chapter 11. The first two analytic levels of the hierarchy are directly applicable to teaching-coaching situations. In addition, they share the same analytic procedures. Therefore, noncinematographic and basic cinematographic analyses receive the emphasis in this chapter. Specifically, basic cinematographic skill analyses are presented *as examples* of how they should be conducted: (1) by kinesiology students during the professional preparation process, and (2) by practicing physical educators working with physical education classes and/or athletic teams.

It should be understood that virtually all performance skills can be divided logically into five general sequential phases for analytic purposes. These five phases with applicability to most skills are: (1) a stance, (2) preparatory phase, (3) movement phase, (4) follow-through phase, and (5) recovery phase. These terms are used because they have general application to numerous skills. Obviously, other descriptive terms can be utilized which connote specific meaning to the coach and athlete. As an example, the movement phase of a dive might be more aptly described as the "flight phase" of the performance. *Phase terminology should be used which facilitates communication in the teaching process.*

While conducting noncinematographic and basic cinematographic analyses of a sport skill, each of the performer's motions at each joint should be evaluated critically several times during each phase. This type of discipline on the part of the physical educator will help define the performer's movement problems accurately.

Skill analysis phases

Stance

Movement from stationary and moving stances is absolutely essential in many sports, among which are tennis, volleyball, football, baseball, wrestling, golf, swimming, track, field, and badminton. The appropriate stance in the same skill differs for each individual, depending upon the length of the limbs and trunk (anthropometric measurements) and other factors related to technique and skill objectives. The stance allows the performer to assume a relatively comfortable body position with joint angles set to place muscle groups on optimum stretch.

This is necessary to allow these muscles to contract with force sufficient to overcome inertia and move body segments into position during the next performance phase. Some skills combine the stance and preparatory phases; sprint starts in track and swimming are examples.

The stance of a tennis player ready to receive a serve, as an example, usually includes a slight knee flexion, hip flexion, and lumbar-thoracic flexion with gravity. The muscles most involved for controlling the extent of flexion at these joints are contracting eccentrically, because these flexions are with gravity. A tennis player must be prepared to move in any direction once the serve is put into its trajectory by the opponent. Therefore, the muscles on stretch during the stance are the ones which will contract concentrically as the joints move into varying degrees of extension to overcome inertia and put the player in position on the court to return the serve. Therefore, a stance or position of readiness is absolutely essential to tennis and many other sport skills.

A stance is not an integral aspect of every performance skill a physical educator would analyze. Choreographed events such as modern dance, free floor exercise in gymnastics, and rebound tumbling competition are composed of several skills performed in sequence. Each skill or component part would be analyzed, and few would have stance phases. Swimming and running have stances only in the form of their starts. Sprint starts in track and swimming are individual skills which must be analyzed separately from running form and swimming strokes. A skill such as the flip turn in swimming would not have a stance phase, and would have to be analyzed by the swimming coach independent from as well as integrated with the swimming stroke. The reader can undoubtedly think of numerous skills which do not utilize a stance per se.

A stance should be analyzed quantitatively and qualitatively by measuring the joint angles. It should be determined if the angles are appropriate for the individual to move effectively to meet the performance objective. If not, joint angles during the static stance would need to be adjusted. If the stance is not appropriate, the total skill could be adversely effected.

Preparatory phase

This is the most important phase of a skill for the physical educator to analyze. The joint motions which occur at this time are very important in terms of preparing the performer to execute the critical movement phase which follows. Joint motion mistakes in terms of extraneous motions, limited ranges-of-motion of joint movements, or too much joint motion could be detrimental to body positioning, equilibrium, summation of motion for force application and many other biomechanic related problems.

The preparatory phase motions are directly related to and dependent upon the requirements of each skill in terms of the skill objective and the stereotype of perfect mechanics for the skill. The joint motions can be more subtle during the preparatory phase than in the movement phase. This is one reason the average sport fan misses them and the good coach observes these motions. *If mistakes are made in the movement phase, they were preceded by joint motion errors during the stance and/or preparation phases.* Logically, the good teacher who recognizes preparatory phase motion problems usually attempts to correct them first.

Motion between figures 12.1 and 12.2 shows the important preparatory phase for softball hitting. A golfer's preparatory phase is the complete backswing movement. A ski jumper uses a moving stance and prepares for the jump during the motion down the ramp by setting the correct angles at the ankles, knees, hips, and lumbar-thoracic spine. All motions of the javelin thrower up to the time the throwing limb moves into diagonal adduction prior to release are in the preparatory phase. The same is true for shot putters, discus throwers, baseball pitchers, and for other throwing and striking skills of a ballistic nature. Consequently, preparatory phase motions differ considerably, but they are all essential for effective skill execution.

Myologically, the preparatory phase is the critical stage for application of the muscle length-force ratio principle. Muscle groups are placed on stretch, i.e., the tension within muscles is increased during this phase. That has critical implications for the movement phase effectiveness which follows. The importance of this was discussed earlier in terms of the Serape Effect for ballistic skills. The preparatory phase is analogous to "cocking a pistol" in the shooting process. If the tension in the spring of the pistol is great enough, the pulling of the trigger (movement phase) will be effective to discharge the weapon.

Movement phase

The movement phase includes the critical outcome or end result of the skill. It includes the release in throwing events, point of impact in striking skills, movement into the air in jumping or diving events, and any other culminating portion of a skill.

Several examples will help visualize typical movement phases. The movement phase for the volleyball spiker is from the time ankle, knees, hips, and lumbar spine start to extend to move the body vertically until the ball has been spiked. The same would be the case for the basketball rebounder, except the movement phase would end with control of the ball off the backboard. The movement phase for the swimming start would be joint and body motions from the starter's gun until the swimmer starts the stroke in the water. At that time, the movement phase would start for the swimming stroke.

The movement phase includes "the action" from the standpoint of the average fan or coach who is not professionally prepared in physical education. It is an important aspect of the skill, but probably not as important as the preparatory phase. The movement phase is the "effect," and the preparatory phase is the "cause" in terms of the cause and effect relationship for total skill execution. That which follows the movement phase is also important, because not all performances conclude with the movement phase. Consequently, performers must have concluding phases to protect their own joints and bodies from injuries and to react, if necessary, to their opponents or sport objects.

Follow-through phase

Most sport performances require some type of follow-through phase. The most common use of the follow-through is to bring about negative acceleration in a limb after release of a sport object during a ballistic skill. This is a joint protection mechanism. Follow-through is also used to help maintain body position and equilibrium, dissipate force of the total skill over a wide area, and assist in the mental concentration aspects of the performance.

If the follow-through phase is started prematurely or superimposed on the movement phase, skill will be impeded. This is a common phenomenon of unskilled performers in throwing skills. They will start to negatively accelerate or slow the velocity of the throwing limb prior to release instead of following release. This will reduce linear and angular velocities of the thrown object. The two principal causes for this are: (1) soreness in the throwing limb, or (2) inability on the part of the performer to give an "all out effort," perhaps caused by inhibition. In the latter case, youngsters either consciously or subconsciously believe they will injure their arms if they throw hard. The irony of this lies in the fact that they are *less* susceptible to injury if they go "all out" and let the natural myological mechanisms control the body segments during the movement and follow-through phases. This is true *if* they are in good physical condition and throw through a high diagonal plane of motion instead of the transverse plane using joint motions which only impart backspin to the sport object.

The follow-through phase starts immediately upon release of the thrown sport object or after impact of a sport implement with a sport object. The falls of the rebounder, spiker, high jumper, and pole vaulter are all part of their follow-through phases. Follow-through in the sport of archery simply means holding the release position until the arrow is in the target. Thus, this phase takes many forms depending upon the skill objectives and stereotype of perfect mechanics for the skill under analysis.

Recovery phase

Some sport skills conclude with the follow-through phase, but most require some type of recovery phase. Recovery means that the performer must make several motions to prepare for whatever motion demands are immediately forthcoming in the contest or performance.

A baseball pitcher must have a recovery phase after the follow-through, because he may be required to field a bunt or ground ball, cover a base, or back up a base. His job is not necessarily finished with the release of the ball. On the other hand, a javelin thrower does not have a recovery phase after the follow-through. The reason for this lies in the fact that he or she does not have to worry about someone throwing the javelin back! The recovery following execution of a skill is critical. If the performer is constantly out of position or in a state of disequilibrium at the conclusion of the follow-through and cannot recover, the physical educator must make joint motion adjustments. The beginning or intermediate performer has recovery phase problems in court sports such as handball, tennis, or squash. The player will often make what he or she believes to be a good forehand, backhand, or "kill" shot. Time will be taken to admire it for a fraction of a second instead of recovering both body and court positions. In the meantime, the opponent has hit a return shot which passes the beginner who remained in the follow-through position. Recovery of body position to the point where total movement of the body can be made in any direction is important to good performance.

A basic cinematographic analysis undertaken for the first time by a student during the professional preparation process differs considerably from the same type of analysis by a professional physical educator working with a class or athletic team. *The first analysis by the student should be used to reinforce learning of subject matter from anatomic kinesiology and biomechanics.* It is recommended that the student undertake a detailed written analysis comparing and contrasting two performers on film with each other and against the stereotype of perfect mechanics for the skill under analysis. The practicing physical educator, who has already learned the anatomic kinesiology and biomechanic principles, does not have time to go into the same written detail during the analytic process. However, the essential elements of the basic cinematographic analysis are very similar for students and physical educators. *Examples* of these two analytic styles are presented in this chapter. The procedure for conducting noncinematographic and basic cinematographic analyses are the same, except that film is available for the latter analysis.

Basic cinematographic analysis for students

The written basic cinematographic analysis by a student should contain the following chapters:

1. Introduction
2. Review of Related Literature
3. Anatomic Analyses
4. Biomechanic Analyses
5. Discussion
6. Summary, Major Findings, and Teaching-Coaching Recommendations

A bibliography should be included, along with pertinent tabular material and figures. (McKinney 1975), (McKinney and Logan 1977), (Dillman and Sears 1978).

Stereotype of perfect mechanics determination

Before any analysis can be made, the analyzer must know what constitutes the stereotype of perfect form or mechanics for the skill to be analyzed. This means knowing what the "experts" have to say regarding the skill from technical and scientific standpoints. The technical and scientific literature must be reviewed. This means reading everything available related to the skill being analyzed—in journals, books, theses, and dissertations. Examples of appropriate journal articles related to analyses are included in the selected references and recommended reading at the conclusion of the various chapters in this book. In addition, the Bibliography includes reference books in anatomic kinesiology and biomechanics.

Attendance at professional conventions and athletic clinics where performance areas are discussed is also recommended. Materials and information gained from these meetings add to understanding skills and their variations. Also, interviews with recognized experts, performers, and coaches are ways of gathering information about a skill. These are all examples of professional awareness and involvement. Professional involvement is necessary if one wishes to remain up-to-date. This practice should start at the undergraduate level and continue through retirement.

The understanding of current and accepted stereotype of perfect mechanics, along with variations for any given skill, should come from a variety of sources. It must not be based on the opinion of any one "expert" or a few sources. If, for example, one accepts the opinion of an expert performer regarding his or her interpretation of the stereotype of perfect mechanics for the skill, it could be erroneous in nature. If expert performers have no professional background in physical education, they often cannot identify and describe what they actually are doing during their performances. They do not understand cause and effect relationships between their joint motions and performance outcomes. What they say they do and what they actually do may not be the same! This is also true regarding most motion descriptions by television and radio sport announcers.

Once the physical educator has a good grasp of what constitutes the stereotype of perfect mechanics for a skill, this should serve as a basis for teaching-coaching suggestions. However, it should not be assumed that the stereotype can be automatically superimposed on all students. *Teaching-coaching is an art based upon a scientific understanding of humans in motion.* Therefore, to practice this art, the physical educator must make allowances and adjustments for individual differences in performers, such as limb lengths, movement times, reaction times, body builds, and other genetic and anthropometric factors. The stereotype of perfect mechanics is for the "ideal performer"; but not too many performers meet those criteria. A critical element of the art of teaching is to help performers reach their potential skill levels. If this is done, both teacher and performer can gain satisfaction, even if the performance outcome is something less than "world class."

It must also be recognized that the stereotype of perfect mechanics for any skill has the potential to be changed. It is not a rigid concept. Skill execution needs constant scientific and technical evaluation. This is an ongoing process on the part of sport scientists, coaches, and athletes, to perceive possible changes of stereotypes of perfect mechanics for skills. *These do change.* As an example, during the last twenty-five years there have been significant modifications in ideas related to the stereotype of perfect mechanics for high jumping and the shot put. The skill stereotypes have been altered, and the performance outcomes have improved dramatically. Over the years, the same thing has occured regarding the mechanics of hurdling, swimming starts, long jumping, basketball shooting techniques, baseball pitching, pole vaulting, and others. Therefore, the existing stereotype of perfect mechanics should be defined by using a variety of expert scientific and technical opinions, and it should be understood that a more efficient way to perform the skill may, in fact, exist and be defined in the future. *That is one purpose of research in the analysis hierarchy for sport motion.*

Finally, knowledge about a skill can be gained by the student undertaking the analysis when he or she performs a skill. Consequently, it is recommended that the first basic cinematographic analysis written by the student include the analyzer as one performer on film. This is one of the best ways to gain insight into the complexities of learning and teaching the skill.

All of this information should be included in the "Review of Related Literature" chapter of the project. *When all aspects of the skill along with variations are understood in technical and scientific detail, the analysis can begin.*

Determination of skill phases

The film should be viewed many times to: (1) make preliminary observations of the overall performance, (2) determine whether or not the performer attained the skill objective, (3) determine the most logical way to divide the skill into phases for analysis, and (4) draw contour and/or point and line drawings of the performers.

Analysis of two softball hitters with differing levels of ability are presented here to serve as examples of basic cinematographic analysis. The left-handed male performer, Bonus Frost, was named to the All-World softball team as an outfielder and performed in many Amateur Softball Association National Championships. The right-handed female performer, Sue Schuble, was a member of an intercollegiate softball team. At the time the film was taken, she was experiencing difficulties in hitting.

The male performer in this analysis adheres closely to the stereotype of perfect mechanics for hitting in softball. The major emphasis in the example is to analyze the motions of the female performer, attempt to determine her major faults, and describe drills to remove these motion problems to improve her ability as a softball hitter (Schuble 1969).

Four critical phases were chosen for analysis: (1) the stance, (2) preparatory phase, (3) movement phase, and (4) follow-through phase. A recovery phase is also needed in hitting if the ball is hit. The recovery was not included in the example analysis.

Figures 12.1 through 12.9 are contour drawings of the two performers showing the phases chosen for analysis. These drawings were taken directly from sixteen-millimeter film by projecting the images on paper and tracing. (No artistic ability is needed for this.) Four contour drawings of the male performer were made to illustrate the phases. An extra contour drawing of the female performer was made during her movement phase, to focus on a major fault in her hitting form. The selection of frames for contour drawings is an arbitrary matter. In this example, the selection was based on the logical sequence of the skill as dictated by the skill stereotype. The drawings can also be made at equal time intervals, as discussed previously in chapter 11.

Motion between contour drawings is the important factor for study. Each contour drawing is selected from a film frame to show an efficient flow of motion during the execution of the skill under study. In essence, the arbitrarily selected phases or illustrations by contour drawings serve only as *reference points* for the total motion. *They are not the only frames to be analyzed.* The physical educator must be concerned primarily with the motion throughout the total skill performance instead of focusing attention on the static illustrative phases. This is essential to an understanding of complex body motions seen in a skill such as softball-hitting. The physical educator must deal with the *total* motion of any skill from phase to phase.

In the softball-hitting examples, joint motions are described from the preparation phase to the movement phase, and these motions are indicated under the *preparatory heading.* Joint motions from the movement phase to the follow-through phase are described under the *movement heading.* Joint motions during the follow-through or recovery phase are described under the *follow-through* heading.

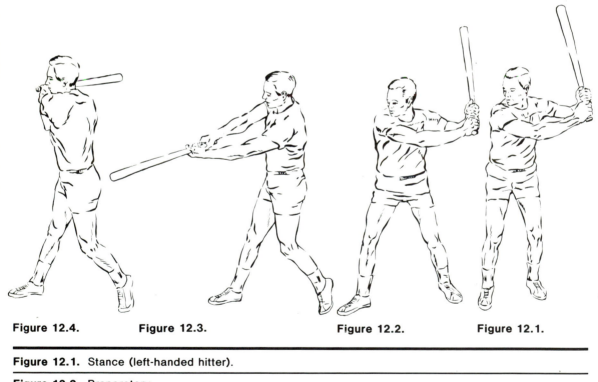

Figure 12.4.   **Figure 12.3.**   **Figure 12.2.**   **Figure 12.1.**

Figure 12.1. Stance (left-handed hitter).

Figure 12.2. Preparatory.

Figure 12.3. Movement—point of impact.

Figure 12.4. Follow-through.

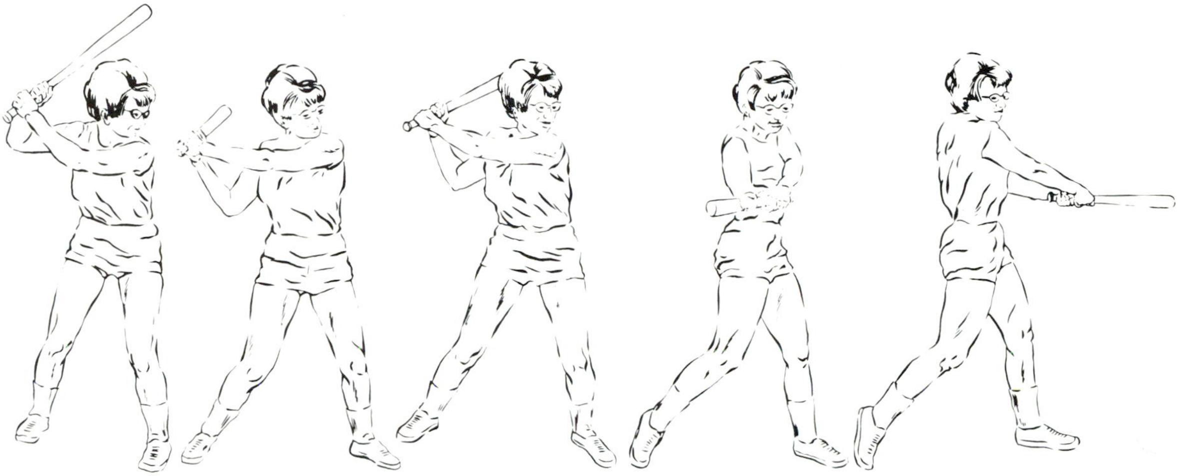

Figure 12.5.   Figure 12.6   Figure 12.7.   Figure 12.8.   Figure 12.9.

Figure 12.5.	Stance (right-handed hitter).
Figure 12.6	Preparatory—start of "hitch."
Figure 12.7.	Preparatory—end of "hitch."
Figure 12.8.	Movement—point of impact.
Figure 12.9.	Follow-through.

If a visual presentation is needed to show the comparative speed of movement between body parts, the point-and-line technique for illustrating motion is recommended. This technique is illustrated for both performers in figures 12.10 and 12.11. This technique, which was discussed in chapter 11, allows for greater precision in determining ranges of motion in joints. The point-and-line technique should have a consistent time interval between each darwing. The time interval is taken from the framing rate used in filming.

Contour drawings and point-and-line illustrations should be included in the "Anatomic Analysis" chapter of the written project. These, along with the film, will help to determine the joint motions occurring during and between the phases. Some universities have sophisticated film analyzers in their human performance laboratories which provide electronic readings of joint angles and motion. These, obviously, can be utilized for conducting a kinesiology project if they are available for student use.

Joint motions by phases

The next step in the analysis is to write observations of the performance, phase by phase. These observations can be used later in writing the "Discussion" chapter of the project where the major emphasis is on the *implications* of the motions observed relative to the outcome of the performance. General observations of the phases are included in the example analysis. Notations are also made regarding the joint motions observed. This information helps in writing the "Anatomic Analysis" chapter.

Stance phase

The stances of the two softball hitters are shown in figures 12.1 and 12.5. These are static, nonmoving body positions. When comparing the stances of the two performers, it can be seen that the female performer has an excessive amount of radial flexion in both wrists. This causes the bat to be carried too high and behind her head. She also has an excessive amount of right shoulder abduction. This contributes to the bat being held too high. Both elbows are flexed more than needed for proper execution of the softball swing. These basic faults combined lead to another major fault which is discussed below. There is one other notable difference between the stances of the two performers—in the weight distribution over the lower limbs. The male performer distributes his weight evenly

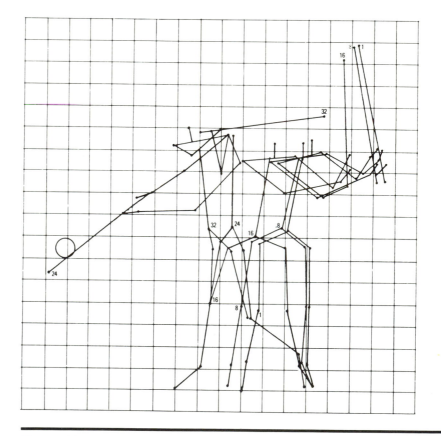

Figure 12.10. Point and line illustration—male performer (numbers indicate film frames—film taken at 32 frames/second), left-handed hitter.

over both lower limbs, whereas the female performer distributes her weight primarily on the right leg.

Since a stance does not involve active joint motion, the student should simply describe the overall body position. This would be accomplished by determining the joint angle settings for each major joint. These angles would be recorded, and the joints would be assumed to be stabilized at those angles prior to the preparatory phase. From a myologic standpoint, all muscles surrounding a joint tend to contribute internal force for stabilization of the joint. Therefore, it would be inappropriate, in most cases, to list the muscles most involved and their contralateral muscles for a stabilized joint.

Once these very general observations have been written, the film should be reviewed again. At that time, calculations should be made regarding the exact extent or range of motion in each joint. Also, notations should be made as to: (1) whether or not joint motions were made with or against gravity, and (2) how much, if any, momentum or velocity contributed to the motion instead of muscle contraction. This information is needed in the writing of the myologic analysis—motion observations follow for each phase:

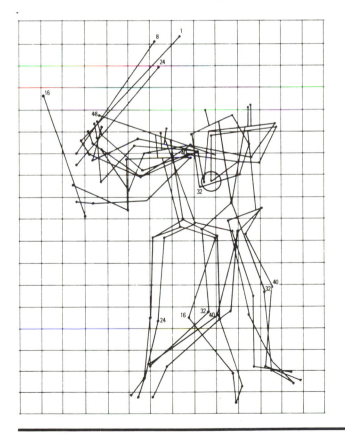

Figure 12.11. Point and line illustration—female performer (numbers indicate film frames—film taken at 32 frames/second), right-handed hitter.

Preparatory phase

Male Performer

Figure 12.2

A. Pelvic girdle motion
  1. Slight right transverse rotation of the pelvic girdle.
B. Rib Cage
  1. Slight left spinal rotation of the lumbar and thoracic spines.
C. Base of support
  1. Right foot has moved approximately twelve inches in the direction of the pitcher.
  2. The toes of the right foot are pointed in the direction of the pitch as a result of right hip lateral rotation.
  3. The left foot remains relatively fixed.
D. Head and shoulders
  1. Slight cervical rotation to the right.
  2. Slight horizontal adduction of the right shoulder joint.

E. Arms and hands
  1. No change in the hands and wrist joints.

  2. The right elbow joint has extended slightly.
F. Knee and hip joints
  1. Slight lateral rotation of the right hip joint.
  2. Slight flexion of the right knee.

  3. Slight abduction at both hips.

Female Performer

Figure 12.6

A. Pelvic girdle motion
  1. Some left transverse pelvic rotation.
B. Rib cage
  1. Slight lumbar and thoracic rotation right.
C. Base of support
  1. Base of support has widened approximately twelve to fourteen inches.
  2. The left foot is moving to the left of the ball's line of flight. Slight lateral rotation and abduction of the left hip.
  3. Right foot remains relatively stable.
D. Head and shoulders
  1. Slight cervical rotation to the left.
  2. Slight left shoulder joint horizontal adduction and flexion.
  3. The right shoulder has adducted approximately twenty to twenty-five degrees. These movements have resulted in a drop of the bat from its original position in the stance.

E. Arms and hands
  1. The hands and wrists have maintained about the same position, but the bat is dropped due to shoulder action.
  2. There has been a slight extension of the left elbow.
F. Knee and hip joints
  1. Marked lateral rotation and flexion of the right knee.
  2. No change appreciable at right hip joint.
  3. Abduction and lateral rotation of the left hip joint.

Male Performer	Female Performer	Movement phase

Figure 12.7

A. (The female performer demonstrated a major fault at this point. Consequently, an extra frame was drawn to illustrate that fault, commonly known as a "hitch." The total "hitch" is illustrated between figures 12.6 and 12.7.)

A. Pelvic girdle movements
  1. Right transverse rotation continues.

B. Rib cage
  1. Marked right lumbar and thoracic spinal rotation.

C. Base of support: no change.

D. Head and shoulders
  1. Slight left cervical rotation.
  2. Slight lateral flexion of the cervical spine.
  3. Increased left shoulder flexion.

E. Arms and hands
  1. Slight left elbow flexion.
  2. Slight right shoulder abduction.
  3. Slight right elbow flexion.
  4. Hands remain the same.

F. Knee and hip joints
  1. Medial rotation, right knee.
  2. Abduction of the right hip.
  3. Slight lateral rotation of the right hip.

Figure 12.3

A. Pelvic girdle motion
  1. Right transverse pelvic girdle rotation.

B. Rib cage
  1. Right thoracic spine rotation.

  2. Slight left lateral flexion of the lumbar spine.

C. Base of support
  1. Weight shift from the left foot to the right foot.
  2. Plantar flexion of the left ankle joint.

Figure 12.8

A. Pelvic girdle motion
  1. Left transverse pelvic girdle rotation with left lumbar rotation.

B. Rib cage
  1. Considerable thoracic and lumbar spine rotation to the left.

C. Base of support
  1. Weight shift to the left foot.

  2. Plantar flexion of the right ankle.
  3. No change in the width of the stance.

Movement phase
continued

Figure 12.3 Continued

D. Head and shoulders
  1. Slight left cervical rotation.
  2. Left shoulder joint, low diagonal adduction and medial rotation.
  3. Right shoulder joint, low diagonal abduction and lateral rotation.
  4. The total motion of the arms and bat is through a low diagonal plane of motion.

E. Arms and hands
  1. Left elbow has moved from flexion to extension.
  2. The right elbow remains about the same.
  3. Both wrists are ulnar flexing.

F. Knee and hip joints
  1. Slight right knee extension.

  2. Marked left knee flexion.
  3. Marked medial rotation of the right hip.

Male Performer

Figure 12.4

A. Pelvic girdle motion
  1. Continuation of right transverse pelvic girdle rotation.
B. Rib cage
  1. Slight right lateral flexion of the lumbar spine.
  2. Continued thoracic spine rotation to the right.

Female Performer

Figure 12.8 Continued

D. Head and shoulders
  1. Right cervical rotation.
  2. Slight cervical flexion.

  3. Marked right shoulder joint diagonal adduction and medial rotation.
  4. Marked left shoulder joint diagonal abduction and lateral rotation. The arms and bat are moving through low diagonal plane of motion.

E. Arms and hands
  1. Excessive left elbow flexion.

  2. Extensive right elbow flexion.

  3. Ulnar flexion starting at both wrists.

F. Knee and hip joints
  1. Moving into left knee extension.
  2. Right knee flexion.
  3. Medial rotation of the left hip.

Female Performer

Figure 12.9

A. Pelvic girdle motion
  1. Continued left transverse pelvic girdle rotation.
B. Rib cage
  1. Continued left thoracic spine rotation.
  2. The spinal column is relatively extended.

Follow-through phase

Male Performer

Female Performer

Figure 12.4 Continued

Figure 12.9 Continued

C. Base of support
   1. Foot placement relatively the same.
   2. Continued weight shift to the right leg.

C. Base of support
   1. Slight weight shift to the left leg.
   2. Left foot is bearing most of the body weight.
   3. Right ankle is plantar flexed.

D. Head and shoulders
   1. Right cervical rotation continued.
   2. Left shoulder continues through low diagonal adduction.
   3. Right shoulder continues through low diagonal adduction.

D. Head and shoulders
   1. Slight cervical extension.
   2. Left shoulder joint diagonal abduction.
   3. Right shoulder joint diagonal adduction.

E. Arms and hands
   1. Left elbow remains extended.
   2. Right elbow is flexed.
   3. Left radio-ulnar joint is pronated.
   4. Right radio-ulnar joint is supinated.

E. Arms and hands
   1. Left and right elbow extension.
   2. Ulnar flexion both wrists.

F. Knees and hips
   1. Right knee in extreme extension
   2. Left knee flexed.
   3. Right hip is at the limit of medial rotation.
   4. Left hip moving toward medial rotation.

F. Knee and hips
   1. Slight flexion of the left knee.
   2. Right knee in relatively the same position.
   3. Continued medial rotation of the left hip joint, but not to the maximum of medial rotation range of motion.
   4. Right hip remains in the same position.

Aggregate muscle action

One way to reinforce learning of anatomic kinesiology subject matter and concepts is to work with and apply the knowledge and ideas during an actual analysis. Therefore, the next step in a basic cinematographic analysis for the student is to determine what internal and external forces are causing or controlling the joint motions noted previously. If the joint motion analysis has been done with precision, this is not a difficult task. The myologic analysis may be completed in outline or paragraph form, and it should include: (1) muscles most involved, (2) contralateral muscles, (3) guiding muscles, and (4) stabilizers and/or dynamic stabilizers where applicable.

For example, during the preparatory and movement phases, the pelvic girdle and rib cage motions of the male performer will be analyzed from a myologic standpoint. In the "Anatomic Analysis" chapter, each body segment and joint would be analyzed in the following manner during each phase:

I. Preparatory Phase—Figure 12.1 to 12.2 Motions
   A. Pelvic Girdle Motion:
      1. Right Transverse Rotation: 5°–7° against resistance; motion initiated in unilateral weight-bearing position
         a) Muscles Most Involved: concentric contraction
            (1) Right external oblique
            (2) Left internal oblique
         b) Contralateral Muscles:
            (1) Left external oblique
            (2) Right internal oblique
         c) Dynamic Stabilizers:
            (1) Right external oblique
            (2) Left external oblique
            (3) Right internal oblique
            (4) Left internal oblique
   B. Rib Cage Motion:
      1. Left Lumbar-thoracic Rotation: 10°–15° against resistance
         a) Muscles Most Involved: concentric contraction
            (1) Right external oblique
            (2) Left internal oblique
            (3) Right erector spinae
         b) Contralateral Muscles:
            (1) Left external oblique
            (2) Right internal oblique
            (3) Left erector spinae
         c) Dynamic Stabilizers:
            (1) Right and left external obliques
            (2) Right and left internal obliques
            (3) Right and left erector spinae
         d) Guiding Muscles:
            (1) Muscles most involved and contralateral muscles' force-counterforce during rotation rules out flexion tendencies.
II. Movement Phase—Figure 12.2 to 12.3 Motions
   A. Pelvic Girdle Motion:
      1. Right Transverse Rotation: 75° against resistance; bilateral weight-bearing position
         a) Muscles Most Involved: concentric contraction
            (1) Right gluteus maximus
            (2) Left tensor fasciae latae
            (3) Left gluteus minimus
            (4) Left gluteus medius—anterior fibers

b) Contralateral Muscles:
  (1) Left gluteus maximus
  (2) Right tensor fasciae latae
  (3) Right gluteus minimus
  (4) Right gluteus medius—anterior fibers
c) Dynamic Stabilizers:
  (1) Muscles most involved and contralateral muscles move the pelvis while helping to stabilize it for hip and spinal column motions
B. Rib Cage Motions:
1. Right Lumbar-thoracic Rotation: 70° against resistance
  a) Muscles Most Involved: concentric contraction and momentum provide the force
    (1) Left external oblique
    (2) Right internal oblique
    (3) Right erector spinae
  b) Contralateral Muscles:
    (1) Right external oblique
    (2) Left internal oblique
    (3) Left erector spinae
  c) Dynamic Stabilizers:
    Muscles most involved and contralateral muscles
  d) Guiding Muscles:
    (1) Muscles most involved and contralateral muscles' force-counterforce rule out flexion tendencies
2. Left Lateral Flexion: 5°–10° with gravity
  a) Muscles Most Involved: eccentric contraction
    (1) Right rectus abdominis
    (2) Right external oblique
    (3) Right internal oblique
    (4) Right erector spinae
  b) Contralateral Muscles:
    (1) Left rectus abdominis
    (2) Left external oblique
    (3) Left internal oblique
    (4) Left erector spinae

Motions are analyzed frame by frame from the film. The contour drawings only represent reference points in the skill sequence. *The motion analysis must not be restricted to the contour drawings.* If this is done, critical motions will be missed. As one example, an observation of figures 12.1 and 12.2 would not give an accurate picture of the weight shift for this performer. The film frames *between* these two contour drawings show the initiation of right transverse pelvic girdle rotation while he is in a unilateral weight-bearing position shifting weight. During a basic cinematographic analysis, all frames of the film are utilized to clarify joint motions.

Basic biomechanic analysis

A course in kinesiology must include a unit of instruction in biomechanics if students have not had a prerequisite course in this subject. *A complete analysis of a sport skill includes anatomic and biomechanic explanations of the performance.* These two areas are distinct, but they do have many interrelated aspects. The comlpete analysis, therefore, will consider functional myology ("Anatomic Analysis" chapter), biomechanics ("Biomechanic Analysis" chapter), and a synthesis of these two scientific areas with the techniques of the skill ("Discussion" chapter). As noted previously, the latter chapter includes a complete discussion of the *implications* of the performance faults in relation to the skill objectives; and these are discussed both pro and con in terms of the expert opinion that has been gathered concerning the skill ("Review of Related Literature" chapter).

The professional physical educator should be able to explain any skill from points of view of anatomic kinesiology, biomechanics, and the techniques of the performance. Once the skill has been thoroughly analyzed, using the subject matter and vocabulary of anatomic kinesiology, the same skill should be explained, using the applicable principles, concepts, and vocabulary of biomechanics. The latter are presented in the "Biomechanic Analysis" chapter dealing with the basic cinematographic analysis, by discussing the biomechanic principles utilized effectively or ineffectively by the performers. The intermediate cinematographic analysis goes one step further by including mathematical calculations to objectify, compare, and contrast the motions observed.

The softball hitters are compared below, for exemplary purposes, by using some general principles from biomechanics. These are general observations of a biomechanic nature which should be made. The example does not include a complete biomechanic analysis, because biomechanic subject matter has not been emphasized within this book.

Preparatory phase

This phase is seen in figure 12.2 and figure 12.6 for the male and female respectively. The muscle length-force ratio has been more effectively applied by the male performer. His muscles most involved for subsequent spinal rotation have been placed on stretch. This means that force exerted by those muscles will be greater, because the force exerted by the muscle group placed on stretch is directly proportional to the length of those muscles. The male performer's base of support equilibrium is adequate between the stance and preparatory phases. On the other hand, the female performer's base of support stability is good in the stance, but it deteriorates considerably as she moves into the preparatory phase. The placement of her left foot is away from the line of flight of the ball. Conversely, the male performer's movement of his right foot is into the line of flight of the ball. Movement of the females's foot in this direction causes some slight equilibrium problems resulting in compensatory and extra motion to her left. This motion also tends to dissipate some of her force.

Movement phase

Figure 12.3 represents the movement phase for the male performer, and figures 12.7 and 12.8 are the movement phase for the female performer. The female performer's slight lateral rotation at the left hip joint and placement of the left foot during the stride has resulted in a compensatory movement in the upper limbs. Thus there is an interruption in the summation of internal forces. This causes a reduction in the amount of force transferred from body part to body part. There is also loss of leverage advantage within the bones acted upon by the muscles most involved. Her arms are held relatively close to the body to maintain equilibrium. This has reduced her muscle length-force ratio within the arm musculature. As can be seen in figure 12.3, the male performer does not have this same problem. It is also obvious that the rib cage of the female performer has not rotated sufficiently to her right to place the abdominal muscles on their greatest stretch in order to initiate the Serape Effect. This also reduces the amount of internal force summated and transferred to the next body segments within the kinetic chain.

The male performer is applying force in the direction of the intended motion. The female performer, however, is moving her body mass away from the direction of intended motion, thus tending to dissipate a percentage of the summated internal forces. The extraneous arm actions noted between figures 12.6–12.7, commonly known as a "hitch," have also caused an interruption within the kinetic chain, resulting in a dissipation of summated internal forces. These factors, combined with the lack of leverage at the point of impact, reduce bat velocity for the female performer. It can be noted that the male performer has little, if any, wasted motion between figures 12.2 and 12.3. His kinetic chain has been continuous and uninterrupted. Thus, his bat velocity at the point of impact has reached its maximum. His leverage advantage at the point of impact can be seen by the effective use of extended elbows. Both performers have maintained an adequate grip at the point of impact. It should be noted that the position of the female's elbow and shoulder joints has a detrimental effect upon the transfer of internal forces through the wrists and the grip action into the sport implement at this point (fig. 12.8). Her leverage advantage is not the same as seen for the male performer in figure 12.3.

Follow-through phase

This phase is seen in figures 12.4 and 12.9 for the male and female performers respectively. The extent of the follow-through is in direct proportion to the intensity of the summation of internal forces. It can be seen that the male performer has summated a greater degree of internal forces for his swing than the female performer. The female performer has a habit of dropping the bat within a fraction of a second after the phase shown in figure 12.9. Also, the follow-through for the female performer indicates that she has not used all potential internal force.

The left knee has remained slightly flexed, and her pelvic girdle has not been brought over the base of support. On the other hand, the male performer's right knee is fully extended and his pelvic girdle is moving over the base of support in the follow-through phase (fig. 12.4).

Improving performance

Any findings from a skill analysis made by a physical educator are intended for use in helping to improve the performance level of the student. Teaching follows analysis and instruction should be based on the objective findings of the physical educator. Therefore, the final step in a basic cinematographic analysis includes ranking the performance faults noted, in the order of their severity, and outlining a plan for the removal of these specific performance problems ("Major Findings and Teaching-Coaching Recommendations" chapter).

In the example analysis of the softball hitters, the objective was to improve the hitting ability of the female performer. The female's major performance problems are placed in rank order as follows:

1. Improper stride—movement of the left foot away from the line of flight of the ball to the performer's left.
2. Limited left transverse pelvic girdle rotation during the movement phase.
3. Lack of elbow extension during the movement phase.
4. Lack of shoulder joint extension in the stance.
5. Lack of left knee extension during the final aspects of the movement phase and during the follow-through phase.

The physical educator must use his or her best professional judgment and extreme care in setting up the priority list for correcting faults of the performer. Experience has indicated that if the major fault is corrected, many of the lesser faults on the priority list will be corrected during the process of eliminating the major skill problem. It is also of importance to deal with the improvement of one fault at a time. Furthermore, all information about the individual, in addition to the kinesiologic analysis, must be used to help improve performance. This type of information is derived over the entire athletic season. Therefore, the coaching suggestions should take into account both the analytic findings of the skill and the sociopsychologic-physiologic characteristics of the individual. This combined approach can lead to more precise and specific recommendations for the improvement of skill for the performer.

Exercise prescription

As noted in chapter 11, the athlete should be given a written exercise prescription designed to (1) ameliorate the most significant skill problem noted in the analyses and (2) improve on the fitness parameters. The prescription should be followed by the performer on a daily basis during the offseason and preseason.

The following is a partial example of an exercise prescription to improve the problem observed in the female's performance. If this were written for a student, the repetition and weight load detail would also be included to clarify intensity, duration, and frequency for all exercises prescribed to improve fitness. The reader is referred to various chapters for background to write those details.

Activities would be included to improve strength, muscular endurance, flexibility, and cardiovascular endurance parameters within the performer. The latter would be of particular importance for the maintenance and development of fitness during the offseason for the athlete. Also, problems like those noted in the female hitter's performance mechanics can best be improved during off-season and preseason work. There is literally more time for concentration on the problem, and the student does not have the pressures of the competitive season (McKinney, Logan, and Birmingham 1968). The following recommendations should be discussed with and demonstrated for the female student in our example:

I. Skill development drills:
    A. The initial stance should be adjusted to lower the bat about four inches. This can be done by slight extension of both shoulder joints.
    B. Stride drill progression:
        1. Striding in front of a mirror fifty to seventy-five times daily. Emphasize movement of the left leg into the line of flight of the pitch—left hip abduction.
        2. Stride and include left transverse pelvic rotation to the extreme of the range of motion.
        3. Stride, left transverse pelvic rotation followed by left and right elbow extension as used in the softball-hitting action.
        4. Perform the actual softball swing in front of a mirror, moving the bat through the low diagonal plane of motion—fifty repetitions.
    C. Hitting practice, with emphasis on the motions practiced above.
        1. *Practice does not make one perfect!* It is common to see students practicing their errors! Practice with specific purpose and direction will improve performance.
II. "Specifics" (see chap. 13):
    Fifty repetitions of the softball swing with the resistance rope of an Exer-Genie Exerciser attached to the bat handle between the hitter's hands. The initial resistance setting on the Exer-Genie Exerciser should be at two pounds to allow a bat velocity of at least 75 percent of bat velocity used during a game.
III. Strength development exercises:
    A. Perform strength development exercises for the antigravity musculature (exercises and procedures are discussed in chap. 9).
    B. Elbow extension and ulnar flexion exercises performed against resistance. (see chap. 13).
IV. Flexibility exercises:
    A. Spinal rotation exercises, slowly sitting, to both sides through the maximum range of motion (see chap. 13).

V. Muscular endurance exercises:
   A. (see chap. 13).
VI. Cardiovascular endurance activities (see chap. 13).

A basic cinematographic analysis as produced by the student involved in the professional preparation process can assist in the learning of subject matter from anatomic kinesiology and biomechanics. And the procedure followed needs only to be modified slightly to be functional in practice. The practical application of basic cinematographic analysis techniques is discussed in the following section.

Skill analysis for practicing physical educators

Time is a critical factor for the physical educator in a secondary school. The teaching load averages five classes per day, with two coaching assignments. This means that one physical educator will work with a minimum of two hundred students per day in an average situation. Numerous skills will be taught in a wide variety of sport and dance activities. The elementary school physical educator usually has more students without the athletic assignment. Knowledge of what is to be taught is a key factor if teaching is to be effective. As implied previously, analytic ability is a functional part of the physical educator's knowledge. Analysis of sport skills is one example of how and where the practicing teacher of physical education applies his or her knowledge. In order to accomplish this, however, one attribute that the physical educator must possess is *organizational ability*.

Noncinematographic analysis must be used in the average class situation where film and videotape are not available. This type of analysis should be *standard operating procedure* every time a physical educator observes a student executing a skill. The physical educator should be disciplined to look at specific segments or joints to see where problems *start* within a performance, instead of looking at the total performance only and observing where they *end!* The latter leads to ineffective teaching.

Once kinesiology subject matter has been learned, it should be applied in the practical situation. *Application is the best way to retain any type of technical or scientific subject matter.* This is one reason for having undergraduate and graduate students write detailed projects in classes dealing with kinesiology subject matter. The physical educator working with a class or athletic team does not have time to write analyses or make extensive notes following observations of students. *Therefore, skill analysis in the average class situation using noncinematographic techniques is primarily a mental process with some written observations.* The techniques of the skill under observation are known, and the probable problem areas for students are understood. During analysis, the physical educator mentally asks and answers relevant questions regarding the performance, in terms of the techniques and scientific subject matter known. Notes may be made during the observation. When the student finishes performing and the relevant questions have been answered, the physical educator should make a *positive teaching recommendation* based on the analysis. This recommendation should be designed to ameliorate the most serious problem noted during the performances observed.

The procedure for a basic cinematographic analysis is the same. However, when film or videotape are utilized more time may be taken for making written observations or notes. This is particularly applicable when coaches analyze game film. Many coaches, in team sports particularly, have a rating system for their athletes following each contest. The basic cinematographic analysis technique can be utilized as the conceptual framework for such a rating system. This helps the coach to focus on the *causative elements* of the athlete's performance as well as the *effect*. This makes the rating more objective, and more important, it should help to improve the level of the performance by isolating the major performance problem. This motion problem would be dealt with in subsequent practices through drills, exercises, or anything else deemed necessary to help the student-athlete improve. This procedure eliminates guesswork and tends to make coaching more personalized; and there are many positive psychological implications to justify this approach, instead of using the dogmatic and negative coaching techniques of the past.

Figure 12.12 shows a film sequence of the sprint start as used in track. It will be utilized as an example of a basic cinematographic analysis, including the type of questions the physical educator must ask and answer during or following the analysis in order to help the performer. The complexity of noncinematographic analysis is better understood when one considers the fact that motion between frames 5 and 22 in figure 12.12 occurs in 0.44 seconds. Film or videotape should be utilized whenever feasible and possible in teaching-coaching situations. Segmental analytic techniques are used in this example.

Observation of the total performance

Film should be viewed numerous times to obtain a general feeling about the execution of the performance. This helps gain insight into the overall timing of the skill. Also, this gives the physical educator an opportunity to compare and contrast the observed performance with what is believed to be the stereotype of perfect mechanics for the sprint start.

Pelvic area and rib cage observations

Motions of the pelvic girdle and lumbar-thoracic spine should be observed. These are appropriate body segments to start with, because they tend to show the line of thrust of the total movement. Also, they are relatively slow-moving areas in all sport skills.

A limitation of film, as cited previously, is that it shows one performance at one angle only. This is the case in figure 12.12. If this were the only view on film, the coach would have to make noncinematographic observations from anterior and posterior views on the track in order to gain total understanding of the motions. For example, the lateral view of this skill is excellent for observing anteroposterior plane motions. However, it is poor for viewing motions through transverse and diagonal planes of motion.

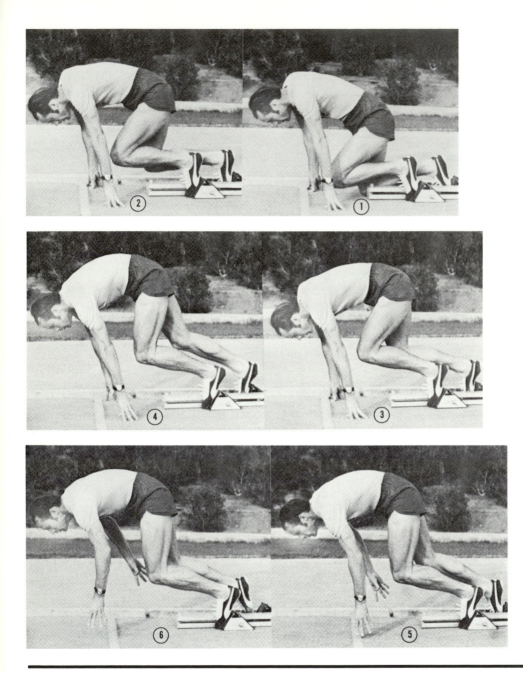

Figure 12.12. The sprint start of Tom Jones, U.S.A. Olympic Team. From Northrip, Logan, and McKinney, *Introduction to Biomechanic Analysis of Sport Skills.* Courtesy Visual Track and Field Techniques, 292 LaCienaga Blvd., Beverly Hills, California 90211.

Figure 12.12. Continued.

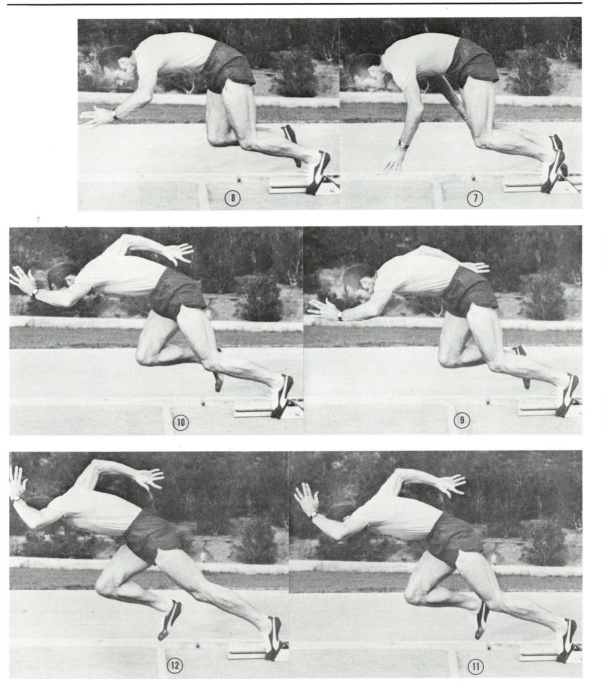

Figure 12.12. Continued.

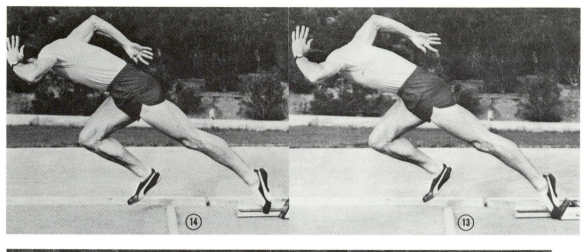

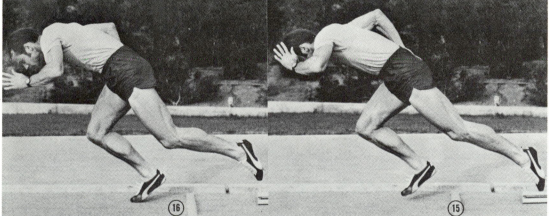

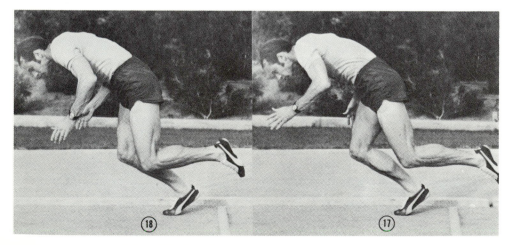

Figure 12.12. Continued.

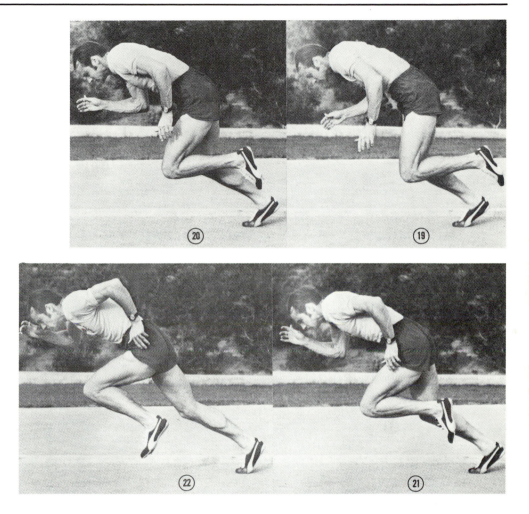

Questions the track-and-field coach might ask himself and attempt to answer while observing the pelvic girdle and rib cage of the athlete during the sprint start are: How high is the center of mass above the base of support throughout the entire skill? Are there any extraneous rotations of the spinal column and pelvic girdle through the transverse plane? Is there an undesired hyperextension of the lumbar spine during the sprint start? Does the path of the pelvic girdle deviate from a straight line at any time during the skill? In the illustration shown, the performer exemplifies ideal pelvic, spinal column, and rib cage position in frames 12 and 13. From frame 5, or the start of the movement phase, the lumbar spine moves from flexion to extension in frame 13. This is accomplished without any extraneous transverse rotations. There are, however, slight lateral rotations of the pelvic girdle when the athlete is in a unilateral weight-bearing position.

This is accomplished without excessive movement while the pelvic girdle, lumbar spine, and thoracic spine remain dynamically stabilized. If the pelvic girdle, for example, were not dynamically stable at this time, force executed through the blocks would not be effective in driving the center of mass linearly.

Base of support observations

The base of support in the stance-preparatory phase for this skill as seen in frames 1–4 consists of hand and feet placements. Several questions must be going through the mind of the physical educator as the film is viewed. Is the weight distribution between the feet and the hands appropriate? Is the block setting for the feet adequate to provide optimum force and range of motion for ankle plantar flexion, knee extension, and hip extension at the start of the movement phase in frame 5? Are there equilibrium problems in the movement phase which cause extraneous motions elsewhere when the hands no longer serve weight-bearing functions? Is there an excessive vertical lift when the left ankle finishes plantar flexing and pushes off of the block? Are the feet too far apart or close together throughout the performance? Are there any extraneous motions within the subtalar and transverse tarsal joints? Are there any extraneous medial or lateral rotations at the hip joints which would cause the feet to "toe-in" or "toe-out" too much?

The answers to these questions relative to this performance actually determine the degree of efficiency the athlete has in transferring internal forces from muscular contractions into accelerating forces for the center of mass. If the coach observes considerable extraneous motion within the bases of support during the spring start, the athlete will not be effective in transferring these forces.

Head and cervical spine observations

Motions of the cervical spine must be observed, because total body motion tends to follow motions within the cervical spine. Cervical spine motions also position the eyes. There are times when eye motions can be maximized to minimize cervical spine motions, and this will have a positive effect on the total performance.

The most important question the coach should ask himself regarding the positions of the head and cervical spine during the sprint start is: How soon does the cervical spine movement occur which allows the athlete to actually look down the track toward the finish line? Any hyperextension of the cervical spine will cause a corresponding reaction in the lumbar spine. These two major movements have a tendency to extend the trunk and greatly increase the resistive or drag force caused by air. Cervical hyperextension also tends to raise the body to the point where the horizontal force component is diminished during the acceleration phase. Both factors contribute to a decreased velocity. In the example, the cervical spine and head are stabilized in an extended position in all three phases of the skill. This adheres to the recognized stereotype of perfect mechanics for this skill.

Arm and hand observations

Motions of the shoulder joints, shoulder girdle, elbows, radio-ulnar joints, and wrists should be made as they relate to the skill undergoing analysis.

The sprinter must utilize strong shoulder joint diagonal adduction and diagonal abduction during the early part of the movement phase. Diagonal adduction of the left shoulder joint is observed in frames 6–14. From the lateral view, it is difficult to determine which plane of motion is being traversed by the right arm. Observations from anterior and posterior views need to be made on the track or on film.

During the sprint start, the arms must provide a powerful counterforce from the end of the movement phase to the start of the recovery phase. In order to be in this position, the arms must be moved to a position as high as possible during the power phase of the sprint start, while the left foot in the example is pushing back against the blocks. The diagonal movements of both upper limbs are made in such a way as to provide an optimum state of equilibrium. It must be remembered that during the sprint start the sprinter is actually in a dynamic state of disequilibrium. He is protected from falling only because he is undergoing extreme acceleration. Movement of the arms through the diagonal plane during the movement phase is extremely important relative to the principle of equilibrium. Movement through the diagonal plane provides a greater moment of inertia than movements at the shoulder joints through anteroposterior planes. Movements of the hands and fingers are of interest. Are the fingers flexed or extended? If the sprinter has a flexed hand, this would be an indicator of stress and extraneous muscle tension within the extrinsic musculature of the hand. That would be the type of muscle contraction a coach would want to eliminate, because it ultimately leads to increased energy cost and decreased linear velocity. The athlete in figure 12.12 demonstrates excellent hand and arm motions.

Leg observations

Motions at the hip, knee, and ankle joints must be observed to determine their overall contributions to the skill. The hip joint motions are very important in getting out of the blocks. Are the left hip extension and right hip flexion ranges of motion and velocity adequate at the start of the movement phase in frames 5–14? Are there any extraneous transverse plane motions at the hip and knee joints? Are the extensor motions at the three major left leg joints performed throughout their complete ranges of motion prior to the time the sprinter leaves the blocks? Are the flexions at the hips and knees great enough to functionally conserve angular momentum?

These, and other, questions should be answered during the analysis of the sprint start. Any teaching or coaching would follow and be based upon the objective findings of the basic cinematographic analysis. This type of analysis is not too time-consuming; it is, therefore, functional in practice, especially in athletic situations where film is available.

Summary

There is one basic difference between a kinesiologic analysis of a sport skill as conducted by students involved in the professional preparation process, and that of physical educators doing analyses in the field. The undergraduate should do an extensive series of written *academic exercises* dealing with the myologic and biomechanic subject matter. Those activities are performed to help reinforce the learning of kinesiologic subject matter. Physical educators in the field analyze the performers noncinematographically and cinematographically, using those same techniques and answering the same types of questions related to the performances. Their skill evaluations or grading of game film performances are accomplished without using extensive written reports. The analytic techniques based on kinesiologic principles can help improve performances. And this is the major objective for professional preparation in kinesiology.

Recommended readings

Alderman, Richard B. "A Comparative Study of the Effectiveness of Two Grips for Teaching Beginning Golf." *Research Quarterly* 38 (March 1967) :3–9.

Alexander, John F., et al. "Effect of Strength Development on Speed of Shooting of Ice Hockey Players." *Research Quarterly* 35 (May 1964) :101–6.

Anderson, Margaret B. "Comparison of Muscle Patterning in the Overarm Throw and Tennis Serve." *Research Quarterly* 50 (December 1979) :541–553.

Arensen, Arne U. "Analyzing the Pole Vault." *Athletic Journal* 39 (1959) :28.

Blievernicht, Jean Gelner. "Accuracy in the Tennis Forehand Drive: Cinematographic Analysis." *Research Quarterly* 39 (October 1968) :776–78.

Breen, James L. "What Makes a Good Hitter?" *Journal of Health, Physical Education and Recreation* 38 (April 1961) :36–39.

Budney, David R. and Bellow, Donald G. "Kinetic Analysis of a Golf Swing." *Research Quarterly* 50 (May 1979) :171–179.

Chandler, Joe; Langley, Thomas D.; and Blair, Steven N. "Movement Times for Jab and Cross-over Steps by High School Football Players." *Research Quarterly* 46 (May 1975) :147–52.

Collins, M. R. "Research on Sprint Running." *Athletic Journal* 32 (1952) :30.

Counsilman, J. E. "Forces in Swimming Two Types of Crawl Strokes." *Research Quarterly* 26 (May 1955) :127.

Dainis, A. "Cinematographic Analysis of the Handspring Vault." *Research Quarterly* 50 (October 1979) :341–349.

Dillman, Charles J. and Sears, Ronald G. (Eds.). *Kinesiology: A National Conference on Teaching.* Urbana-Champaign: University of Illinois, 1978.

Edwards, Donald K. "Effects of Stride and Position on the Pitching Rubber on Control in Baseball Pitching." *Research Quarterly* 34 (March 1963) :9-14.

Elbell, E. R. "Measuring Speed and Force of Charge of Football Players." *Research Quarterly* 23 (October 1952) :295.

Elftman, Herbert. "The Basic Pattern of Human Locomotion." *Annals of the New York Academy of Science* 51 (1951) :1207-12.

Ganslen, Richard V. "High Hurdling Mechanics." *Scholastic Coach* 18 (February 1949) :11.

————. "A Form Study of Don Laz." *Scholastic Coach* 20 (February 1951) :9.

————. "The Hop, Step and Jump." *Athletic Journal* 35 (April 1955) :12, 14, 16, 67-70.

————. "Style in the Hop, Step and Jump." *Athletic Journal* 36 (May 1956) :12-14.

Ganslen, Richard V., and Jarvinen, Matti. "Finnish Javelin Throwing." Scholastic Coach 19 (February 1950) :8.

Hay, James G. "Pole Vaulting: A Mechanical Analysis of Factors Influencing Polebend." *Research Quarterly* 38 (March 1967) :34-40.

————. "An Investigation of Take-off Impulses in Two Styles of High Jumping." *Research Quarterly* 39 (December 1968) :983-92.

Jackson, Andrew S., and Cooper, John M. "Effects of Hand Spacing and Rear Knee Angle on the Sprint Start." *Research Quarterly* 41 (1970) :378-92.

Johnson, Joan. "The Tennis Serve of Advanced Women Players." *Research Quarterly* 28 (May 1957) :123.

King, W. H., and Irwin, L. W. "A Time and Motion Study of Competitive Backstroke Swimming Turns." *Research Quarterly* 28 (October 1957) :257.

Lanoue, Fred. "Analysis of the Basic Factors in Fancy Diving." *Research Quarterly* 11 (March 1940) :102-9.

Lapp, V. W. "A Study of Hammer Velocity and the Physical Factors Involved in Hammer Throwing." *Research Quarterly* 6 (October 1935) :134.

Macmillan, M. B. "Determinants of the Flight of the Kicked Football." *Research Quarterly* 46 (1975) :48-57.

McKinney, Wayne C. "A Syllabus for Writing a Basic Cinematographic Analysis." Mimeographed. Springfield, Mo.: Health and Physical Education Department, Southwest Missouri State University, 1975.

McKinney, Wayne C., and Logan, Gene A. "A Syllabus for the Undergraduate Kinesiology Project." Mimeographed. Springfield, Mo.: Health and Physical Education Department, Southwest Missouri State University, 1977.

McKinney, Wayne C.; Logan, Gene A.; and Birmingham, Dick. "Training Baseball Pitchers in the Off-Season." *Athletic Journal* 47 (January 1968) :58, 84–86.

Maglischo, Cheryl W., and Maglischo, Ernest. "Comparison of Three Racing Starts Used in Competitive Swimming." *Research Quarterly* 39 (October 1968) :604–9.

Mann, Ralph and Sprague, Paul. "A Kinetic Analysis of the Ground Leg During Sprint Running." *Research Quarterly for Exercise and Sport* 51 (May 1980) :334–348.

Marshall, S. "Factors Affecting Place Kicking in Football." *Research Quarterly* 29 (October 1958) :302.

Menely, Ronald, and Rosemier, Robert A. "Effectiveness of Four Track Starting Positions on Acceleration." *Research Quarterly* 39 (March 1968) :161–65.

Mortimer, E. M. "Basketball Shooting." *Research Quarterly* 22 (May 1951) :234.

Mowerson, G. R., and McAdam, R. E. "A Comparison of Two Methods of Performing the Racing Start in Competitive Swimming." *Swimming World* 5 (February 1964) :4.

Northrip, John W., Logan, Gene A. and McKinney, Wayne C. *Introduction to Biomechanic Analysis of Sport* (Second Edition). Dubuque, Ia: Wm. C. Brown Company, 1979.

Owens, Jack A. "Effect of Variations in Hand and Foot Spacing on Movement Time and on Force Charge." *Research Quarterly* 31 (March 1960) :66–76.

Peterson, H. D. "A Scientific Approach to Shooting in Basketball." *Athletic Journal* 40 (October 1959) :32.

Plagenhoef, Stanley. "Biomechanical Analysis of Olympic Flatwater Kayaking and Canoeing." *Research Quarterly* 50 (October 1979) :443–459.

Purdy, Bonnie J., and Stallard, Mary L. "Effect of Two Learning Methods and Two Grips on the Acquisition of Power and Accuracy in the Golf Swing of College Women." *Research Quarterly* 38 (October 1967) :480–84.

Race, Donald E. "Cinematographic and Mechanical Analysis of External Movements Involved in Hitting a Baseball Effectively." *Research Quarterly* 32 (October 1961) :394–404.

Rehling, C. H. "Analysis of Techniques of the Golf Drive." *Research Quarterly* 26 (March 1955) :80.

Schuble, Sue. "Comparative Kinesiologic Analyses of Two Softball Hitting Styles." Unpublished paper, Southwest Missouri State University, Springfield, 1969.

Seymour, Emery W. "Comparison of Base Running Methods." *Research Quarterly* 30 (October 1959) :321–25.

Slater-Hammel, A. T. "Action Current Study of Contraction-Movement Relationships in the Golf Stroke." *Research Quarterly* 19 (October 1948) :164.

――――. "An Action Current Study of Contraction-Movement Relationships in the Tennis Stroke." *Research Quarterly* 20 (December 1949) :424.

Smith, Karl U., et al. "Analysis of the Temporal Components of Motion in Human Gait." *American Journal of Physical Medicine* 39 (August 1960) :142-51.

Stock, Malcolm. "Influence of Various Track Starting Positions on Speed." *Research Quarterly* 33 (December 1962) :607-14.

Van Huss, W. D., et al. "Effect of Overload Warm-up on the Velocity and Accuracy of Throwing." *Research Quarterly* 33 (October 1962) :472-75.

White, R. A. "Effect of Hip Elevation on the Starting Time of the Sprint." *Research Quarterly Supplement* 6 (1935) :128-33.

Zimmerman, Helen M. "Characteristic Likeness and Differences Between Skilled and Non-Skilled Performance of Standing Broad Jump." *Research Quarterly* 27 (October 1956) :352-62.

13 Improving the Individual through Exercise

Ability to execute skills effectively is enhanced considerably if the performer is "in shape"; that is, the performer who has excellent levels of strength, muscular endurance, cardiovascular endurance, and flexibility is more likely to reach his or her potential than someone who has not attained a similar level of athletic conditioning. However, exercise goes beyond the scope of athletics and other performance areas. *Physical fitness* is a responsibility of physical education teachers in instructional as well as athletic program assignments. The skill levels of the students in these two programs may differ, but their individual requirements for attaining optimum levels of physical fitness and scientific knowledge about physical conditioning are the same. This knowledge is important, because it will endure long after the class or athletic season has come to an end. As such, it has the potential of making a significant contribution to the individual student's value system and life-style. This part of the physical education process should be available to everyone. Every physically educated individual should know what muscular activity can and cannot do for the human organism.

Exercises should be prescribed by physical educators to meet fitness requirements of the individuals within the instructional and athletic programs. When prescribing any exercise, there should be a thorough kinesiologic understanding of the desired outcome of each exercise or activity. There is a professional obligation to each student to meet this criterion. Furthermore, the physical educator is morally, ethically, and legally obligated to know what effects each exercise or activity will have on the students. If a thorough understanding of *why* the students are subjected to an exercise or activity is not documented technically and scientifically, it should not be included in the program.

Some exercises are potentially dangerous, and others waste the time of the performers. The potentially dangerous exercises must be eliminated. This can be accomplished *if* the physical educator takes time to analyze kinesiologically each exercise *before* giving it to students, instead of using an exercise because it is a "traditional activity." An example of a very poor "traditional activity" is the double leg raise (left and right hip flexion with knees extended and ankles plantar flexed) while lying supine. This exercise is potentially dangerous because of the action of the psoas major on the lumbar spine during the double hip flexion. The psoas major contracts with the iliacus as a muscle most involved for hip flexion. The psoas major also attaches on the bodies of the lumbar vertebrae; therefore, as the hips flex, the psoas major causes excessive lumbar hyperextension in individuals who cannot counteract the effect of the psoas by strong contraction of the abdominals. This hyperextension can cause some spinal problems for individuals who have tight erector spinae and weak abdominal muscles. This type of exercise should never be given to a general physical education class.

The four physical fitness parameters of strength, muscular endurance, cardiovascular endurance, and flexibility are important to skill development, regardless of the skill level of the performer. They are just as significant to the "recreational athlete" as they are to the "superstar," because these are the undergirding elements for the development of skill.

They are also essential to the health and well-being of the individual. All types of performers learning sport or dance activities are developing skill. In addition, fitness development activities also possess sufficient versatility to be used independently, as avocational activities completely separated from skill development. Many people enjoy fitness activities as an end in themselves, leading to better well-being. These individuals are not interested in fitness activities because they are a means to an end, i.e., that end being an increased skill level. Therefore, the way in which fitness activities are presented will depend, in part, on the desired objectives or outcomes expected by the individual, class, athletic team, or group being taught.

The development of strength, muscular endurance, cardiovascular endurance, and flexibility is based on the application of the SAID principle: *Specific Adaptation to Imposed Demands* (Wallis and Logan 1964). The demands imposed on the human organism to bring about change in any of the aforementioned factors and to subsequently improve performance must supersede or be progressively more intense than previous demands. As a result of this type of overloading of the organism, specific adaptations result in these performance factors. The imposed demand must be applied specifically to bring about the desired results. The term *specifics,* as used in this chapter, is an application of the SAID principle. *Specifics is defined as application of resistance allowing limb velocities not less than 75 percent of maximum velocity through the exact plane of motion, ranges of motion, and at precise joint angles used by the athlete while performing skills in the athletic contest* (Logan and McKinney 1969).

Strength is the ability to overcome resistance. It can be developed by isometric as well as isotonic techniques. Due to numerous inherent traumatic effects associated with isometric strength techniques, that form of strength development is not recommended for general use. It can be utilized safely and effectively at some joints, e.g., to increase strength at a specific angle in knee extension, but it should be prescribed by qualified exercise scientists who fully understand the merits and limitations of isometric strength development procedures.

Isotonic strength development procedures are recommended for general use by physical educators. Some of the guidelines for strength programs were discussed in chapter 9. *If the objective of a weight training exercise is to develop*

Strength development

strength, it is recommended that a maximal weight load be slowly moved concentrically and eccentrically through the desired range of motion of the joint for eight repetitions. That is a functional, safe weight load which will produce strength and minimizes potential trauma to the performers. A maximal weight load for one or two repetitions is vastly different; and this could create some of the same traumatic problems inherent in "all out" isometric exercise.

The guideline of the maximum weight for eight repetitions for strength development needs to be qualified in terms of intensity for an exercise prescription for a normal performer. A series of weight training exercises must be prescribed to work the anteroposterior antigravity muscles, their contralateral muscles (see chapter 9), and various other joint musculature in need of strength—examples follow in this chapter. This series of strength exercises is called a set. The performer needs to complete three sets each day of the strength exercises recommended by the physical educator who develops the exercise prescription. Strength exercises can be performed daily without ill effects. This works effectively with highly motivated athletes. On the other hand, it has been found pragmatically that an alternate day strength program works better for less motivated performers and people with general fitness as their goal. However, in the case of the latter groups, they should be given other activities on days when they are not doing strength work. They should not be completely sedentary half of the week!

With athletic populations, the duration of the strength development program should be for the full year. The year should be divided into: (1) post season, (2) preseason, and (3) in season blocks of time. Strength work should be prescribed for each athlete in each of these time periods, with short, strategically placed "rest periods" at intervals, to facilitate motivation. The number one fundamental in athletics is conditioning. It is a mistake for a physical educator not to emphasize this throughout the year. This daily approach to fitness activities should also be stressed for people who are interested in exercise for its potential preventive medicine objectives.

Shoulder and arm strength exercises

The exercises in this section also utilize the SAID principle to develop strength in the muscle groups within the shoulders and arms. These exercises are recommended for general strength development programs. Although the discussion focuses on the muscles most involved for each motion, it must be remembered that other muscles also benefit from the exercise. Muscle groups are working as contralateral muscles, stabilizers, dynamic stabilizers, and guiding muscles. A simple exercise for the shoulder joints as shown in figure 13.1 works the shoulder joint adductors against resistance, shoulder girdle downward rotators (dynamically stabilizing), and the musculature surrounding the lumbar-thoracic spine and pelvic girdle (stabilizing).

Figure 13.1 shows an exercise for shoulder adduction and downward rotation of the shoulder girdle against resistance. The bar may be pulled down behind the head, in front of the head, or in front of the body with the elbows fully extended. Changing the angle of the pull in this manner provides movement through different ranges of motion. The spine should remain extended during the pulling of the bar.

Figure 13.2 shows the bench press exercise. This isolates the horizontal adductors and elbow extensor for work during the press. The spinal column is stabilized and the shoulder girdle dynamically stabilizes as it upwardly and downwardly rotates to maintain the positioning of the glenoid fossa of the scapula with the head of the humerus.

Figure 13.3 shows the overhead press exercise combining shoulder joint abduction, upward rotation of the shoulder girdle, and elbow extension against resistance. This exercise can be performed while standing; however, it is recommended that a seated position be taken as shown. This results in less strain in the lumbar area if the stool is placed directly under the bar. The performer should have the spinal column stabilized in an extended position during the overhead press.

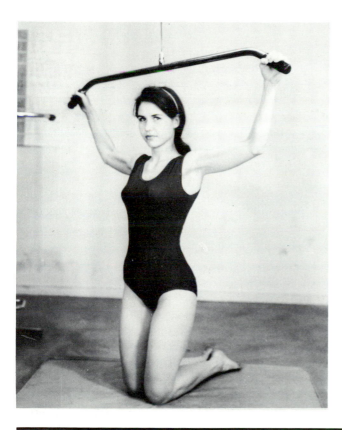

Muscles most involved
- *LATISSIMUS DORSI*
- *TERES MAJOR*
- *PECTORALIS MAJOR (LOWER FIBERS)*
- *RHOMBOIDS*
- *PECTORALIS MINOR*

Figure 13.1. Latissimus pull—shoulder adduction and downward rotation of the shoulder girdle (Ruth Miller).

Muscles most involved
- *DELTOID (ANTERIOR FIBERS)*
- *PECTORALIS MAJOR*
- *CORACOBRACHIALIS*
- *TRICEPS BRACHII*

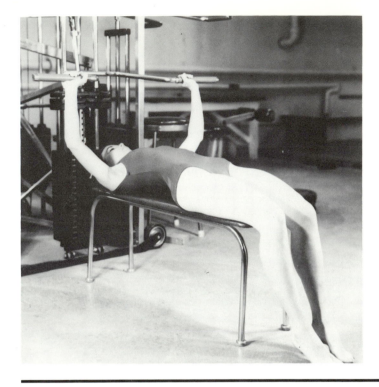

Figure 13.2. Bench press—horizontal adduction and elbow extension.

Figure 13.4 shows an exercise to work the elbow flexors against resistance. The radio-ulnar joints are sulpinated. At the end of the range-of-motion for elbow flexion on each repetition, the wrists may be flexed against resistance. The lumbar-thoracic spine should remain in stabilized extension throughout the exercise. This position becomes increasingly difficult to maintain as the performer becomes tired; therefore, it is a good idea to place the performer against a wall if possible.

The common push-up exercise is shown in figure 13.5. Body weight is utilized as the resistance, and this weight load may not be enough for many people in terms of strength development. This is a good strength exercise for the muscles indicated if the individual can only perform eight to twelve repetitions of the push-up. This exercise is usually used to develop muscular endurance in elbow extensors and shoulder flexors by performing maximum repetitions until fatigued. The major joints should remain stabilized and extended as shown on every repetition, i.e., there should be no extraneous flexions of the hip joints and lumbar-thoracic spine. The latter motions are usually incorporated by the performer when fatique starts.

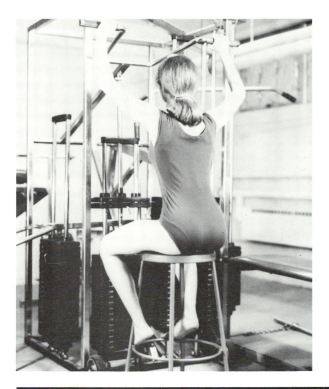

Muscles most involved
• *DELTOID*
• *SUPRASPINATUS*
• *TRAPEZIUS*
• *SERRATUS ANTERIOR*
• *TRICEPS BRACHII*

Figure 13.3. Overhead press—shoulder abduction, upward rotation, and elbow extension.

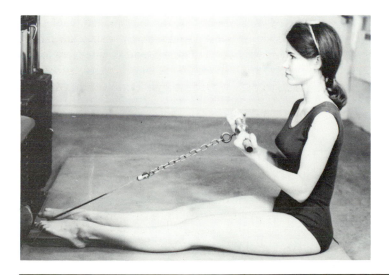

Muscles most involved
• *BICEPS BRACHII*
• *BRACHIALIS*
• *BRACHIORADIALIS*

Figure 13.4. Biceps curl—elbow flexion (Ruth
Miller).

The exercises presented in this section are intended to be examples of shoulder and arm exercises only. There are numerous isotonic exercises with a wide variety of equipment which can provide strength in the muscle groups cited. Free weights, as one example, are recommended in preference to weight machines while working with small groups, such as most athletic squads. Weight machines are desirable, especially from the standpoint of safety control, for large groups and classes.

Regardless of what overload technique is used, it must be remembered always to work muscles on both sides of a joint during the sets of exercise. This is demonstrated in figures 13.4 and 13.5.

Flexibility development

Of the major factors contributing to the development of skill, flexibility is most commonly overlooked in training programs for sports. *Flexibility is the range of motion through which body parts move at joints.* Joint flexibility can be increased by properly applied exercises, and is decreased through disuse or inactivity. For normal individuals, flexibility in any joint can be increased appreciably through proper stretching exercises if performed continuously over a period of time. Too often sport performance is inhibited by a lack of flexibility.

The SAID principle applies to the development of flexibility. To develop flexibility, the performer must steadily increase the demand on the joint undergoing training in order to enhance the joint's range of motion. Contrary to common belief, flexibility is specific to given joints (Holland 1968). As an example, an individual's right elbow might be capable of a full range of motion while the left elbow remains relatively inflexible. This condition may be directly related to the work habits of the individual; that is, flexibility is related to the daily demands placed upon the specific body part. This example indicates that the adaptation of the body part may be positive or negative in response to the demands made on it. Physical educators have an obligation to impose exercise demands on joints for purposes of improving flexibility and thus improving skill.

Muscles most involved
- *TRICEPS BRACHII*
- *DELTOID (ANTERIOR FIBERS)*
- *PECTORALIS MAJOR (UPPER FIBERS)*

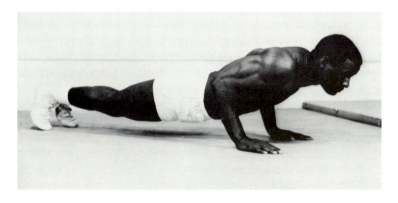

Figure 13.5. Push-up—elbow extension and shoulder flexion (Ardie McCoy).

The optimum degree of flexibility in joints, however, is specific to each activity. Some activities, such as dance and gymnastics, require that performers be highly flexible in many joints. On the other hand, certain sport skills require only limited ranges of motion.

There are many misconceptions regarding flexibility. The strong, muscular individual may have extreme flexibility in all major joints. Strength and flexibility are independent of each other. Strength involves the state of the *contractile tissue* within the muscle; whereas, flexibility involves the status of the *noncontractile tissue* surrounding the muscle fiber as well as in the joint involved. *Therefore, judicious stretching to develop flexibility cannot impede strength development.* Conversely, strength development will not have a detrimental effect on flexibility, providing the individual is working through a full range of motion for each motion possible for the joint.

It is recommended that flexibility exercises be done *slowly* and under control without the development of momentum. (Falls, Baylor, Dishman 1980). The use of "bobbing" exercise with momentum while warming up may be a predisposing factor to injury of connective tissues during an "all-out" or ballistic athletic performance. It is highly possible that many injuries occur or are "set up" during the stretching phase of the warm-up prior to football games and track meets, due to a stretching of the posterior thigh area as a result of "bobbing" with uncontrolled momentum. It has been observed that athletes often limp off the field or track with an injury in the area which has been stretched previously as a result of using this undesirable technique. Flexibility exercises should be done with the center of mass on or near the ground when possible.

To avoid possible injury during flexibility exercises, "slow stretch to one's limit" is recommended. At the end of the stretch, a static position should be held for twenty to thirty seconds. Each flexibility exercise should be performed five to ten times on a daily basis. It is recommended that the exercise prescription integrate flexibility exercises with strength exercises. (examples follow).

The slow stretch should be continued to the individual's tolerance point for pain. If pain persists throughout a twenty-four-hour period in the body area being stretched, however, the flexibility exercises have been too strenuous. Furthermore, it is advised that the muscles contralateral to the area being stretched should be actively contracted concentrically during the lengthening process. This has a neurologic benefit in dampening the stretch reflex within the musculature being stretched.

There are several body areas requiring special consideration in terms of flexibility. These are the posterior thigh, anterior hip region, lumbar spine area, cervical spine, and the pectoral region of the chest. Connective tissue in these areas tends to shorten adaptively in the inactive individual. The student-athlete is particularly vulnerable because he or she is generally sedentary during the day. The crucial joint movements to analyze for flexibility are hip joint flexion when the knees are extended, lumbar flexion, cervical flexion, and diagonal abduction at the shoulder joint.

It appears beneficial to precede flexibility exercises with muscular and/or cardiovascular endurance exercises. The rationale for this lies in the assumption that flexibility is more likely to be improved when there is an elevation in the internal temperature of the body. A temperature elevation is a common bodily adaptation which results from endurance exercise.

Figures 13.6 and 13.7 show one exercise which may be used to increase flexibility in the posterior hip joint and lumbar spine regions. The knee and hip joints are flexed to start the exercise (fig. 13.6). The hip joints are extended slowly while the abdominal musculature contracts concentrically. Figures 13.8 and 13.9 show an alternate exercise to increase flexibility within the same body segments. The latter are better exercises, because the body is in a more stable position.

Flexibility exercises for the lumbar spine are shown in figures 13.10 and 13.11. The knees are flexed to eliminate the action of the biceps femoris, semitendinosus, and semimembranosus on the posterior hip region. The objective in this exercise is to slowly flex the lumbar-thoracic spine as much as possible, while maintaining a strong concentric contraction of the abdominal musculature. The exercise may be performed on the floor or in a chair as shown.

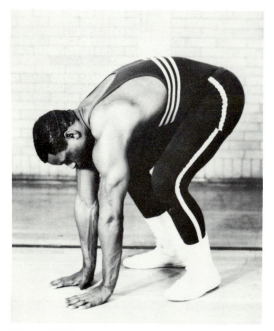
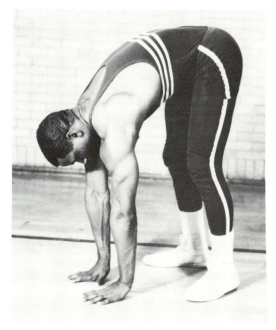

Figure 13.6.   **Figure 13.7.**

Figure 13.6. Hamstring stretch, standing—start.

Figure 13.7. Hamstring stretch, standing—finish.

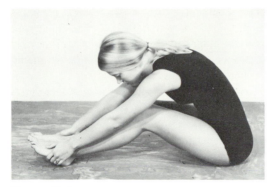

Figure 13.8.

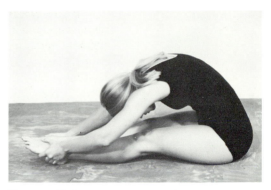

Figure 13.9.

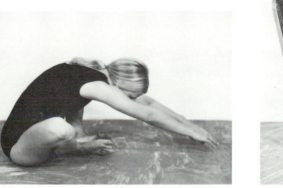

Figure 13.10.

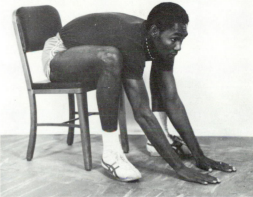

Figure 13.11.

Figure 13.8. Hamstring stretch, sitting—start (Jan Stevenson). From Logan, *Adapted Physical Education.*

Figure 13.9. Hamstring stretch, sitting—finish. From Logan, *Adapted Physical Education.*

Figure 13.10. Lumbar stretch. From Logan, *Adapted Physical Education.*

Figure 13.11. Lumbar stretch. From Logan, *Adapted Physical Education.*

Exercises to stretch the hamstrings and lumbar area should be performed with the body stable as shown in figures 13.8–13.11. Flexibility exercises for these areas performed while standing are not recommended.

Figure 13.12 is a flexibility exercise for the thoracic spine. The hands are pressed against the floor as shown, and the abdominals are strongly contracted as the legs are brought back over the head with the knees flexed. The knees remain extended throughout the stretch.

Figures 13.13 and 13.14 show a flexibility exercise for increasing transverse plane ranges of motion in the cervical, thoracic, and lumbar spinal areas. Spinal rotation is aided by pressing forcefully against the lateral aspect of the thigh. An attempt should be made to look over one shoulder and see as far as possible in the opposite direction.

The flexibility exercise shown in figures 13.15 and 13.16 is used primarily for the anterior pectoral region. With the elbows and wrists extended, the hands grip the back of a chair. The cervical spine is flexed slowly. The abdominal muscles are contracted concurrently. The knee and hip joints remain stabilized as shown throughout the exercise. This also facilitates stretching the posterior knee and hip musculature. This, and other flexibility exercises in this section, should be repeated five to ten times daily.

Muscular endurance development

Although strength and muscular endurance are developed concurrently, they are discussed here as separate entities. The two factors were separated in order to convey more clearly ideas concerning the kinesiologic aspects of strength and muscular endurance development.

A strength-endurance continuum has been hypothesized (Logan and Foreman 1961). This hypothesis regarding the existence of a strength-endurance continuum has been supported in the literature (Yessis 1963). The development of strength and muscular endurance involves a ratio between the amount of resistance and the number of repetitions. Greater resistance and fewer repetitions

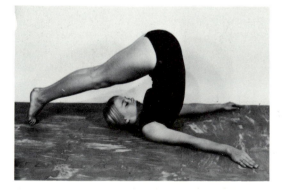

Figure 13.12. Thoracic and cervical spine stretch (Jan Stevenson). From Logan, *Adapted Physical Education.*

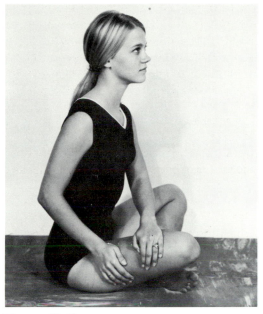

Figure 13.13.

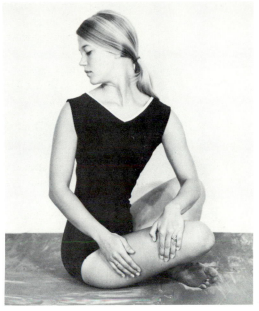

Figure 13.14.

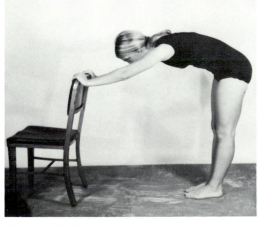

Figure 13.15.

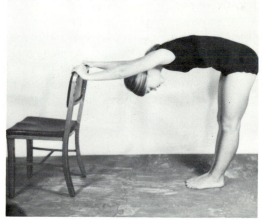

Figure 13.16.

Figure 13.13. Spinal rotation stretch, sitting—start (Jan Stevenson). From Logan, *Adapted Physical Education.*

Figure 13.14. Spinal rotation stretch, sitting—finish. From Logan, *Adapted Physical Education.*

Figure 13.15. Pectoral stretch—start. From Logan, *Adapted Physical Education.*

Figure 13.16. Pectoral stretch—finish. (Jan Stevenson). From Logan, *Adapted Physical Education.*

will produce strength and some muscular endurance. On the other hand, a greater number of repetitions with low resistance tends to produce muscular endurance and some strength. *Muscle endurance is the ability of a muscle group to make sustained contractions against relatively light resistance.*

An efficient technique, circuit training, for the development of muscular endurance with some reciprocal strength benefits has been advanced by Morgan and Adamson (1958). Circuit training involves the use of the station method. The circuit can be designed to fulfill the specific objectives of training. Generally, there are six to ten stations in a circuit training program. The following principles should serve as the bases for the development of a circuit: (1) There should be exercises for the antigravity musculature; (2) The stations should be established to work alternate body segments as the individual moves from one station to the next; and (3) The exercise stations, in addition to the antigravity stations, should be designed to develop muscular endurance for a specific sport, provided that the circuit is used in an athletic situation.

The example of a circuit training program presented below is designed for athletes involved with throwing skills. There are exercises for the antigravity musculature, shoulder and arm musculature, and a specific throwing exercise station through the high diagonal plane of motion against resistance. Resistance loads in a circuit training program are arbitrarily established, depending upon the strength and endurance levels of the individuals involved in the group. The strength and muscular endurance levels of the weakest and strongest individuals in the group are taken into consideration when establishing resistance loads. Arbitrarily, the repetition range in a circuit training program should be between ten and thirty repetitions at each station. If the individual with a low level of strength and muscular endurance cannot complete ten repetitions, he or she should perform at a maximum level at the station. On the other hand, if the individual with a high level of strength and muscular endurance can do more than thirty repetitions at a given station, a duplicate station with a higher level of resistance should be provided to allow this person to work between the ten and thirty repetition range.

Circuit training program

The example circuit training program below consists of seven stations: (1) upright rowing, (2) half squat, (3) bench press, (4) flexed knee sit-up, (5) pull-up, (6) back-raise, and (7) throwing.

Station 1, figure 13.17, shows the upright rowing exercise. The muscles most involved in this exercise are the deltoid, supraspinatus, serratus anterior, biceps brachii, brachialis, brachioradialis, and trapezius.

Station 2, figure 13.18, is an exercise to develop muscular endurance primarily in the quadriceps femoris muscle group. The muscles most involved in the half-squat exercise are the gluteus maximus, rectus femoris, vastus medialis, vastus intermedius, and vastus lateralis muscles. The feet should be shoulder-width apart, with heels placed on a two-inch board as shown. Also, for safety purposes, a chair should be placed behind the athlete to insure half-knee flexion only. Spotters are necessary for this particular exercise to remove the weight from the participant's shoulders if a weight rack is not available.

Station 3, figure 13.19, is the bench press. This exercise was discussed previously. It is recommended that spotters be utilized for the bench press if weights are used as shown in figure 13.19.

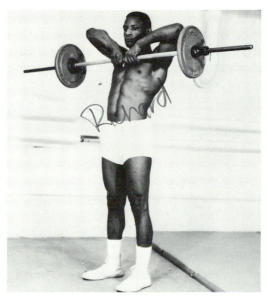

Figure 13.17.

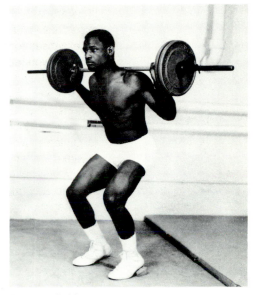

Figure 13.18.

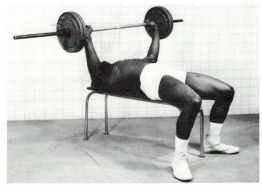

Figure 13.19.

Figure 13.17. Upright rowing—station one (Ardie McCoy).

Figure 13.18. Half squat—station two.

Figure 13.19. Bench press—station three.

Station 4, figure 13.20, shows the flexed knee sit-up on an incline board. The muscles most involved are the rectus abdominis, external oblique, and internal oblique. The resistances for this exercise are applied by changing the angles of the incline board and/or placing additional weight behind the head. Both of these resistances can be increased periodically during the training program. Care should be taken to place the buttocks from six to ten inches from the heels. It should be noted that this exercise is performed by flexing the cervical and lumbar spines in a "curling fashion." The abdominal station can be done more safely in the circuit as a "curl up" exercise involving lumbar-thoracic flexion from the supine position.

Station 5, figure 13.21, is a pull-up. This exercise can be done with the radio-ulnar joints either pronated or supinated, depending upon the desired outcome. The muscles most involved in the pull-up are the biceps brachii, brachialis, brachioradialis, lower and middle pectoralis major, pectoralis minor, rhomboids, lattisimus dorsi, and teres major. The resistance for this exercise is provided by the individual's body weight. If the individual cannot perform ten repetitions of this exercise, maximum repetitions should be done at this station.

Station 6, figure 13.22, shows the back-raise. The muscles most involved in the back-raise are the erector spinae muscle group, gluteus maximus, biceps femoris, semitendinosus, and semimembranosus. It is recommended that individuals with a relatively low-strength level refrain from lumbar hyperextension. They should move through a range of motion bringing them to the level of the

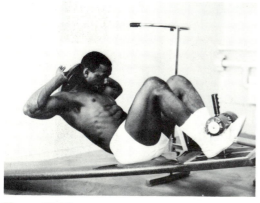

Figure 13.20.

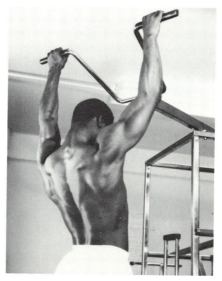

Figure 13.21.

Figure 13.20. Hook-lying sit-up—station four.

Figure 13.21. Pull-up—station five.

table. Resistance for this exercise is derived from the trunk weight of the individual as well as the weight plate held behind the individual's head. The feet may be held down by a strap, as shown, or by another individual. Once average strength has been attained in the erector spinae, the back raise should be done through a complete anteroposterior range of motion including lumbar hyperextension.

Station 7, figure 13.23, shows an exercise designed specifically for throwing. The muscles most involved in this throwing exercise are the pectoralis major, teres major, latissimus dorsi, coracobrachialis, short head of the biceps brachii, and triceps brachii. The resistance at this station must be 1–3 pounds on the Exer-Genie Exerciser, because this station is primarily concerned with developing local muscular endurance in order to improve throwing skill. A greater resistance could cause trauma to the rotary cuff. *The principle to follow in regard to the amount of resistance is that limb velocity during the application of specific resistance should not be reduced more than one-fourth of limb speed without resistance during the actual athletic performance* (Logan and McKinney 1967). A greater resistance causes an undesirable change in the athlete's throwing mechanics. Generally, resistances of more than three pounds tend to cause a distinct change in throwing form. It is essential that the athlete concentrate on throwing mechanics for a particular position. This should include footwork as well as arm and trunk movements.

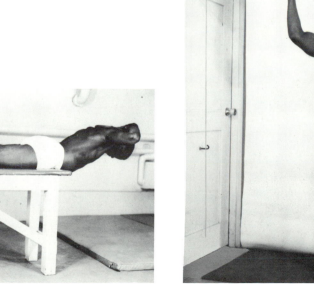

Figure 13.22.   **Figure 13.23.**

Figure 13.22. Back raise—station six.

Figure 13.23. Specifics—throwing—station seven.

Starting a circuit training program

To start a circuit training program, the squad or class is divided into equal groups based on the number of stations in the circuit. Since the circuit is designed to work different body segments in sequence, it is not necessary for everyone to start at station one. Therefore, the groups can be distributed evenly throughout the seven stations to initiate the training program. On the first day, all participants complete maximum repetitions at the seven stations on the circuit. These are recorded, and the repetition number is reduced by one-third for each station for each performer. On subsequent training days, the groups move in sequence through the circuit three times per workout. It is essential to the development of muscular endurance that the groups move through the circuit as rapidly as possible while executing the exercises properly. An example of one individual starting at station one follows: Eighteen repetitions were performed on the first day for upright rowing. This figure is reduced by one-third for subsequent work-outs. Consequently, twelve repetitions would be completed each time station one is reached. The same number of repetitions would be repeated three times (three sets per workout), making a total of thirty-six repetitions during the workout period of approximately forty-five minutes.

The overload demands should be increased as the circuit training program proceeds. This may be done in the following ways: (1) decrease the allotted time for the completion of the three circuits, (2) increase the arbitrarily established resistances at the various stations, or (3) increase the number of repetitions to be performed at each station on the circuit. The maximum repetition self-test should be performed periodically to reestablish the individual's workout repetitions. It is important to emphasize that each repetition of each exercise should be performed at a relatively low rate of speed.

Cardiovascular endurance development

Development and maintenance of cardiovascular endurance is the most important aspect of physical fitness for the average adult. Regular attention to this fitness parameter on a year-round basis is essential. Cardiovascular endurance will regress faster than any other aspect of physical fitness, and the degenerative aspects of sedentary living on the cardiorespiratory mechanisms have many negative effects on the well-being of the individual.

The intensity of the workouts is very important if one expects to develop cardiovascular endurance. The intensity level can be calculated by using the maximum heart rate to determine the threshold level at which a training effect will occur. Research indicates that most people can expect some cardiovascular training effect if the intensity of the exercise elevates the pulse rate to approximately 75 percent of the individual's maximum heart rate capacity. The threshold heart rates adjusted for age to produce a cardiovascular training effect are shown in figure 13.24.

The threshold rates shown in figure 13.24 are for those individuals with normal resting heart rates between 55–75 beats/minute. The threshold rates must be adjusted for those individuals with resting pulse rates below and above 55–75 beats/minute. If the resting heart rate taken at the wrist while lying in bed

AGE GROUP	MAXIMAL HEART RATE	THRESHOLD RATE
10–14	210	158
15–19	200	150
20–24	195	146
25–29	190	142
30–34	185	138
35–39	180	135
40–44	175	131
45–49	170	127
50–54	165	123
55–59	160	120
60–64	155	116
65–69	150	112
70–74	145	108

Figure 13.24. Age adjusted threshold heart rates needed to produce a cardiovascular training effect during exercise for individuals with normal resting heart rates. The standard deviation in maximal heart rate is ± 10 beats/minute in all age groups.

in the morning before arising is *above* 75 beats/minute, a training effect can be expected if the pulse rate is at 65 to 70 percent of the age-adjusted maximal heart rate. For example, the threshold rate for such an individual in the 15–19 age group would be 130 beats/minute instead of 150 beats/minute. If the resting heart rate is *below* 55 beats/minute, the intensity of the cardiovascular workout must be increased to 80 to 85 percent of the age-adjusted maximal heart rate. This would mean a threshold level of 160 beats/minute instead of 150 beats/minute for the person meeting that criterion in the 15–19 age group (Falls, Baylor, Dishman 1980).

While many activities can be utilized as aerobic exercise to develop cardiovascular endurance, running is very effective for most athletic populations. It is recommended that athletes be prescribed cardiovascular exercise with enough intensity to have them working at or above the aforementioned threshold heart rate levels for 30 to 60 minutes daily. To maintain cardiovascular efficiency, workouts which elevate the heart rates at or above the individual's threshold level should be performed at least three to four days per week throughout the year.

The type of running can vary from day-to-day to increase motivation, reduce boredom, and develop skill. As an example, the portion of the exercise prescription for development of cardiovascular endurance for a flanker back in American football could show these variations during the offseason:

Sunday: Five mile jog—country, hill course; forty minutes.
Monday: *Continuous* fast and slow pass patterns for 45 minutes on the marked football field.

Tuesday:	Nine mile road run in one hour.
Wednesday:	*Continuous* fast and slow pass patterns for 45 minutes on the marked football field.
Thursday:	Six mile road run in forty minutes.
Friday:	*Continuous* fast and slow pass patterns for 45 minutes on the marked football field.
Saturday:	Twelve Minute Test; 7½ laps in 12 minutes, no additional running; less than 7½ laps, jog 5 mile country, hill course.

Individuals interested in cardiovascular endurance exercise should be taught to monitor their pulse rate periodically during workouts. The performer needs to determine whether or not the exercise intensity is great enough to maintain his or her threshold heart rate, based on the factors presented above. The pulse should be taken at the wrist. It should be taken *immediately* when one stops during the run, and the runner should remain standing. The heart rate count is taken for six seconds and multiplied by ten, or for ten seconds and multiplied by six. If the heart rate is below the threshold rate, the pace would need to be increased during the workout. If the heart rate is above the threshold rate, the intensity of effort could be decreased somewhat.

The Balke Field Test is an excellent and efficient measurement tool for determining the individual's level of cardiovascular fitness. This test consists of running as far as possible within a twelve-minute period of time (Balke 1954; Balke and Ware 1959). Balke's original work has been modified by Kenneth H. Cooper, whose modification appears in *Aerobics* (Cooper 1968). Cooper's norms are based on the average male adult in a United States Air Force population. Consequently, it is expected that the athlete in excellent cardiovascular condition should exceed the standards established in Cooper's excellent rendition of the twelve-minute field performance test.

Maximal cardiac output is the best indicator of cardiovascular efficiency, but it requires sophisticated procedures for measurement. Maximal oxygen consumption or uptake (Max O_2) correlates favorably to maximal cardiac output, and that parameter can be estimated with relatively good accuracy based on the twelve minute run performance (Falls, Baylor, Dishman 1980). For this reason, physical educators need to use the Balke Field Performance Test extensively as one indicator to determine the level of cardiovascular fitness in their students and student-athletes.

Any exercise designed to improve cardiovascular endurance should involve the large musculature of the lower limbs. This is essential since the lower limb musculature acts as an auxiliary pump for the heart. It has been estimated that approximately one-third of the circulatory function during activity is performed by the lower limb musculature. This means that running should be a supplementary feature of any weight training or circuit training program.

Running can be incorporated very effectively into a circuit training program. First, prior to starting the actual work on the circuit, the physical educator can have the squad run as far as possible during a predetermined period of time. A predetermined time allows for individual differences, and each individual's distance per workout is recorded. Second, a short run can be introduced following each trip through the circuit. Finally, the training period might be concluded with a second run following the three trips through the circuit.

A thorough discussion of cardiovascular endurance is beyond the scope of a basic kinesiology textbook. The reader is referred to exercise physiology textbooks for a more thorough discussion of cardiovascular endurance (Falls 1968; Astrand and Rodahl, 1977; DeVries 1974).

Specifics

The traditional weight-training exercises utilize movements primarily through the three conventional planes of motion. From an athletic standpoint, this appears to be very unrealistic. For example, some coaches advocate the military press as a beneficial exercise for shot-putters. How many shot-putters put the shot through a transverse plane of motion? A shot is put through a low diagonal plane of motion involving the shoulder joint! Consequently, it is more logical to have the shot-putter use the "Specifics" concept plus traditional resistance training. This is not to say that conventional weight training is not beneficial to athletic performance (Thompson and Martin 1964). However, Specifics are more effective in the actual athletic situation (Logan and McKinney 1967, 1969; Logan, McKinney, Rowe and Lumpe 1966).

The following steps, for example, would be used prior to placing a shot-putter on a Specifics program: (1) analyze his shot-putting style cinematographically to determine major joint angles used during performance; (2) design a weight-training program to emphasize strength development of the antigravity musculature, and (3) determine specific resistance exercises through the low diagonal plane of the shoulder, precise joint ranges of motion, and the accurate joint angles utilized during the putting of the shot. The athlete would be given an *exercise prescription* which would include *written details* for eight *strength exercises* for the anteroposterior antigravity muscles; traditional *strength exercises* for the shoulder and elbow joints; a "specifics" exercise for *muscle endurance* based on the above criteria; *flexibility* exercises through the transverse plane of the lumbar-thoracic spine and the low diagonal plane for the shoulder of the "throwing limb;" *cardiovascular endurance* work for thirty minutes daily; and a *skill drill* based on cinematographic analyses of past performances which would be designed functionally to remove the major fault and improve performance.

If the performer is motivated by the physical educator to work on such an exercise prescription diligently all year, the performance level should improve. The exercise prescription is designed to do that, because it is based on the specific needs of the individual to reach his or her potential as a performer. It is based on numerous kinesiologic analyses, noncinematographic and cinematographic, throughout at least one competitive season. It is also based on personal and academic insights regarding the performer. As such, if the prescription for improvement is written by a *professional* physical educator who can utilize these extensive kinesiologic evaluations and analyses, it will help the performer, enabling him or her to focus on what actually needs to be done as contrasted with what a technician type of coach *guesses* regarding what ought to be done to improve performance. The professional puts kinesiology theory into practice.

The athlete should work on skill development concurrently with resistance training. It is illogical, especially with athletes involved in accuracy skills, to disregard individual skill development while gaining strength, muscular endurance, cardiovascular endurance, and flexibility. It is recommended that a daily workout program include skill drills as well as resistance training. *This is important because it gives the athlete the opportunity to adjust skills gradually to anatomic and physiologic changes occurring as a result of the training regimen.* Specifics have the distinct advantage of allowing the athlete to concentrate on mechanics while attempting to increase strength and flexibility during resistance training. In addition to the development of these factors, the athlete should also concentrate on other skill elements such as footwork and timing.

Specific conditioning can be accomplished by using conventional weight-training exercises and equipment, but there are limitations. For example, a traditional pull-over may be modified by using a dumbbell in a motion diagonal to the body. This would appear to be the same type of throwing motion used by a pitcher or outfielder. The principal disadvantage is that the athlete is in a back-lying position while doing the pull-over. If he were standing, gravity would do most of the work. The pull-over is unlike throwing in the standing position. The motion, although it resembles throwing, differs myologically from a baseball throw. The athlete must use muscle action to stop the momentum of the dumbbell before it strikes his body. This muscular effort is performed at a point far beyond the normal release position of the ball. In addition, the athlete must recover the weight and return it to the starting position or move the weight back through diagonal abduction. Motion against resistance in this case is in direct opposition to the follow-through action of the arm during the throwing process. Also, in the back-lying position no opportunity is present for rotation of the spine or "opening of the hips" (transverse pelvic rotation), one of the most important sources of internal force required for throwing with any degree of velocity.

In order to duplicate closely the pitch or throw in this example, the resistance must be carried through the complete range of motion for the throw. This will allow normal striding, medial and lateral rotations at the hip joint, medial rotation of the throwing limb, and movement through the high diagonal plane at the shoulder. There should be no resistance at the conclusion of the follow-through. One isotonic resistance device which allows for the application of Specifics is the Exer-Genie Exerciser.[1]

Specific resistance can be used for conditioning athletes in a wide variety of sport skills. It is essential to use basic cinematographic analysis prior to establishing a program of Specifics. Cinematographic analysis is appropriate for the more skilled athlete for purposes of determining Specifics, than for lower-level performers. Ideally, the basic cinematographic analysis should be made from game film rather than practice film. As skill increases, a unique or individual style of motion is usually observed. This individuality of the athlete must be

1. Exer-Genie Exerciser is a registered trademark of Exer-Genie Inc. which identifies this exerciser.

considered when planning training programs for improvement. From the basic cinematographic analysis, the physical educator should determine the important planes of motion, ranges of motion, joint angles and body or limb velocity to use as a base for the subsequent specific training program. This information is used subsequently when attempting to alter performance, especially in the athlete's preseason and off-season conditioning programs.

Figures 13.25 and 13.26 show two examples of the application of the Specifics concept. When using a unilateral shoulder joint exercise as shown in figure 13.25, a very low resistance load of from one to four pounds must be used to protect the rotary cuff. This must be a muscle endurance exercise instead of a strength exercise. A strength weight load for eight repetitions is not indicated because of the undesirable changes in form which it will cause. Furthermore, there is also the possibility of muscle and joint damage owing to the fact that joints during ballistic actions are often in positions of mechanical disadvantage. This is also the reason for never applying an "isometric hold" at a point within a throwing or kicking range of motion. In addition to the injury potential of the "isometric hold," the movement pattern of the skill is changed. In terms of "Specifics," this is contraindicated for the improvement of skill. *Improvement of skill is one of the major purposes of kinesiology.*

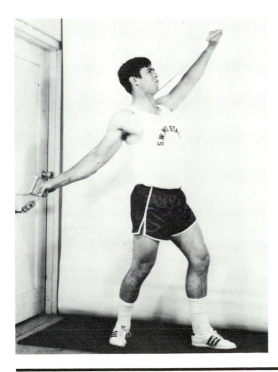

Figure 13.25. Specifics—discus throw through the low diagonal plane (the late Bill Lamberson, NCAA Division II Discus Champion).

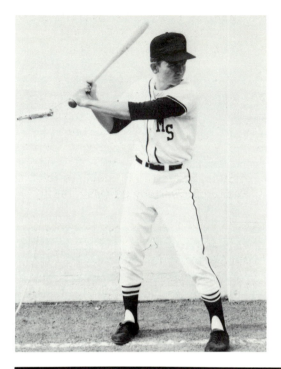

Figure 13.26. Specifics—baseball hitting (Tom Hodge).

Recommended readings

Astrand, Per-Olof, and Rodahl, Kaare. *Textbook of Work Physiology.* St. Louis: McGraw-Hill, Inc., 1977.

Balke, Bruno. "Optimal Working Capacity, Its Measurement, and Alteration as Effect of Physical Fatigue." *Arbeitsphysiologie* 15 (1954) :311.

Balke, Bruno, and Ware, Ray W. "The Present Status of Physical Fitness in the Air Force." Air University, Randolph Air Force Base, Texas. School of Aviation Medicine, U.S.A.F., May, 1959.

Bender, Jay A., and Kaplan, Harold M. "The Multiple Angle Testing Method for the Evaluation of Muscle Strength." *Journal of Bone and Joint Surgery* 45-A (January 1963) :135-40.

Berger, Richard A. "Comparison Between Resistance Load and Strength Improvement." *Research Quarterly* 33 (December 1962) :637.

Brose, Donald E., and Hanson, Dale L. "Effect of Overload Training on Velocity and Accuracy in Throwing." *Research Quarterly* 38 (December 1967) :528-33.

Clarke, David H., and Henry, Franklin M. "Neuromotor Specificity and Increased Speed from Strength Development." *Research Quarterly* 32 (October 1961) :315-25.

Cooper, Kenneth H. *Aerobics.* New York: M. Evans & Co., Inc., 1968.

Cooper, Kenneth H. et al. "An Aerobics Conditioning Program for the Fort Worth, Texas, School District." *Research Quarterly* 46 (October 1975) 345-50.

Cotten, Doyce J. "A Comparison of Selected Trunk Flexibility Tests," *American Corrective Therapy Journal* 26, no. 1, (January-February 1972) :24.

Daugherty, G. "The Effects of Kinesiological Teaching on the Performance of Junior High School Boys." *Research Quarterly* 16 (March 1945) :26.

De Vries, Herbert A. "Evaluation of Static Stretching Procedures for Improvement of Flexibility." *Research Quarterly* 33 (May 1962) 230-35.

————. *Physiology of Exercise for Physical Education and Athletics.* Dubuque, Iowa: Wm. C. Brown Company Publishers, 1974.

Dickinson, R. V. "The Specificity of Flexibility." *Research Quarterly* 39 (October 1968) :792-93.

Doolittle, T. L., and Logan, Gene A. "A Device for Measuring Simultaneous Flexion Strength of Both Wrists." *Perceptual and Motor Skills* 21 (August 1965) :121-22.

Egstrom, Glen H.; Logan, Gene A.; and Wallis, Earl L. "Acquisition of Throwing Skill Involving Projectiles of Varying Weights." *Research Quarterly* 31 (October 1960) :420-25.

Falls, Harold B., Jr. ed. *Exercise Physiology.* New York: Academic Press, Inc., 1968.

Falls, Harold D., Baylor, Ann M. and Dishman, Rod K. *Essentials of Fitness.* Philadelphia: Saunders College, 1980.

Gardner, Gerald W. "Specificity of Strength Changes of the Exercised and Nonexercised Limb Following Isometric Training." *Research Quarterly* 34 (March 1963) :98-101.

————. "Effect of Isometric and Isotonic Exercise on Joint Motion." *Archives of Physical Medicine and Rehabilitation* 47 (January 1966): 24-30.

Gettman, L. R. et. al. "The Effect of Circuit Weight Training on Strength, Cardiorespiratory Function, and Body Composition of Adult Men." *Medicine and Science in Sports* 10 (Fall 1978): 171-176.

Henry, Franklin M., and Smith, Leon. "Simultaneous vs. Separate Bilateral Muscular Contractions in Relation to Neural Overflow Theory and Neuromotor Specificity." *Research Quarterly* 32 (March 1961) :42-46.

Holland, George. "Specificity of Flexibility." In *Kinesiology Review— 1968.* Washington, D.C.: National Education Association, 1968.

Howell, Maxwell L.; Kimoto, Ray; and Morford, W. R., "Effect of Isometric and Isotonic Programs Upon Muscular Endurance." *Research Quarterly* 33 (December 1962) :536-40.

Hupprich, F. L., and Sigerseth, P. O. "The Specificity of Flexibility in Girls." *Research Quarterly* 21 (March 1950) :25.

Leach, Robert E.; Stryker, William S.; and Zohn, David A. "A Comparative Study of Isometric and Isotonic Quadriceps Exercise Programs." *Journal of Bone and Joint Surgery* 47A (October 1965) :1421-26.

Leighton, Jack R. "Flexibility Characteristics of Three Specialized Skill Groups of Champion Athletes." *Archives of Physical Medicine and Rehabilitation* 38 (September 1957): 580-83.

————. "A Comparison of the Flexibility Characteristics of Weight Training Perfectionists with the Flexibility Characteristics of Four Specialized Skill Groups of College Athletes." *Journal of the Association for Physical and Mental Rehabilitation* 19 (March-April 1965) :47-51.

Linderburg, Franklin A. "Leg Angle and Muscular Efficiency in the Inverted Leg Press." *Research Quarterly* 35 (May 1964) :179-83.

Lloyd, B. B. "The Energetics of Running: An Analysis of World Records." *Advancement of Science* 515-30, January 1966.

Logan, Gene A. "Comparative Gains in Strength Resulting from Eccentric and Concentric Muscular Contraction." Master's thesis, University of Illinois, 1952.

————. "Differential Applications of Resistance and Resulting Strength Measured at Varying Degrees of Knee Extension." Ph.D dissertation. University of Southern California, 1960.

Logan, Gene A., and Egstrom, G. H. "Effects of Slow and Fast Stretching on the Sacro-Femoral Angle." *Journal of the Association for Physical and Mental Rehabilitation* 15 (May-June 1961) :85-86, 89.

Logan, Gene A., and Foreman, Kenneth E. "Strength-Endurance Continuum." *The Physical Educator* 18 (October 1961) :103.

Logan, Gene A., and Lockhart, Aileene. "Contralateral Transfer of Specificity of Strength Training." *Journal of the American Physical Therapy Association* 42 (October 1962) :658-60.

Logan, Gene A.; Lockhart, Aileene; and Mott, Jane A. "Development of Isometric Strength at Different Angles Within the Range of Motion." *Perceptual and Motor Skills* 20 (June 1965) :858.

Logan, Gene A., and McKinney, Wayne C. "Effect of Progressively Increased Resistance Through a Throwing Range of Motion on the Velocity of a Baseball." *Journal of the Association for Physical and Mental Rehabilitation* 21 (1967) :11-12.

————. "Cinematographic Analysis of Varying Resistances on Batting Form and Velocity." Unpublished paper. Springfield: Southwest Missouri State College, 1969.

————. "Weight Training in Athletics." Unpublished report. Springfield: Southwest Missouri State College, 1969.

Logan, Gene A.; McKinney, Wayne C.; Rowe, Wm.; and Lumpe, Jerry. "Effect of Resistance Through a Throwing Range of Motion on the Velocity of a Baseball." *Perceptual and Motor Skills.* 23 (1966) :55-58.

Lotter, Willard S. "Specificity or Generality of Speed or Systematically Related Movements." *Research Quarterly* 32 (March 1961) :55-62.

McKinney, Wayne C. "Transfer of a Learned Neuromuscular Performance to the Ipsilateral and Contralateral Limbs: Dynamic Steadiness and Speed." Ph.D. dissertation. The University of Southern California, 1963.

Mathews, Donald K.; Stacy, Ralph W.; and Hoover, George N. *Physiology of Muscular Activity and Exercise.* New York: Ronald Press Company, 1964.

Morgan, R. E., and Adamson, G. T. *Circuit Training.* New Rochelle, N.Y.: Sportshelf and Soccer Associates, 1958.

Munroe, Richard A., and Romance, Thomas J. "Use of the Leighton Flexometer in the Development of a Short Flexibility Test Battery," *American Corrective Therapy Journal* 29 (January-February 1975) :22.

Pierson, William R., and Rasch, Philip J. "Strength and Speed." *Perceptual and Motor Skills* 14 (February 1962) :144.

Shelton, Robert. Personal Correspondence with Gene A. Logan, 1960.

Straub, William F. "Effect of Overload Training Procedures Upon Velocity and Accuracy of the Overarm Throw." *Research Quarterly* 39 (May 1968) :370-79.

Taylor, D. E. "Human Endurance—Mind or Muscle?" *British Journal of Sports Medicine* 12 (January 1979): 179-184.

Thompson, C. W., and Martin, E. T. "Weight Training and Baseball Throwing Speed." *Journal of the Association for Physical and Mental Rehabilitation* 19 (November-December 1965): 194-96.

Wallis, Earl L., and Logan, Gene A. *Figure Improvement and Body Conditioning Through Exercise.* Englewood Cliffs, N.J.: Prentice-Hall, 1964.

Watkins, David L. "Motion Pictures as an Aid in Correcting Baseball Batting Faults." *Research Quarterly* 34 (May 1963) :228-33.

Williams, Marian, and Stutzman, Leon. "Strength Variation Through the Range of Joint Motion." *Physical Therapy Review* 39 (March 1959) :145-52.

Yessis, Michael. "Relationships Between Varying Combinations of Resistances and Repetitions in the Strength-Endurance Continuum." Ph.D. dissertation, University of Southern California, 1963.

Zajaczkowska, A. "Constant Velocity in Lifting as a Criterion of Muscular Skill." *Ergonomics* 5 (April 1962) :337-56.

Zorbas, W. S., and Karpovich, P. V. "The Effect of Weight Lifting Upon the Speed of Muscular Contractions." *Research Quarterly* 22 (May 1951) :145.

Bibliography

Adrian, M.; Tipton, C. M.; and Karpovich, P. *Electrogoniometry Manual.* Springfield, Mass.: Springfield College, 1965.

Alhabashi, Z. *Kinesiology in the Field of Physical Education.* Maktabet: Al-Kahira Al-Haditha, 1964.

Amar, Jules. *The Human Motor.* New York: E. P. Dutton and Co., 1920.

American Academy of Orthopedic Surgeons. *Measuring and Recording of Joint Motion.* Chicago: The Academy, 1965.

American College of Sports Medicine (ed.) *Guidelines for Graded Exercise Testing and Exercise Prescription* (Second Edition). Philadelphia: Lea and Febiger, 1980.

Anderson, T. McClurg. *Human Kinetics and Analyzing Body Movements.* London: William Heinemann Medical Books, Ltd., 1951.

Aristotle. *Progressions of Animals* 9. Translated by E. S. Forster. Cambridge: Harvard University Press, 1945.

Asmussen, Erling and Jorgensen, Kurt (eds.). *International Congress of Biomechanics.* Baltimore: University Park Press, 1978.

Bade, Edwin. *The Mechanics of Sport.* Kingswood: Glade House, 1962.

Barham, Jerry N. *Mechanical Kinesiology.* St. Louis: C. V. Mosby Co., 1978.

Barham, Jerry N., and Thomas, William L. *Anatomical Kinesiology.* New York: Macmillan Co., 1969.

Barham, Jerry N., and Wooten, Edna P. *Structural Kinesiology.* New York: Macmillan Co., 1973.

Barnett, C. H.; Davies, D. V.; and MacConaill, M. A. *Synovial Joints, Their Structure and Mechanics.* Springfield, Ill.: Charles C Thomas, Publisher, 1961.

Barrow, Harold M. *Man and Movement: Principles of Physical Education.* Philadelphia: Lea and Febiger, 1977.

Basmajian, J. V. *Muscles Alive. Their Functions Revealed by Electromyography.* Baltimore: The Williams and Wilkins Co., 1962.

Beevor, C. *The Croonian Lectures on Muscular Movements.* London: Macmillan, Ltd., 1903.

Bernstein, N. A. *Investigations on the Biodynamics of Walking, Running, and Jumping.* Moscow: Central Scientific Institute of Physical Culture, 1940.

———. *The Co-ordination and Regulation of Movements.* New York: Pergamon Press, 1967.

Birdshistell, R. L. *Introduction to Kinesics: An Annotation System of Analysis of Body Motion and Gesture.* Washington, D.C.: U.S. Foreign Service, 1952.

Bleustein, J., ed. *Mechanics and Sport.* New York: The American Society of Mechanical Engineering, 1976.

Bootzin, David, and Muffley, Harry C. *Rock Island Arsenal Biomechanics Symposium.* New York: Plenum Press, 1969.

Borelli, G. A. *De Motu Animalium.* Ludguni Batavorum, 1680–81.

Bourne, G. H. B., ed. *The Structure and Function of Muscle.* New York: Academic Press, 1960.

Broer, M. R. *An Introduction to Kinesiology*. Englewood Cliffs, N.J.: Prentice-Hall, 1968.

————. *Efficiency of Human Movement*. Philadelphia: W. B. Saunders Company, 1973.

————. *Laboratory Experiences: Exploring Efficiency of Human Movement*. Philadelphia: W. B. Saunders Company, 1973.

————, and Houtz, Sara J. *Patterns of Muscular Activity in Selected Sport Skills: An Electromyographic Study*. Springfield, Ill.: Charles C Thomas, Publisher, 1967.

Broer, Marion R. and Zernicke, Ronald F. *Efficiency of Human Movement* (Fourth Edition). Philadelphia: Saunders Company, 1979.

Brown, Roscoe C., and Kenyon, Gerald S., eds. *Classical Studies on Physical Activity*. Englewood Cliffs, N.J.: Prentice-Hall, 1968.

Brunnstrom, Signe. *Clinical Kinesiology*. Philadelphia: F. A. Davis Co., 1972.

Bunn, John W. *Scientific Principles of Coaching*. Englewood Cliffs, N.J.: Prentice-Hall, 1972.

Campbell, E. J. M. *The Respiratory Muscles and the Mechanics of Breathing*. London: Lloyd-Luke (Medical Books) Ltd., 1958.

Canna, D. J., and Loring, E. *Kinesiography*. Fresno, Calif.: The Academy Guild Press, 1955.

Cerquiglini, S.; Venerando, A.; and Wartenweiler, J., eds. *Biomechanics III*. Basel, Switzerland: S. Krager AG, 1973.

Chesterman, W. D. *The Photographic Study of Rapid Events*. London: Oxford University Press, 1951.

Clarke, Harrison H. *Muscular Strength and Endurance in Man: International Research Monograph*. Englewood Cliffs, N.J.: Prentice-Hall, 1966.

Clarys, J., and Lewillie, L. *Swimming II*. Baltimore: University Park Press, 1975.

Close, J. R. *Motor Function in the Lower Extremity: Analyses by Electronic Instrumentation*. Springfield, Ill.: Charles C Thomas, Publisher, 1964.

————. *Functional Anatomy of the Extremities*. Springfield, Ill.: Charles C Thomas, Publisher, 1973.

Cochran, Alastair, and Stobbs, John. *The Search for the Perfect Swing*. New York: J. B. Lippincott Company, 1968.

Cooper, John M., ed. *C.I.C. Symposium on Biomechanics*. Chicago: Athletic Institute, 1971.

————, and Glasgow, Ruth B. *Kinesiology*. St. Louis: The C. V. Mosby Company, 1976.

————, and Siedentrop, D. *The Theory and Science of Basketball*. Philadelphia: Lea and Febiger, 1969.

Counsilman, James E. *The Science of Swimming*. Englewood Cliffs, N.J.: Prentice-Hall, 1968.

Crouch, J. E. *Functional Human Anatomy*. Philadelphia: Lea and Febiger, 1972.

Cureton, T. K. *Physics Applied to Health and Physical Education*. Springfield, Mass.: International YMCA College, 1936.

Daish, C. B. *The Physics of Ball Games*. London: The English Universities Press Ltd., 1972.

Daniels, L., and Worthingham, C. *Muscle Testing Techniques of Manual Examination*. Philadelphia: W. B. Saunders Co., 1972.

Donskoi, D. D. *Biomechanik der Korperübungen*. Berlin: Sportverlag, 1961.

DuBois, J., and Santschi, W. R. *The Determination of the Moment of Inertia of Living Human Organisms*. New York: John Wiley & Sons, 1963.

Duchenne, G. B. A. *Physiology of Motion*. Translated by E. B. Kaplan. Philadelphia: W. B. Saunders Company, 1959.

Duvall, Ellen Neall. *Kinesiology: The Anatomy of Motion*. Englewood Cliffs, N.J.: Prentice-Hall, 1959.

Dyson, Geoffrey H. G. *The Mechanics of Athletics*. London: University of London Press, 1973.

Elftman, H. *Skeletal and Muscular Systems: Structure and Function in Medical Physics*. Chicago: Year Book Publications, 1944.

Esch, D., and Lepley, M. *Evaluation of Joint Motion: Methods of Measuring and Recording*. Minneapolis: University of Minnesota Press, 1974.

————. *Musculoskeletal Function: An Anatomy and Kinesiology Laboratory Manual*. Minneapolis: University of Minnesota Press, 1974.

Eshkol, N., and Wachman, A. *Movement Notation*. London: Weidenfeld and Nicolson, 1958.

Evans, F. Gaynor, ed. *Biomechanical Studies of the Musculoskeletal System*. Springfield, Ill.: Charles C Thomas, Publisher, 1961.

————. *Studies on the Anatomy and Function of Bone and Joints*. New York: Springer-Verlag, 1966.

————. *Mechanical Properties of Bone*. Springfield, Ill.: Charles C Thomas, Publisher, 1973.

Feather, N. *An Introduction to the Physics of Mass, Length, and Time*. Edinburgh: University Press, 1959.

Fetz, F. *Bewegungslehre der Leibesubungen*. Frankfurt a.M.: Wilhelm Limpert-Verlag GmbH, 1972.

Finley, F. Ray. *Kinesiological Analysis of Human Locomotion*. Eugene: University of Oregon Press, 1961.

Fischer, O. *Theoretische Grundlagen fuer eine Mechanik der lebenden Koerper*. Berlin: B. G. Teubner, 1906.

————. *Kinematik organischer Gelenke*. Braunschweig: F. Vieweg & Sohn GmbH, 1907.

Frankel, Victor H., and Burstein, Albert H. *Orthopaedic Biomechanics*. Philadelphia: Lea and Febiger, 1970.

Frankel, Victor H. and Nordin, Margareta. *Basic Biomechanics of the Skeletal System*. Philadelphia: Lea and Febiger, 1980.

Frost, Harold M. *An Introduction to Biomechanics*. Springfield, Ill.: Charles C Thomas, Publisher, 1967.

————. *Orthopaedic Biomechanics*. Springfield, Ill.: Charles C Thomas, Publisher, 1973.

Fung, Y. C.; Perrone, N.; and Anliker, M., eds. *Biomechanics: Its Foundations and Objectives*. Englewood Cliffs, N.J.: Prentice-Hall Inc., 1972.

Gage, Howard (ed.). *Biomechanical and Human Factors Conference*. New York: American Society of Mechanical Engineers, 1967.

Gans, Carl. *Biomechanics: An Approach to Vertebrate Biology*. Philadelphia: J. B. Lippincott Company, 1974.

Ganslen, R. V., and Hall, K. G. *The Aerodynamics of Javelin Flight*. Fayetteville: University of Arkansas Press, 1960.

Ganslen, R. V. *Mechanics of the Pole Vault*. St. Louis: John S. Swift Co., 1963.

George, Gerald S. *Biomechanics of Women's Gymnastics*. Englewood, N.J.: Prentice-Hall, Incorporated, 1980.

Goldsmith, Werner. *Impact*. New York: St. Martin's Press, 1961.

Govaerts, A. *Biomechanics: A New Method of Analyzing Motion*. Brussels: Brussels University Press, 1962.

Gowitzke, Barbara A. and Milner, Morris. *Understanding the Scientific Bases of Human Movement* (Second edition). Baltimore: The Williams and Wilkins Company, 1980.

Gray, Henry. *Anatomy of the Human Body*. Philadelphia: Lea and Febiger, 1973.

Gray, J. *How Animals Move*. London: Cambridge University Press, 1960.

Grieve, D. W., et al. *Techniques for the Analysis of Human Movement*. London: Lepus Books, 1975.

Groves, Richard, and Camaione, David N. *Concepts in Kinesiology*. Philadelphia: W. B. Saunders Company, 1975.

Hall, Michael C. *The Locomotor System: Functional Anatomy*. Springfield, Ill.: Charles C Thomas, Publisher, 1965.

Halliday, D., and Resnick, R. *Physics for Students of Science and Engineering*. Part I. New York: John Wiley & Sons, 1965.

Harris, Ruth W. *Kinesiology Workbook and Laboratory Manual*. Boston: Houghton and Mifflin Co., 1977.

Hawley, Gertrude. *An Anatomical Analysis of Sport*. Cranbury, N.J.: A. S. Barnes & Co., 1940.

————. *The Kinesiology of Corrective Exercise*. Philadelphia: Lea and Febiger, 1949.

Hay, James G. *The Biomechanics of Sports Techniques*. Englewood Cliffs, N.J.: Prentice-Hall, 1978.

———. *A Bibliography of Biomechanics Literature*. Ames: Department of Physical Education for Men, University of Iowa, 1977.

Hemming, George W. *Billiards Mathematically Treated*. London: Macmillan, 1899.

Hertel, Heinrich. *Structure-Form-Movement*. New York: Reinhold Publishing Corp., 1966.

Hickman, C. N.; Nagler, F.; and Klopsteg, Paul E. *Archery: The Technical Side*. Redlands, Calif.: National Field Archery Association, 1947.

Higgins, Joseph R. *Human Movement*. St. Louis: C. V. Mosby Co., 1977.

Hill, A. V. *Muscular Movements in Man*. New York: McGraw-Hill Book Co., 1927.

———. *Living Machinery*. New York: McGraw-Hill Book Co., 1927.

———. *First and Last Experiments in Muscle Mechanics*. Cambridge: University Press, 1970.

Hinson, Marilyn M. *Kinesiology*. Dubuque, Iowa: Wm. C. Brown Company, Publishers, 1977.

Hochmuth, G. *Biomechanik sportlicher Bewegungen*. Frankfurt a.M.: Wilhelm Limpert-Verlag GmbH, 1967.

Hollinshead, H. W. *Functional Anatomy of the Limbs and Back*. Philadelphia: W. B. Saunders Company, 1960.

Hopper, B. J. *Notes on the Dynamical Basis of Physical Movement*. Twickenham, Middlesex, England: St. Mary's College, 1959.

———. *The Mechanics of Human Movement*. New York: American Elsevier Publishing Co., Inc., 1973.

Howard, I. P., and Templeton, W. B. *Human Spatial Orientation*. New York: John Wiley & Sons, 1966.

Howell, A. Brazeir. *Speed in Animals: Their Specialization for Running and Leaping*. New York: Hafner Publishers, 1965.

Hoyle, G. *The Nervous Control of Muscular Contraction*. New York: Cambridge University Press, 1958.

Hyzer, William G. *Engineering and Scientific High Speed Photography*. New York: Macmillan Co., 1963.

International Society of Electrophysiological Kinesiology. *Proceedings: Fourth Congress of the International Society of Electrophysiological Kinesiology*. Boston: C. J. DeLuca, 1979.

Jensen, Clayne R., and Schultz, Gordon W. *Applied Kinesiology*. New York: McGraw-Hill Book Co., 1977.

Johnson, Warren R., and Buskirk, E., eds. *Science and Medicine of Exercise and Sports*. New York: Harper & Row, Publishers, 1974.

Jones, F. W. *Structure and Function as Seen in the Foot*. London: Bailliere, Tindall and Cox, Ltd., 1949.

Joseph, J. *Man's Posture: Electromyographic Studies*. Springfield, Ill.: Charles C Thomas, Publisher, 1960.

Karas, V., and Stapleton, A. *Application of the Theory of the Motion System in the Analysis of Gymnastic Motions*. New York: S. Karger, 1968.

Katz, B. *Nerve, Muscle, and Synapse*. New York: McGraw-Hill Book Co., 1966.

Kelley, David L. *Kinesiology: Fundamentals of Motion Description*. Englewood Cliffs, N.J.: Prentice-Hall, 1971.

Kendall, M. B. *Muscles: Testing and Function*. Baltimore: Williams and Wilkins, 1971.

Kenedi, R. M., ed. *Symposium on Biomechanics and Related Bioengineering Topics*. New York: Pergamon Press, 1955.

Klopsteg, P. E., and Wilson, P. V., eds. *Human Limbs and Their Substitutes*. New York: McGraw-Hill Book Co., 1954.

Knuttgen, H. G. *Neuromuscular Mechanisms*. Baltimore: University Park Press, 1976.

Komi, P. V., ed. *Biomechanics V–A and V–B*. Baltimore: University Park Press, 1976.

Krause, J. V., and Barham, Jerry. *The Mechanical Foundations of Human Motion: A Programmed Text*. St. Louis: The C. V. Mosby Company, 1975.

Kreighbaum, Ellen and Barthels, Katherine. *Biomechanics: A Qualitative Approach for Studying Human Movement*. Minneapolis: Burgess Publishing Company, 1980.

Krogman, W. M., and Johnston, F. E. *Human Mechanics (Four Monographs Abridged)*. AMRL Technical Documentary Report 63–123. Wright-Patterson Air Force Base, Ohio: 6570th Aerospace Medical Research Laboratories, December, 1963.

Kuel, J., et al. *Energy Metabolism of Human Muscle*. Baltimore: University Park Press, 1972.

Lam, C. R. *An Introduction to Biomechanics*. Springfield, Ill.: Charles C Thomas Publishing Co., 1967.

Landry, Fernand and Orban, William (eds.). *Biomechanics of Sports and Kinanthropometry*. Miami: Symposia Specialists, 1978.

Larson, L. *Foundations of Physical Activity*. New York: Macmillan Publishing Co., 1976.

LeVeau, Barney. *Biomechanics of Human Motion*. Philadelphia: W. B. Saunders Co., 1977.

Levens, Alexander. *Graphical Methods in Research*. New York: John Wiley & Sons, 1965.

Lewille, L., and Clarys, J. P., eds. *International Symposium on Biomechanics in Swimming, Water Polo, and Diving*. Brussels, 1971.

Lipovetz, F. J. *Basic Kinesiology*. Minneapolis: Burgess Publishing Co., 1952.

Logan, Gene A. *Adapted Physical Education*. Dubuque, Iowa: Wm. C. Brown Company Publishers, 1972.

———, and McKinney, Wayne C. *Kinesiology*. Dubuque, Iowa: Wm. C. Brown Company Publishers, 1970.

———, and McKinney, Wayne C. *Anatomic Kinesiology*. Dubuque, Iowa: Wm. C. Brown Company Publishers, 1977.

Long, C. *Normal and Abnormal Motor Control in the Upper Extremities*. Washington: Social and Rehabilitation Services, 1970.

Lucas, D. B., and Inman, V. T. *Functional Anatomy of the Shoulder Joint*. Berkeley: University of California Medical School, 1963.

MacConaill, M. A., and Basmajian, J. V. *Muscles and Movement: A Basis for Human Kinesiology*. Baltimore: The William and Wilkins Co., 1969.

McCormick, E. J. *Human Factor Engineering*. New York: McGraw-Hill Book Co., 1970.

Maquet, Paul G. J. *Biomechanics of the Knee*. New York: Springer-Verlag, 1976.

Marey, Etienne J. *Movement*. Translated by Eric Pritchard. London: William Heinemann, Limited, 1895.

Margaria, Rodolfo. *Biomechanics and Energetics of Muscular Exercise*. Oxford: Clarendon Press, 1976.

Martin, Thomas P., ed. *Biomechanics of Sport, Selected Readings*. Brockport, N.Y.: T. P. Martin, 15 Beverly Dr., 1976.

Mascelli, Joseph V., and Miller, Arthur. *American Cinematographer Manual*. Hollywood: American Society of Cinematographers Holding Corporation, 1966.

Massey, Benjamin H., et al. *The Kinesiology of Weight Lifting*. Dubuque, Iowa: Wm. C. Brown Company Publishers, 1959.

Metheny, Eleanor. *Body Dynamics*. New York: McGraw-Hill, Inc., 1952.

Miller, Doris, and Nelson, Richard C. *The Biomechanics of Sport*. Philadelphia: Lea and Febiger, 1973.

Montagu, M. F. A. *A Handbook of Anthropometry*. Springfield, Ill.: Charles C Thomas, Publisher, 1960.

Morehouse, L. E., and Cooper, J. M. *Kinesiology*. St. Louis: The C. V. Mosby Company, 1950.

Morris, Roxie. *Correlation of Basic Sciences with Kinesiology*. New York: American Physical Therapy Association, 1955.

Morton, D. J., and Fuller, D. D. *Human Locomotion and Body Form*. Baltimore: The Williams and Wilkins Co., 1952.

Muybridge, Eadweard. *The Human Figure in Motion*. New York: Dover Publications, Inc., 1955.

Naylor, T. H. *Computer Simulation Techniques*. New York: John Wiley & Sons, 1966.

Nelson, Richard, and Morehouse, Chauncey, eds. *International Seminar on Biomechanics.* Baltimore: University Park Press, 1974.

Nemessuri, M. *Funktionelle Sportanatomie.* Berlin: Sportverlag, 1963.

Northrip, John W.; Logan, Gene A.; and McKinney, Wayne C. *Introduction to Biomechanic Analysis of Sport.* Dubuque, Iowa: Wm. C. Brown Company Publishers, 1979.

O'Connell, Alice L., and Gardner, Elizabeth B. *Understanding the Scientific Bases of Human Movement.* Baltimore: The Williams and Wilkins Co., 1972.

Ostyn, Michel, Beunen, Gaston and Simons, Jan (eds.). *International Seminar on Kinanthropometry.* Baltimore: University Park Press, 1979.

Peterson, A. P. G., and Gross, E. E. *Handbook of Morse Measurements.* Concord, Mass.: General Radio Co., 1974.

Piscopo, John and Baley, James. *Kinesiology: The Science of Movement.* New York: John Wiley and Sons, 1981.

Plagenhoef, Stanley. *Fundamentals of Tennis.* Englewood Cliffs, N.J.: Prentice-Hall, 1970.

————. *Patterns of Human Motion: A Cinematographic Analysis.* Englewood Cliffs, N.J.: Prentice-Hall, 1971.

Posse, N. *The Special Kinesiology of Educational Gymnastics.* Boston: Lothrop, Lee and Shepard Co., Inc., 1890.

Rasch, Philip J., and Burke, Roger K. *Kinesiology and Applied Anatomy.* 5th ed. Philadelphia: Lea and Febiger, 1978.

Rebikoff, Dimitri, and Cherney, Paul. *A Guide to Underwater Photography.* New York: Greenberg, 1955.

Rodahl, K., and Horvath, S. M. *Muscle as a Tissue.* New York: McGraw-Hill, Inc., 1962.

Ruch, T. C., and Patton, H. D., eds. *Physiology and Biophysics.* Philadelphia: W. B. Saunders Company, 1965.

Scott, M. Gladys. *Analysis of Human Motion.* New York: Appleton-Century-Crofts, 1963.

Sharpley, F. *Biomechanics for Beginners.* Ardmore, New Zealand: Ardmore Teacher's College, 1968.

Simons, E. N. *Mechanics for the Home Student.* London: Iliffe and Sons Ltd., 1950.

Skalak, Richard and Nerem, Robert M. (eds.). *Biomechanics Symposium.* New York: American Society of Mechanical Engineers, 1975.

Skalak, Richard and Schultz, Albert (eds.). *Biomechanics Symposium.* New York: American Society of Mechanical Engineers, 1977.

Skarstrom, W. *Gymnastic Kinesiology.* Springfield, Mass.: F. A. Bassette Co., 1909.

————. *Kinesiology of Trunk, Shoulders and Hip.* Springfield, Ill.: Charles C Thomas, Publisher, 1946.

Slocum, D. B., and Bowerman, William. *The Biomechanics of Running.* Clinical Orthopaedics No. 23. Philadelphia: J. B. Lippincott Co., 1962.

Spence, D. *Essentials of Kinesiology.* Philadelphia: Lea and Febiger, 1975.

Squire, P. J. *Biomechanics of Sport and Human Movement: A Reference Bibliography.* Edinburgh: Dufermline College of Physical Education, 1977.

Stapp, J. P. *Jolt Effects of Impact on Man.* San Antonio, Tex.: Brooks Air Force Base, 1961.

Steindler, Arthur. *Mechanics of Normal and Pathological Locomotion in Man.* Springfield, Ill.: Charles C Thomas, Publisher, 1935.

————. *Kinesiology of the Human Body under Normal and Pathological Conditions.* Springfield, Ill.: Charles C Thomas, Publisher, 1973.

Stoddard, J. T. *The Science of Billiards.* Boston: Butterfield, 1913.

Strasser, H. *Lehrbuch der Muskel and Gelenkmechanik.* Berlin: J. Springer, 1913.

Streeter, V. L. *Fluid Mechanics.* New York: McGraw-Hill, 1966.

Terauds, Juris (ed.). *International Symposium of Science in Weightlifting.* Del Mar, CA: Academic Publishers, 1979.

————. *Science in Biomechanics Cinematography*. Del Mar, CA: Academic Publishers, 1979.

Terauds, Juris and Dales, George G. (eds.). *International Symposium of Science in Athletics*. Del Mar, CA: Academic Publishers, 1979.

Terauds, Juris and Danials, Dayna (eds.). *International Symposium of Science in Gymnastics*. Del Mar, CA: Academic Publishers, 1979.

Thompson, Clem W. *Kranz Manual of Kinesiology* (Eighth edition). St. Louis: The C. V. Mosby Company, 1977.

Tichauer, E. R. *The Biomechanical Basis of Ergonomics: Anatomy Applied to the Design of Work Situations*. New York: Wiley and Sons, 1978.

Tricker, R. A. R. and Tricker, B. J. K. *The Science of Movement*. New York: American Elsevier Publishing Company, 1967.

VanVeen, F. *Handbook of Stroboscopy*. Concord, Mass.: General Radio Co., 1977.

Vredenbregt, J., and Wartenweiler, J., eds. *International Seminar on Biomechanics*. Baltimore: University Park Press, 1971.

Waddell, J. H., and Waddell, J. W. *Photographic Motion Analysis*. Chicago: Indust. Lab. Publ., 1955.

Wartenweiler, J.; Jokl, E.; and Hebbelnick, M., eds. *International Seminar on Biomechanics*. New York: S. Krager, 1968.

Webster, F. A. M. *Why? The Science of Athletics*. London: John F. Shaw and Co., Ltd., 1936.

Wells, Katharine F., and Luttgens, K. *Kinesiology*. Philadelphia: W. B. Saunders Co., 1976.

Wickstrom, Ralph L. *Fundamental Motor Patterns*. Philadelphia: Lea and Febiger, 1977.

Widule, Carol J. *Analysis of Human Motion*. Lafayette: Balt Publishers, 1977.

Williams, M., and Lissner, H. R. *Biomechanics of Human Motion*. Philadelphia: W. B. Saunders Company, 1962.

Wilt, Fred. *Mechanics Without Tears*. Tucson, Ariz.: United States Track and Field Federation, 1970.

Winter, David. *Biomechanics of Human Movement*. New York: John Wiley and Sons, 1980.

Woolridge, D. E. *Mechanical Man: The Physical Bases of Intelligent Life*. New York: McGraw-Hill Book Co., 1968.

Wright, W. *Muscle Function*. New York: Paul B. Hoeber, Inc., 1928.

Yamada, Hiroshi. *Strength of Biological Materials*. Baltimore: The Williams and Wilkins Co., 1970.

Name Index

Sport Index

Arm wrestling, 234

Badminton, 54
Baseball, 46-47, 55, 58, 60, 69, 108, 109, 162, 177-178, 196, 257, 290, 291, 312, 313, 325, 326, 328
Basketball, 60, 109, 131, 133, 191, 196, 216, 218, 225, 230, 231, 248, 325, 326, 328

Circuit training, 368-373
Cross country skiing, 190

Dance, 50, 59, 70, 127, 179, 182, 324
Discus, 48, 49, 237, 238, 325
Diving, 36, 42, 43, 50, 57, 147, 325

Field hockey, 196
Football, 55-56, 72-73, 105-107, 123-124, 153-154, 162, 175-176, 191, 196, 285, 299-302, 373-374

Golf, 49, 58, 118-119, 177, 325
Gymnastics, 38-43, 50, 58, 59, 60, 179, 196, 197, 198, 199, 200, 217, 219, 279, 324

Handball, 60, 327
High jumping, 127, 192-193, 326
Hurdling, 159, 160, 328

Ice hockey, 196

Javelin, 48, 290, 292-299, 325, 326

Kicking, 164, 299-302

Long Jump, 37-38, 328

Pike's Peak Marathon, 275, 276, 277
Pole vaulting, 182, 183, 326, 328

Rowing, 190
Running, distance, 100-101, 115, 116, 120, 134, 146, 177, 181, 182, 272, 273, 274, 275, 276, 277

Shooting, pistol, 325
Shot put, 232, 233, 234, 325
Ski jumping, 152, 153, 325
Soccer, 50, 55, 57, 59, 158, 161-162, 196, 299-302
Softball, 46, 49, 60, 325, 329-344
Sprinting, 115, 116, 120, 134, 142, 143, 146, 164, 177, 225, 226, 230, 272, 273, 275, 277, 324, 345-351
Squash, 327
Swimming, 40, 50, 55-56, 60, 75, 131, 133, 158, 216, 232, 279, 311, 312, 324, 325, 328

Tennis, 92, 194, 235, 258, 324, 327

Volleyball, 5, 191, 199, 200, 252, 253, 325, 326

Weight lifting, 43, 99-100
Weight training, 138-142, 150, 153, 156, 157, 159, 161, 196, 212, 214, 229, 232, 239, 240, 245, 248, 249, 259, 260, 279-285, 357-362, 366-372
Wrestling, 72, 179

Subject Index